The Radiology AI Handbook

The Radiology AI Handbook

EDITED BY

ADAM E. M. ELTORAI, MD, PhD
Brigham & Women's Hospital
Harvard Medical School
Boston, Massachusetts

JAMES M. HILLIS, MBBS, DPhil
Director of Clinical Operations
Mass General Brigham AI
Assistant Neurologist
Department of Neurology
Massachusetts General Hospital
Assistant Professor of Neurology
Harvard Medical School
Boston, Massachusetts

RAJAT CHAND, MD
Interventional Radiologist
Vascular and Interventional Radiology
Independent Contractor
Austin, Texas

SUDHEN B. DESAI, MD, FSIR
Principal
MedTech Consultant, Interventional Radiologist
ASKD Medical, LLC
Paradise Valley, Arizona

KATHERINE P. ANDRIOLE, PhD, FACR, FSIIM, FSPIE
Director of Academic Research and Education
Mass General Brigham AI
Associate Professor of Radiology
Brigham and Women's Hospital
Harvard Medical School
Boston, Massachusetts

ELSEVIER

Elsevier
1600 John F. Kennedy Blvd.
Ste 1800
Philadelphia, PA 19103-2899

THE RADIOLOGY AI HANDBOOK ISBN: 978-0-323-87760-2

Content Strategist: Melanie Tucker
Content Development Specialist: Puneet Bharadwaj
Publishing Services Manager: Deepthi Unni
Project Manager: Prasanna Kalyanaraman
Design Direction: Margaret Reid

Printed in India

Last digit is the print number: 9 8 7 6 5 4 3 2 1

CONTRIBUTORS

Rasheed Majeed Abdullah, MD
Resident Physician
Department of Radiology and Molecular Imaging
Corewell Health William Beaumont University Hospital
Royal Oak, Michigan

Nadeen Aladham, BS
Medical Student
Ross University School of Medicine
Miramar, Florida

Katherine P. Andriole, PhD, FACR, FSIIM, FSPIE
Director of Academic Research and Education
Mass General Brigham AI
Associate Professor of Radiology
Brigham and Women's Hospital
Harvard Medical School
Boston, Massachusetts

John Axerio-Cilies, PhD
Chief Data Technology Officer
Tempus AI, Inc.
Chicago, Illinois

Mustafa Azam, BS
Medical Student
School of Medicine
Oakland University William Beaumont School of Medicine
Rochester, Michigan

Ashley M. Carter, BA
Medical Student
School of Medicine
Eastern Virginia Medical School
Norfolk, Virginia

Rajat Chand, MD
Interventional Radiologist
Vascular and Interventional Radiology
Independent Contractor
Austin, Texas

Adrian Coscia, BS, MS
MD/PhD Student
Department of Cell Biology
Harvard Medical School
MD/PhD Student
Department of Biological Chemistry and Molecular Pharmacology
Harvard Medical School
Boston, Massachusetts

Harrison Dai, BS
Medical Student
School of Medicine
Eastern Virginia Medical School
Norfolk, Virginia

Dania Daye, MD, PhD
Assistant Professor
Department of Radiology
Massachusetts General Hospital
Boston, Massachusetts

Sudhen B. Desai, MD, FSIR
Principal
MedTech Consultant, Interventional Radiologist
ASKD Medical, LLC
Paradise Valley, Arizona

Yuval Duchin, MSc
Senior Algorithm Developer
AI
Viz.ai, Inc.
Tel-Aviv, Israel

Adam E. M. Eltorai, MD, PhD
Brigham & Women's Hospital
Harvard Medical School
Boston, Massachusetts

Marvee Espiritu, MD, MSPAS
Physician
Department of Interventional Radiology
Mount Sinai Hospital
New York, New York

Sijing Feng, MBChB, FRANZCR, BBioMedSci, PGDipSurgAnat
Attending Radiologist
Lake Imaging
Integral Diagnostics
Founder & CEO
Radiology Expertly PTY LTD
Geelong, Australia

Reid Fursmidt, MD, MS
Resident Physician
Department of Radiology
Zucker School of Medicine at Hofstra/Northwell
Manhasset, New York

Michael M. Gilbert Bodell, MD, MS
Resident Physician
Department of Radiology
The Ohio State University College of Medicine
Columbus, Ohio

David Golan, PhD
Co-founder
Viz.ai, Inc.
Tel-Aviv, Israel

Sazid Mohammed Hasan, BS, MD
Resident Physician
Department of Orthopaedic Surgery
University of Toledo
Toledo, Ohio

James M. Hillis, MBBS, DPhil
Director of Clinical Operations
Mass General Brigham AI
Assistant Neurologist
Department of Neurology
Massachusetts General Hospital
Assistant Professor of Neurology
Harvard Medical School
Boston, Massachusetts

Alice Hou, MA, MA
Resident Physician
Department of Psychiatry
Case Western Reserve University
Cleveland, Ohio

Anna Hu, MD
Surgical Intern
Department of Interventional Radiology
Rush University Medical Center
Chicago, Illinois

Michael Karsy, MD, PhD, MSc, FAANS, FCNS
Assistant Clinical Professor of Neurosurgery
Department of Neurosurgery
University of Michigan
Ann Arbor, Michigan

Vishaal Kondoor, MD, MBA
Vascular Interventional Radiology Resident
BayCare Health System
Tampa, Florida
Rochester General Hospital
Rochester, New York

Robert Lauritzen
CEO
Cerebriu A/S
Copenhagen, Denmark

Martin Lillholm, PhD
COO
Cerebriu A/S
Professor
Department of Computer Science
University of Copenhagen
Copenhagen, Denmark

Brandon Lucke-Wold, MD, PhD, MCTS
Neurosurgery Resident
Department of Neurosurgery
University of Florida
Gainesville, Florida

Srikanth Mahankali, MD
CEO & Founder
Shree Advisory & Consulting, LLC
Cleveland Heights, Ohio

Marlee Mason-Maready, BS, MD
Resident Physician
Department of Radiology
Oregon Health & Science University
Portland, Oregon

Heather Mattie, PhD
Lecturer on Biostatistics
Co-Director, Health Data Science Master's Program
Department of Biostatistics
Harvard T.H. Chan School of Public Health
Boston, Massachusetts

Christopher McMahan, DO
Diagnostic Radiology Resident
University of Massachusetts Chan Medical School
Worcester, Massachusetts

Shahrukh Naseer, BS
Medical Student
William Beaumont School of Medicine
Oakland University
Rochester, Michigan

Michel Christian Nèmery, MD
Clinical Advisor
Clinical Research
Cerebriu A/S
Copenhagen, Denmark

Maria Bach Nielsen, Cand Scient MSc in Techno-Anthropology
Senior Project Manager
Department of Clinical Development
Cerebriu A/S
Industrial PhD Fellow
Department of Sustainability and Planning, Techno-Anthropology and Participation (TAPAR)
Aalborg University Copenhagen
Copenhagen, Denmark

Janus Uhd Nybing, MSc
CTO
Radiological AI Testcenter
Bispebjerg and Frederikberg Hospitals
Copenhagen, Denmark

Simran Phuyal, BSc, MS
Medical Student
Eastern Virginia Medical School
Sterling, Virginia

Kevin Pierre, MD
Diagnostic Radiology Resident
Department of Radiology
University of Florida
Gainesville, Florida

Gregory M. Ramina, MS
Director, Regulatory Affairs
Department of Quality Assurance and Regulatory Affairs
Viz.ai, Inc.
San Francisco, California

Ehab S. Saleh, MD
Pediatric Orthopedic Surgeon
Department of Orthopedics
William Beaumont University Hospital
Royal Oak, Michigan

Robert Short, MD, PhD
Section Chief, Interventional Radiology
Department of Therapeutic and Diagnostic Imaging
Dayton VAMC
Dayton, Ohio

Jonathan Antony Stone, BS
Medical Student
Oakland University William Beaumont School of Medicine
Rochester, Michigan

Tulasi Talluri, BS, MPH
Medical Student
Oakland University
William Beaumont School of Medicine
Rochester, Michigan

Satvik Tripathi, BS
Research Assistant
Department of Radiology
Massachusetts General Hospital
Boston, Massachusetts

PREFACE

This book is intended as a practical guide for artificial intelligence (AI) in radiology. Written by clinical and data science experts, *The Radiology AI Handbook* is organized into sections covering fundamental technology concepts, interpretive AI applications, noninterpretive AI applications, and a how-to manual for developing AI applications—starting from idea, data curation, model development, testing, regulatory, through commercialization. Organized by radiology subspecialty, chapters include currently approved AI applications, existing companies, applications under development, as well as unmet opportunities and clinical needs. For radiologists, engineers, data scientists, and entrepreneurs interested in AI and the advancement of radiology, *The Radiology AI Handbook* will be a foundational resource.

ACKNOWLEDGMENTS

The editors thank the authors for their contributions as well as the Elsevier team for their support.

CONTENTS

PART I

Background

PART OUTLINE

CHAPTER 1

AI in Radiology—Past and Present

Nadeen Aladham ■ Katherine P. Andriole

KEY POINTS

- Artificial intelligence (AI) is revolutionizing radiology with applications such as computer-aided diagnosis, image quantification, and workflow automation.
- Nearly 1000 AI healthcare tools have been approved by the FDA, with the largest percentage in radiology.
- Although AI has multiple potential benefits, concerns include medical-legal responsibility, algorithm transparency and explainability, cost, potential job displacement, and ethical considerations, including bias and fairness of models. Seamless integration into point-of-care systems must be addressed in order for tools to be broadly adopted.

GLOSSARY OF TERMS AND DEFINITIONS

Machine Learning (ML): A subset of artificial intelligence that involves the use of algorithms and statistical methods to enable computer systems to learn from data and improve their performance on a specific task without being explicitly programmed (Fig. 1.1).

Deep Learning (DL): A subset of machine learning that utilizes convolutional neural networks with multiple hidden layers to process and analyze data and is especially well suited for complex tasks like image analysis, enabled by current computational capabilities (Fig. 1.1).

Convolutional Neural Network (CNN): A type of machine learning architecture designed for processing grid-like data, such as images and videos, by applying convolution operations to mathematically extract relevant features in data.

Computer-Aided Detection/Diagnosis (CADe/x): A system that employs computer algorithms to assist radiologists in interpreting medical images and providing diagnostic support by identifying potential abnormalities. Some CAD systems use classical machine learning with human-defined features, whereas others use data-driven CNN architectures.

Natural Language Processing (NLP): A branch of artificial intelligence that focuses on the interaction between computers and human language, enabling machines to understand, interpret, and generate human language.

Software as a Medical Device (SaMD): Software intended to be used for one or more medical purposes that perform these purposes without being part of a hardware medical device.[5]

Reference Standard: The correct or true label (sometimes called ground truth) used for training and evaluating AI systems, against which their accuracy and performance are measured.

Transparency: The degree to which the inner workings of an AI system can be understood by humans, including how decisions are made and the rationale behind those decisions.

Explainable AI: AI systems designed to provide clear and comprehensible explanations for their decision-making processes, enhancing trust and accountability.

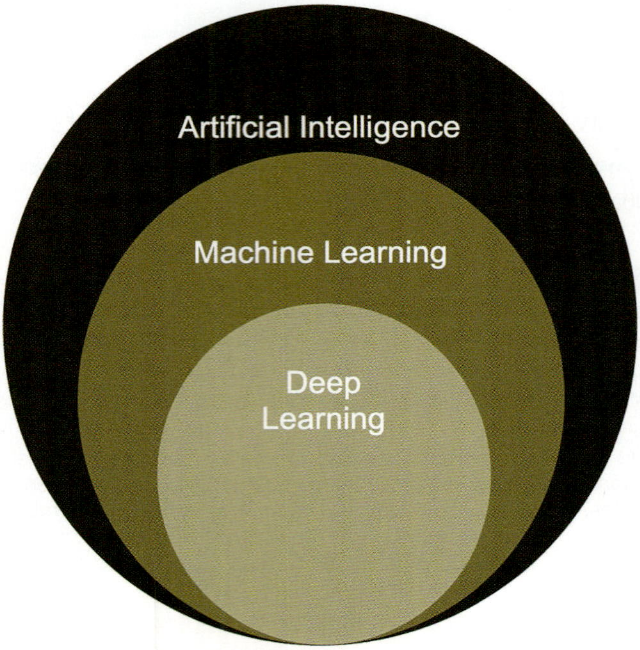

Fig. 1.1 The relationship between artificial intelligence (AI), machine learning (ML), and deep learning (DL).

Introduction

Artificial intelligence (AI) is a tool that is advancing rapidly, and its use in radiology is increasing. Early rule-based machine learning systems have largely been replaced by data-driven deep learning, notably convolutional neural network architectures. More recently, foundation models, large language models, and generative AI applications have appeared on the horizon, with some in clinical use today.

Convolutional neural networks are a building block component of machine learning in which features are mathematically calculated from imaging data. These learned features are used to aid in object recognition, localization and segmentation, feature quantitation, and image classification.[1] More than 750 FDA-approved AI imaging tools[2] now provide clinical decision support to radiologists for interpreting mammograms, chest X-rays, chest CT for lung nodules, and head CT for stroke, improving efficiency and outcomes. AI use cases also encompass tumor measurement and characterization via radiomics, predicting tumor subtypes and providing prognosis.[3] Generative AI will revolutionize data and information search and analysis. In medical education, AI can track individual radiology residents and assist in personalizing residency training.[4] In general, the role of AI in radiology promises to enhance diagnostics, reduce radiologists' workload, and enable large-scale data analysis. Despite AI's great potential and promise to revolutionize patient care and healthcare delivery, ethical concerns such as medical-legal responsibility, issues of algorithm transparency and bias, job displacement, and cost remain. Provider and patient trust is vital for widespread adoption into clinical practice.

AI Past

This chapter provides a brief overview of early AI in radiology, a review of fundamental terms, a snapshot of the present state describing the types of applications of AI in radiology today, and current challenges to widespread adoption.

One of the earliest forms of AI in radiology was the development of rule-based systems designed to aid in the interpretation of medical images.[6] These systems operated on a set of predefined rules explicitly programmed, allowing for the identification of specific patterns or features in images.

Among the earliest classical machine learning algorithms used clinically in radiology were the computer-aided detection (CADe) tools approved by the FDA in 1998[7] to detect calcifications on screening mammograms.[3] These systems evaluate mammograms and highlight areas of concern for radiologists to examine further. Although these early systems had limitations including high false-positive rates, they marked a crucial advancement in the integration of AI in radiology. CADe has since been approved for use in other modalities, including x-rays, computed tomography (CT) scans, ultrasound, and magnetic resonance imaging (MRI).

Fundamental Concepts

The development of deep learning models has revolutionized the field of AI in radiology,[8] made possible by availability of healthcare data in digital format including images, advancements in computational capabilities via graphics processing units (GPUs), and advancements in algorithms. DL models are a type of machine learning model, typically including a convolutional neural network (CNN), with multiple hidden layers that aim to replicate the functioning of the human brain, and have been used to develop tools for image classification and segmentation.[9]

The majority of FDA-approved machine learning (ML)/deep learning (DL) models have been developed using supervised learning in which a mathematical model is trained on a labeled or annotated training set of data. CNNs are a building block component of machine learning models in which features such as edges, size, shape, and texture are mathematically calculated from imaging data much like the human visual system does with light signals received via the retinal photoreceptors that are then passed to the ganglion cells. In a CNN the output of a preceding layer becomes the weighted input to the succeeding layer, with the mathematical model iterating until the learned model weights are optimized to minimize a loss function[9,10] (Fig. 1.2). The loss function is the difference between what the model predicts as the output label or answer versus the true label or answer.

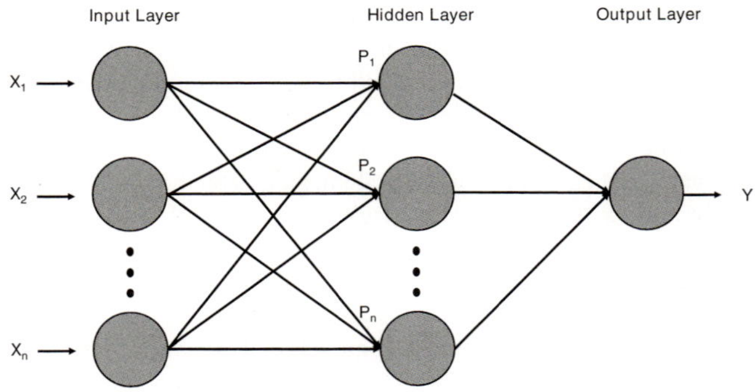

Fig. 1.2 Machine learning model convolutional neural network architecture with a single hidden layer. *P*, Input parameter; *X*, input; *Y*, output parameter. (Based on Brooks H, Tucker N. Electrospinning predictions using artificial neural networks. *Polymer*. 2015;58:22–29.)

Clinical Application of AI Present

There are many AI tools that have been developed to assist in the interpretation of medical images. Currently, multiple FDA-approved AI applications in radiology aid in detection of breast, lung, and other types of cancer. In 2018, the FDA approved the first digital tomosynthesis AI system for breast cancer screening, which utilizes deep learning to analyze tomosynthesis and identify suspicious abnormalities.[11] This system, named ProFound AI (iCAD, Nashua, NH), has demonstrated enhanced accuracy in breast cancer screening by detecting a greater number of cancers while simultaneously reducing false positives and unnecessary callbacks for patients.[12]

Other early FDA-approved applications include stroke detection on brain CT, lung nodule detection and quantification on chest CT, pneumothorax detection on chest x-ray, and prostate cancer assessment on MRI to name a few examples.[13] Many companies large and small, including traditional imaging companies (e.g., GE Healthcare, Chicago; IL Philips, Amsterdam, Holland; Siemens Healthineers, Erlangen, Germany) and computing companies (e.g., NVIDIA, Santa Clara, CA; Microsoft, Redmond, WA; Google, Mountain View, CA; IBM Watson, Yorktown Heights, NY), are involved in developing AI tools in healthcare.[14]

AI can assist radiologists by automating image quantification and measurement to support decision-making.[15] This is especially beneficial in oncology, where it may help identify radiologic characteristics that can predict specific tumor subtypes, grades, and even patient prognosis.[16] Quantitation of disease findings such as tumor size and volume can aid in change detection and monitoring of disease.[11]

AI's integration with augmented reality (AR) and virtual reality (VR) is advancing navigation in interventional radiology. AI enhances procedure planning and real-time monitoring during procedures, supporting precision interventions, identifying potential complications in real time, and improving patient outcomes.[17]

AI tools extend beyond diagnostics and include assistance with test ordering, scheduling, image protocoling, acquisition and reconstruction, report generation, and results communication with potential to reduce radiologist workload and increase efficiency.[14]

As AI continues to advance in radiology, it holds significant potential to influence the education and training of radiologists.[4] AI can monitor and assess the performance of radiology residents, leading to more personalized and efficient training programs. Additionally, AI tools can assist residents in identifying knowledge gaps and areas requiring further clinical exposure. However, it is essential to ensure that AI does not replace residents in the interpretation process during educational activities. A balanced approach to integrating AI is crucial, allowing residents to gain valuable hands-on experience while utilizing technology to enhance their learning.[3]

The market for AI in radiology is rapidly growing, with various companies and startups offering a wide range of AI-based products and services. According to a market research report by MarketsandMarkets, the global AI in healthcare market size was valued at USD 20.9 billion in 2024 and is estimated to reach USD 148.4 billion by 2029, registering a CAGR of 48.1% during the forecast period.[18] The radiology segment is expected to hold the largest share of the AI in healthcare market during the forecast period. The increasing adoption of AI in radiology is driven by factors such as the increasing volume of medical imaging data, the shortage of radiologists, and the need for efficient and accurate diagnostic imaging.

Challenges and Limitations

Challenges in the development of supervised ML models include the need for well-labeled and/or annotated datasets for training and diverse outside testing sets. Annotation of data is tedious and time-consuming, requiring radiology expertise. Further, the "ground truth" can often be subjective based on radiology reports and manual annotation.[19]

Large diverse training data cohorts are required to create models that are unbiased and generalize to broad patient populations. But patient privacy and data security are concerns when sharing data with developers. Federated learning involves a decentralized machine learning approach in which models are trained across multiple devices or servers holding local data samples that do not leave local security firewalls. Only the model weights are passed to participating sites, thus enhancing privacy and security by keeping data localized.

A challenge in adopting AI in radiology is making tools accessible in the point-of-care tools used by radiologists and others including in imaging modality acquisition devices, in picture archiving and communication systems (PACS), reporting systems, and the electronic medical record (EMR). Proper use of integration standards and implementation profiles such as DICOM (Digital Imaging and Communications in Medicine), HL7 FHIR (Health Level 7, Fast Healthcare Interoperability Resources), and IHE (Integrating the Healthcare Enterprise) protocols are essential.[20]

Concerns about AI's impact on jobs in radiology exist, but experts argue that AI will assist rather than replace radiologists. The overall demand for radiologists in the United States and elsewhere is increasing, and practicing radiologists are experiencing a significant increase in professional burnout, further supporting the need for the adoption and integration of AI into the imaging workflow. A hybrid model in which radiologists work together with AI tools will be necessary to maximize benefit of workflow efficiency and patient outcomes.

The current volume-based economic model remains a challenge for creating reimbursement paths, and medicolegal uncertainty is a concern. Who will be responsible when AI tools fail is still an unknown.

The lack of transparency in how AI systems make decisions can undermine trust among both providers and patients. To address this, efforts have focused on developing explainable or transparent AI, designed to offer insights into the algorithms' decision-making processes.[1] Ethical concerns also remain, including the risk of biased decision-making and the potential for job displacement as AI automates tasks traditionally performed by radiologists and other healthcare personnel.[6,14]

Despite these challenges, AI's ability to enhance efficiency and accuracy in radiology remains promising. Collaborative efforts between radiologists, data and computer scientists, and healthcare professionals are essential for unlocking AI's full potential.

References

1. LeCun Y, Bengio Y, Hinton G. Deep learning. *Nature.* 2015;521(7553):436–444. https://doi.org/10.1038/nature14539.
2. FDA. Artificial Intelligence and Machine Learning (AI/ML)—Enabled Medical Devices. 2024. FDA. https://www.fda.gov/medical-devices/software-medical-device-samd/artificial-intelligence-and-machine-learning-aiml-enabled-medical-devices.
3. Rezazade Mehrizi MH, Khameneh MH. Applications of artificial intelligence (AI) in diagnostic radiology: a technography study. *Eur Radiol.* 2020;31(4):1805–1811. https://doi.org/10.1007/s00330-020-07230-9.
4. Mun SK, Ko YK, Lee JH. Artificial intelligence for the future radiology diagnostic service. *Front Mol Biosci.* 2021;7:614258. https://doi.org/10.3389/fmolb.2020.614258.
5. Software as a Medical Device (SaMD). (2018). FDA website. https://www.fda.gov/medical-devices/digital-health-center-excellence/software-medical-device-samd.
6. Kobayashi Y, Furuya Y, Yoshida K. How will "Democratization of Artificial Intelligence" change the future of radiologists? *Jap J Radiol.* 2018;37(1):9–14. https://doi.org/10.1007/s11604-018-0793-5.
7. Milam ME, Koo CW. The current status and future of FDA-approved artificial intelligence tools in chest radiology in the United States. *Clin Radiol.* 2023;78(2):115–122. https://doi.org/10.1016/j.crad.2022.08.135.
8. Iezzi R, Campanella G, Maffei M. Artificial intelligence in interventional radiology: a literature review and future perspectives. *J Oncol.* 2019;2019:6153041. https://doi.org/10.1155/2019/6153041.

9. Kapoor N, Harisinghani M, Chatterjee S. Workflow applications of artificial intelligence in radiology and an overview of available tools. *J Am Coll Radiol.* 2020;17(11):1363–1370. https://doi.org/10.1016/j.jacr.2020.08.016.
10. Brooks H, Tucker N. Electrospinning predictions using artificial neural networks. *Polymer.* 2015;58:22–29.
11. Ou WC, Jiang X, Kwan A, Karp J, Bae S. Deep learning in breast radiology: current progress and future directions. *Eur Radiol.* 2021;31(7):4872–4885. https://doi.org/10.1007/s00330-020-07640-9.
12. Mayo RC, Kent D, Sen LC, Kapoor M, Leung JW, Watanabe AT. Reduction of false-positive markings on mammograms: a retrospective comparison study using an artificial intelligence-based CAD. *J Digit Imag.* 2019;32:618–624.
13. Mello-Thoms C, Mello CA. Clinical applications of artificial intelligence in radiology. *Br J Radiol.* 2023;96(1150):20221031.
14. van Leeuwen KG, Schalekamp S, Rutten MJCM, van Ginneken B, de Rooij M. Artificial intelligence in radiology: 100 commercially available products and their scientific evidence. *Eur Radiol.* 2021;31(6):3797–3804. https://doi.org/10.1007/s00330-021-07892-z.
15. Davendralingam N, Wainwright A, Babbitt J. Artificial intelligence in pediatric radiology: future opportunities. *Br J Radiol.* 2021;94(1117):20200975. https://doi.org/10.1259/bjr.20200975.
16. Otjen JP, Ali R, Aroda M. The current and future roles of artificial intelligence in pediatric radiology. *Pediatr Radiol.* 2021;52(11):2065–2073. https://doi.org/10.1007/s00247-021-05086-9.
17. Von Ende E, Ryan S, Crain MA, Makary MS. Artificial intelligence, augmented reality, and virtual reality advances and applications in interventional radiology. *Diagnostics.* 2023;13(5):892. https://www.mdpi.com/2075-4418/13/5/892.
18. MarketsandMarkets. Artificial Intelligence (AI) in healthcare market size: share, trends, Industry Report, statistics (n.d.). https://www.marketsandmarkets.com/Market-Reports/artificial-intelligence-healthcare-market-54679303.html.
19. Rubin DL. Artificial intelligence in imaging: the radiologist's role. *J Am Coll Radiol.* 2019;16(9):1309–1317.
20. Wiggins WF, Magudia K, Sippel-Schmidt TM, et al. Imaging AI in practice: a demonstration of future workflow using integration standards. *Radiol Artif Intell.* 2021;3(6):e210152. https://doi.org/10.1148/ryai.2021210152.

CHAPTER 2

AI in Radiology—Future

Nadeen Aladham ■ Katherine P. Andriole

KEY POINTS

- **AI Advancements:** The future of radiology will rely on self-supervised learning and large-scale models that learn from unlabeled data, enhancing performance across multiple tasks without requiring extensive retraining.
- **Large Language Models:** Models like BERT and GPT improve the analysis of unstructured text in radiology, increasing efficiency in reporting and extracting meaningful insights.
- **Regulatory Challenges:** Despite the FDA approving numerous AI devices, no generative AI models have been authorized yet, highlighting the need for effective evaluation frameworks to address biases and performance issues.

GLOSSARY OF TERMS AND DEFINITIONS

BERT: Bidirectional Encoder Representations from Transformers; is a machine learning model that uses surrounding text to establish context and meaning in unstructured text.

GPT: Generative Pretrained Transformer; is a multimodal large language model created by OpenAI and launched March 14, 2023.

Natural Language Processing (NLP): A field of AI that focuses on the interaction between computers and humans through natural language, enabling machines to understand, interpret, and generate human language.

Generative Adversarial Networks (GANs): A framework in machine learning consisting of two neural networks (generator and discriminator) that compete against each other, allowing the generator to create increasingly realistic images.

Transformers: A type of deep learning model initially designed for NLP that has demonstrated effectiveness in handling sequential data and is now applied in many foundation models for image analysis tasks; based on the multihead attention mechanism.

Introduction

To date, the FDA has authorized nearly 1000 AI-enabled medical devices, with over 750 of these tools dedicated to radiology alone.[1] These narrow AI products predominantly utilize deep learning convolutional neural network architectures, trained in a supervised manner using labeled data. They are designed to perform a limited range of specific tasks, such as detecting the presence of lung nodules on a chest CT scan, but may not identify other conditions like pulmonary fibrosis that could be present. The performance of these AI tools is heavily dependent on the data cohort used for training, which can potentially limit their generalizability across diverse patient populations. Newer methods, including foundation, large language and generative models built upon very large amounts of unlabeled data, show promise for more generalizable algorithms that could improve radiological workflow. But questions regarding performance and regulation remain.

Natural Language Processing

Natural language processing (NLP) is a branch of AI that intersects with machine and deep learning (Fig. 2.1). NLP works to extract meaning from unstructured text by processing text data, such as radiology reports, in a manner analogous to how AI models analyze pixel data in medical images. The process involves extracting features from the text and generating numerical representations of these features, which can include individual words or more complex linguistic structures.[2] The specific steps in NLP processing include tokenization, stop word removal, token normalization, and embedding and vectorization, all of which contribute to the model's ability to discern patterns and make predictions on previously unseen text structures.[2]

Newer AI Methods: Foundation, Large Language, and Generative Models

The evolution of NLP from rule-based approaches in the 1980s to neural network–based methods like Word2Vec in 2013 and BERT (bidirectional encoder representations from transformers) in 2018 has paved the way for more advanced text analysis in radiology[3,4] and for the newer foundation models, including large language and generative models. This progression from feature-centric

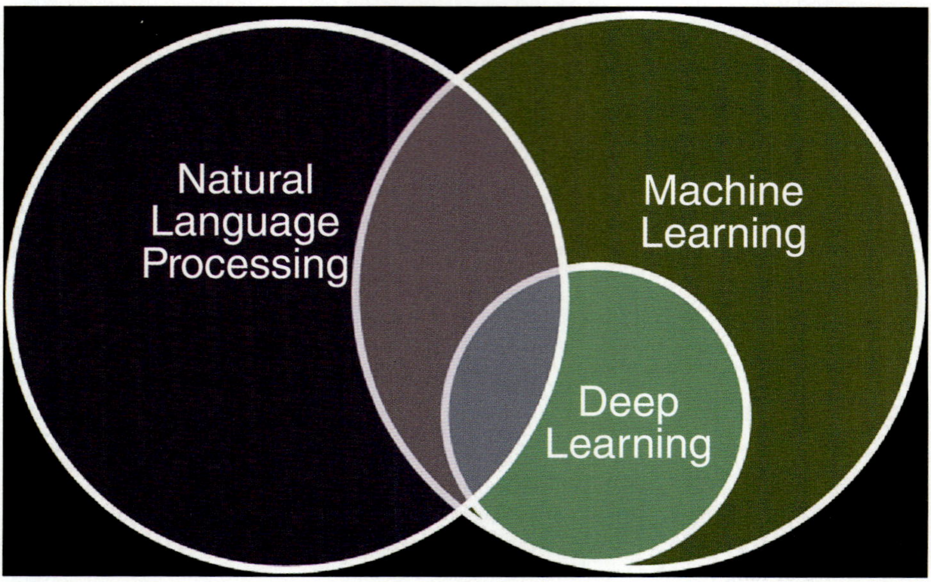

Fig. 2.1 The relationship between natural language processing, machine learning, and deep learning.

machine learning methods to model-centric deep learning models to data-centric foundation models is depicted in Fig. 2.2.

The future of AI in radiology will depend on advancements made in self-supervised learning (SSL) and the development of large-scale, generalized models. These models, pretrained on vast amounts of unlabeled data, including images, text, and language, are capable of learning robust and versatile data representations that can be used as foundations that then can be adapted to multiple downstream tasks in radiology.[5,6] This approach marks a significant departure from traditional supervised learning methods, which rely heavily on labeled datasets. By leveraging SSL,

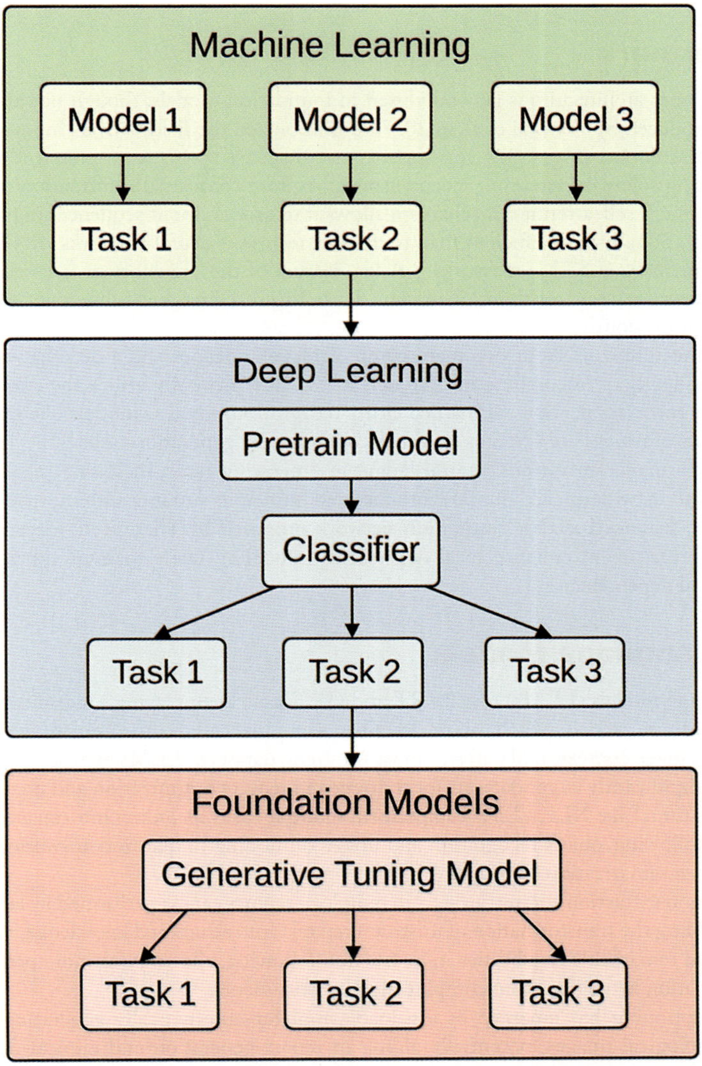

Fig. 2.2 Evolution of artificial intelligence: Progression from feature-centric machine learning to model-centric deep learning and data-centric foundation models.

researchers have demonstrated that models can achieve excellent performance in various radiologic tasks, even outperforming those pretrained on labeled medical datasets in some cases.[5]

The emergence of these adaptable, multitask foundation models represents another frontier in AI-driven radiology. Foundation models, characterized by their immense scale (with some containing over 175 billion parameters[7]) and broad data representations, can be fine-tuned or prompted for domain-specific applications without requiring extensive additional model training. This versatility allows a single model to perform a wide array of tasks, from image classification to text generation, potentially revolutionizing workflow efficiency in radiology departments. The ability to apply these models across diverse radiological tasks through transfer learning and prompting techniques offers a promising solution to the perennial challenge of limited labeled data in medical imaging.[8]

Transformers

The Transformer architecture is generally used in foundation models, though not always. Transformers, introduced by Vaswani et al. in 2017, revolutionized the field with its innovative mechanism of self-attention (Fig. 2.3).[9] This architecture dispensed with recurrence and convolution entirely, relying solely on attention mechanisms to capture contextual information in sequences. The Transformer's self-attention mechanism allows it to process input sequences in parallel, making it computationally more efficient than traditional recurrent neural networks (RNNs) and long short-term memory (LSTM) networks.[10] A key feature of the Transformer is its ability to capture bidirectional context, enabling it to consider both preceding and subsequent elements in a sequence simultaneously.

The architecture consists of two main components: an encoder and a decoder, which can be used independently or in combination. Models like BERT primarily utilize the encoder part for tasks such as text classification and named entity recognition, whereas models like the generative pretrained transformer (GPT) focus on the decoder for text generation tasks.[9] The Transformer's superior performance in various natural language processing tasks, including machine translation, has led to its widespread adoption and inspired numerous variants and improvements.[11] For instance, the distance-based self-attention network proposed by Shen et al. incorporates word distance information to enhance local dependency modeling while maintaining the ability to capture global dependencies.[11]

Large Language Models

Large language models (LLMs) like BERT and GPT have been playing a significant role in AI in radiology. These models, which can be described as sophisticated autocomplete systems, predict text based on given contexts and patterns in vast training datasets.[2] LLMs expand upon NLP concepts using significantly larger datasets for training and require optimization and fine-tuning for a given application. Like NLP, LLMs can perform multiple tasks including information extraction, instruction following, object recognition and image captioning to question answering, sentiment analysis, and summarization (Fig. 2.4).

Information extraction and retrieval from radiology reports can be performed by large language models, enabling the transformation of unstructured text into structured knowledge.[12] LLMs have demonstrated remarkable capabilities in instruction following, allowing for more precise and tailored information extraction from complex medical documents.[13]

Image captioning has emerged as a valuable tool for automatically generating descriptive text for radiological images, potentially aiding in report generation and clinical decision support. Question-answering systems have been developed to assist radiologists in quickly retrieving relevant information from vast databases of medical literature and imaging reports.[14] Sentiment

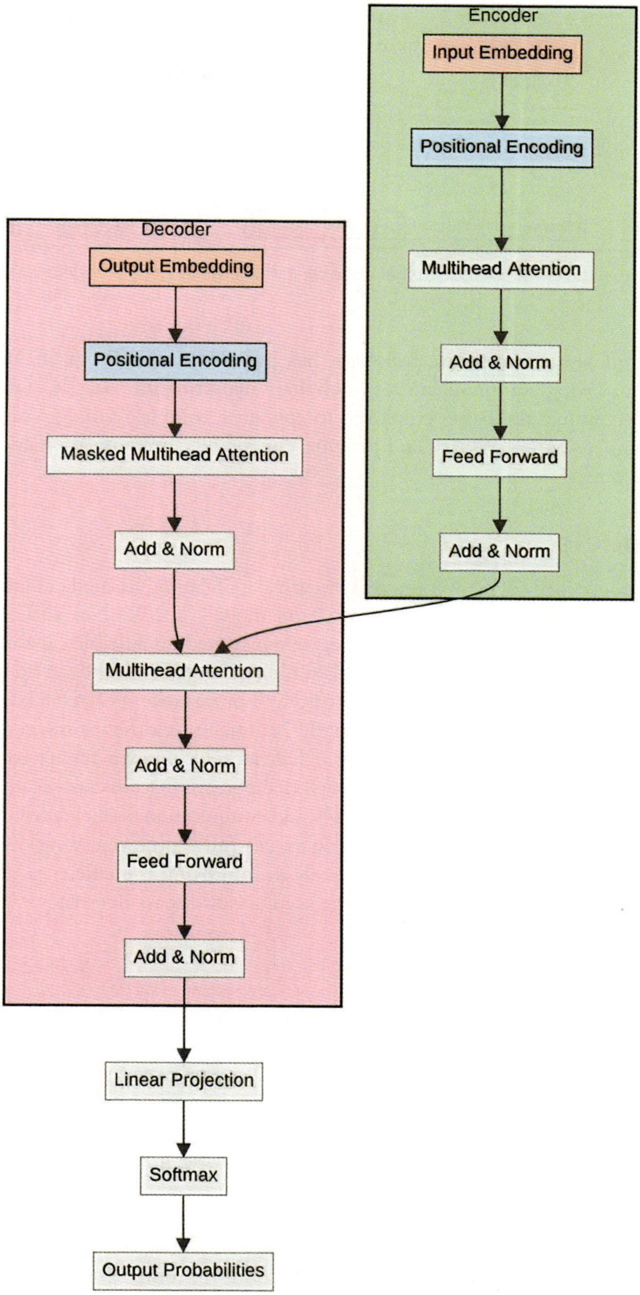

Fig. 2.3 Transformer model architecture. Depicted is the encoder-decoder structure with multihead attention, positional encoding, feed-forward layers, and output probability calculation via softmax.

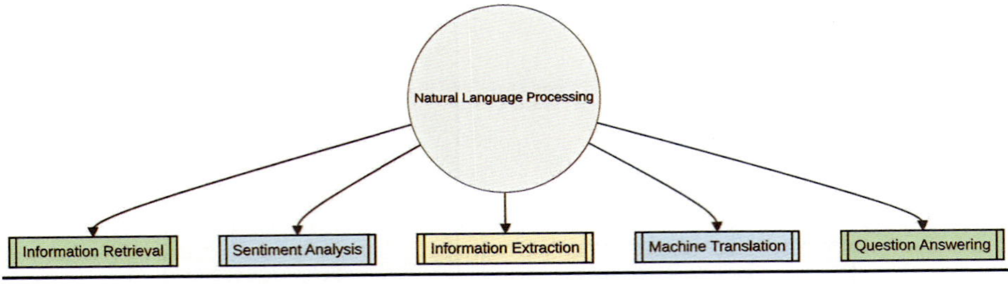

Fig. 2.4 Key tasks—natural language processing and large language models can perform.

analysis, although less common in radiology, has potential applications in analyzing patient feedback and improving communication in radiology departments.[15] Lastly, summarization and simplification techniques are being employed to condense complex radiology reports into more digestible formats for both clinicians and patients, enhancing communication and understanding of diagnostic findings.[12]

Vision Models

Object recognition, organ segmentation, and disease classification via medical imaging have been greatly improved through the application of vision models like ResNet and EfficientNet and YOLO.[16] These deep learning architectures have demonstrated remarkable capabilities in processing complex medical images, including retinal fundus images for diabetic retinopathy detection and MRI scans for Alzheimer's disease classification.[17] For instance, YOLOv8 has shown promise in segmenting and classifying diabetic retinopathy lesions in fundoscopy images, achieving high sensitivity and intersection-over-union scores.[18] EfficientNet, known for its compound scaling method, has been effectively applied in multiclass diabetic eye disease classification, outperforming other pretrained models in terms of accuracy and computational efficiency.[16] ResNet, with its innovative residual learning framework, has been successfully employed in various medical imaging tasks. These models can have a significant role in improving the efficiency of medical image analysis workflows in addition to enhancing the accuracy of disease detection.[17]

Generative Models

Generative adversarial networks (GANs) have emerged as a powerful tool in medical imaging, with their ability to generate synthetic medical images. GANs consist of two neural networks: a generator that creates images and a discriminator that evaluates the synthesized images against real images.[19] This technology has found applications in various aspects of medical imaging, including image generation for training purposes, dataset expansion when real images are limited, creation of educational pathological images,[19] and improving image acquisition. The impact of GANs extends beyond image generation, as they have also shown promise in image classification and segmentation tasks.[20]

Generative models such as GPT, DALL-E, GANs, and VAEs (Variational Autoencoder) have gained significant attention by enabling the creation of novel content, including text and images, rather than merely reproducing existing material.[21] These models have demonstrated remarkable capabilities in tasks such as text-to-text and text-to-image generation, pushing the boundaries of creative AI applications.[22]

LLMs and generative techniques have been employed to automatically generate impressions from radiology report findings, potentially reducing radiologists' workload and improving report

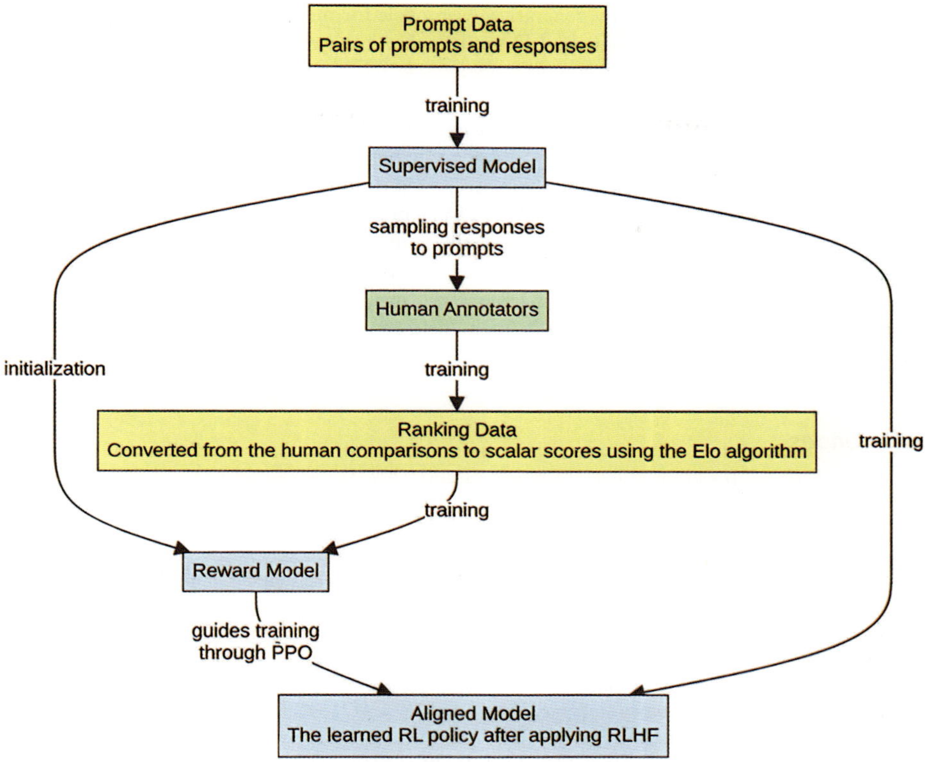

Fig. 2.5 General overview of reinforcement learning from human feedback (*RLHF*).

consistency.[23] Furthermore, efforts have been made to translate complex radiology reports into patient-readable text, enhancing patient understanding and engagement in their healthcare.[24] Similarly, NLP/LLMs have been utilized to simplify preprocedure patient instructions, making them more comprehensible and accessible to patients with varying levels of health literacy.[24] Summarization techniques have been applied to synthesize information from multiple sources, such as radiology reports, electronic health records, and clinical notes, providing a comprehensive overview of a patient's condition and facilitating more informed decision-making by healthcare providers.[24]

However, they are not without limitations. Generative models are prone to hallucinations, sometimes producing plausible but incorrect outputs, and they can propagate biases present in their training data.[25] To improve their performance, these models often require fine-tuning for specific tasks. Researchers and practitioners have found that careful prompt engineering and the application of reinforcement learning from human feedback (RLHF) can significantly enhance the quality and relevance of generated content (Fig. 2.5).[10]

Current Issues

The rapid advancement of artificial intelligence (AI) and machine learning (ML) technologies in healthcare has presented both promising opportunities and significant regulatory challenges. Although the FDA authorized more than 1000 AI/ML-enabled medical devices, as of July 2025 the agency has yet to approve any generative AI models for medical use. This lack of approved models raises questions about how the FDA will evaluate and regulate their performance, especially given the unique challenges posed by generative AI, such as hallucinations and potential biases stemming from training data.[26] The uneven performance of these models and their susceptibility to biases underscore the need for robust regulatory frameworks.

Despite these concerns, there is considerable excitement surrounding the potential benefits of AI applications in healthcare, particularly in areas such as information search and retrieval, data assimilation, and knowledge discovery.[27] The FDA's commitment to developing risk-based guidance for generative AI use in healthcare reflects the agency's recognition of the technology's rapid evolution and the industry's need for greater clarity. The FDA's formation of a Digital Health Advisory Committee and sponsored discussions via open forums aim to provide best practices for technology developers and adopters.[26] As the field continues to advance at an unprecedented pace, striking a balance between fostering innovation and ensuring patient safety remains a critical challenge for regulatory bodies and healthcare stakeholders alike.

References

1. FDA. Artificial Intelligence and Machine Learning (AI/ML)—Enabled Medical Devices. (2024). https://www.fda.gov/medical-devices/software-medical-device-samd/artificial-intelligence-and-machine-learning-aiml-enabled-medical-devices.
2. Klang E, Alper L, Sorin V, Barash Y, Nadkarni GN, Zimlichman E. Advancing radiology practice and research: harnessing the potential of large language models amidst imperfections. *BJR Open*. 2024;6(1):tzae022.
3. Barnard J. What are Word Embeddings? *IBM*. 2024. https://www.ibm.com/topics/word-embeddings.
4. Devlin J, Chang MW, Lee K, Toutanova K. BERT: Pre-training of deep bidirectional transformers for language understanding. *Proceedings of the 2019 conference of the North American chapter of the association for computational linguistics: human language technologies*; 2019;1:4171–4186.
5. Tayebi Arasteh S, Misera L, Kather JN, Truhn D, Nebelung S. Enhancing diagnostic deep learning via self-supervised pretraining on large-scale, unlabeled non-medical images. *Eur Radiol Exp*. 2024;8(1):10.
6. Hendrycks D, Mazeika M, Kadavath S, Song D. Using self-supervised learning can improve model robustness and uncertainty. *Adv Neural Inf Process Syst*. 2019;32. ISBN: 9781713807933.
7. Brown T, Mann B, Ryder N, et al. Language models are few-shot learners. Advances in neural information processing systems, 2020;33:1877–1901.
8. Mei X, Liu Z, Robson PM, et al. RadImageNet: an open radiologic deep learning research dataset for effective transfer learning. *Radiol Artif Intell*. 2022;4(5):e210315.
9. Vaswani A, Shazeer N, Parmar N, et al. Attention is all you need. *Adv Neural Inf Process Syst*. 2017;30. Long Beach, CA.
10. Shah, D. Reinforcement Learning from Human Feedback (RLHF): Bridging AI and Human Expertise. (2024). Lakera.ai. https://www.lakera.ai/blog/reinforcement-learning-from-human-feedback.
11. Im J, Cho S. Distance-based self-attention network for natural language inference. (2017). arXiv preprint arXiv:1712.02047.
12. Reichenpfader D, Müller H, Denecke K. Large language model-based information extraction from free-text radiology reports: a scoping review protocol. *BMJ Open*. 2023;13(12):e076865. https://doi.org/10.1136/bmjopen-2023-076865.
13. Engelbach M, Klau D, Scheerer F, Drawehn J, Kintz M. Fine-tuning and aligning question answering models for complex information extraction tasks. (2023). arXiv preprint arXiv:2309.14805.
14. Lin Z, Zhang D, Tao Q, et al. Medical visual question answering: a survey. *Artif Intell Med*. 2023;143:102611.
15. Jain AP, Dandannavar P. Application of machine learning techniques to sentiment analysis. *2016 2nd International Conference on Applied and Theoretical Computing and Communication Technology (iCATccT)*. IEEE; 2016:628–632.
16. Vadduri M, P. KUPPUSAMY Member I. Enhancing ocular healthcare: deep learning-based multi-class diabetic eye disease segmentation and classification. *IEEE Acc*. 2023;11:137881–137898.

17. Thota NR, Vasumathi D. Wasserstein GAN-gradient penalty with deep transfer learning based Alzheimer disease classification on 3D MRI scans. *i-manager's J Image Proc.* 2022;9(4):9–20.
18. Rizzieri N, Dall'Asta L, Ozoliņš M. Diabetic retinopathy features segmentation without coding experience with computer vision models YOLOv8 and YOLOv9. *Vision (Basel).* 2024;8(3):48. https://doi.org/10.3390/vision8030048.
19. Jeong JJ, Tariq A, Adejumo T, Trivedi H, Gichoya JW, Banerjee I. Systematic review of generative adversarial networks (GANs) for medical image classification and segmentation. *J Digit Imag.* 2022;35(2):137–152. https://doi.org/10.1007/s10278-021-00556-w.
20. Makhlouf A, Maayah M, Abughanam N, Catal C. The use of generative adversarial networks in medical image augmentation. *Neural Comput Appl.* 2023;35(34):24055–24068.
21. Clark K, Jaini P. Text-to-image diffusion models are zero shot classifiers. *Adv Neural Inf Proc Syst.* 2023;36.
22. Brade S, Wang B, Sousa M, Oore S, Grossman T. Promptify: text-to-image generation through interactive prompt exploration with large language models. *Proceedings of the 36th Annual ACM Symposium on User Interface Software and Technology*; 2023:1–14.
23. Silva W, Gonçalves T, Härmä K, et al. Computer-aided diagnosis through medical image retrieval in radiology. *Sci Rep.* 2022;12(1):20732.
24. Casey A, Davidson E, Poon M, et al. A systematic review of natural language processing applied to radiology reports. *BMC Med Inform Decis Mak.* 2021;21(1):179.
25. Bird C, Ungless E, Kasirzadeh A. Typology of risks of generative text-to-image models. *Proceedings of the 2023 AAAI/ACM Conference on AI, Ethics, and Society*; 2023:396–410.
26. FDA. Executive Summary for The Digital Heath Advisory Committee Meeting: Total Product Lifecycle Considerations for Generative AI- Enabled Devices. (2024). https://www.fda.gov/media/182871/download.
27. Zegarelli B, Hawana J, Tikhonovsky M. FDA and CTTI Hold Joint Workshop on AI in Drug Development—AI: The Washington Report. *Mintz.* 2024. https://www.mintz.com/insights-center/viewpoints/2791/2024-08-09-fda-and-ctti-hold-joint-workshop-ai-drug-development-ai.

CHAPTER 3

Technical Principles

Adrian Coscia ■ Satvik Tripathi ■ Dania Daye

KEY POINTS

The typical arc of artificial intelligence (AI) tool development in radiology proceeds in three phases:

- *Data Curation*—model training requires a properly curated and well-labeled and/or annotated dataset
- *Model Development*—choice of model design and learning method is context dependent
- *Implementation*—proper technical operation must also be subject to ethical stewardshipIn this chapter, we outline each of these phases and consider practical aspects particular to applications in clinical radiology.

Introduction

This chapter introduces professionals across the healthcare industry—clinicians, scientists, researchers, healthcare administrators—to the technical principles behind the AI most used in clinical radiology. Specifically, the core phases of AI development—data curation, modeling, and implementation—are discussed and key considerations described (see Fig. 3.1). Radiologic dataset curation and labeling/annotation are discussed, noting key challenges including de-identification and data cohort bias. Next, deep learning and convolutional neural networks are described, as well as other established and emerging learning methods often applied in clinical radiology (Table 3.1). Finally, the technical and ethical aspects of model implementation in the clinical setting are discussed. Understanding the principles underlying AI in clinical radiology empowers healthcare professionals to work more effectively with AI systems, to critically interpret their results, and to make more informed clinical decisions.

Data Curation

The first key phase of AI development involves curating the dataset needed to train and evaluate a machine learning model. The lack of large, diverse medical image datasets is a major limitation for the training of AI algorithms. Small, unrepresentative, or imbalanced datasets can introduce data bias, compromising the accuracy of AI models. Although a growing number of open-source datasets are improving data access to research developers, quality and annotation is nonstandard, and in many cases sample size and representation remain limited.[1] Furthermore, because most open-source datasets are strictly for research use, commercial developers must undergo the costly process of compiling new datasets. This section reviews how datasets are curated and annotated, giving particular attention to data cohort bias, and a brief description of data content.

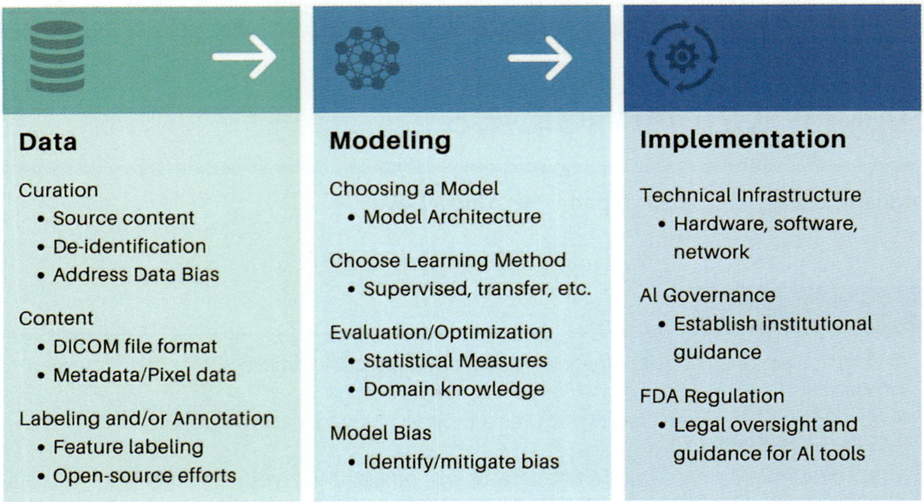

Fig. 3.1 Artificial intelligence development workflow. Key phases of artificial intelligence tool development comprising data, modeling, and implementation stages. The data stage tasks include curating a dataset, labeling and/or annotating the dataset, and understanding data content. The modeling stage involves choosing a model architecture, selecting a learning method to train the model, and optimizing model performance. The implementation stage requires technical infrastructure and dedicated technical support and must be subject to varying aspects of institutional and FDA oversight.

DATA CONTENT

In clinical radiology, the Digital Imaging and Communications in Medicine (DICOM) file format serves as the worldwide standard for medical imaging data. DICOM images contain both pixel data and metadata that describes the image data, including instrument specifications, acquisition parameters, and patient demographic information. AI algorithms process and analyze the pixel data from different imaging modalities (e.g., CT, MRI, nuclear imaging, x-ray, ultrasound, etc.) and preprocessing techniques such as noise reduction, gray-level normalization, and image enhancement are often applied to improve the accuracy and performance of AI algorithms.

CURATION

Before compiling, patient data must be de-identified. Several tools are available for the automated de-identification of DICOM metadata, but de-dentification of image data requires context-specific preprocessing before it can be used.[2,3] For example, ultrasound images often contain patient demographic data burned into the pixel data that must be located in the image and blackened out for de-identification. For CT or MRI scans of the head, defacing techniques are often used so that patients cannot be identified by 3D reconstructions of the data. Access to large, high-quality source data is also a challenge, as patient data protection and management in the United States are decentralized. Open data initiatives like The Cancer Imaging Archive (TCIA) and the Radiological Society of North America (RSNA) Medical Imaging and Data Resource Center (MIDRC) provide researchers with large amounts of data for algorithm development, and the NIH has released datasets specifically for training machine learning models.[4,5]

ANNOTATION

Data must be labeled and annotated for both training and testing of machine learning models, and standardized labeling is critical for ensuring consistency and interoperability of AI algorithms.

and annotation into routine clinical work.[6] The ACR-DSI has also launched ACR Connect and AI-Lab—a free, cloud-based platform that provides access to large datasets for AI algorithm development and validation.[7]

DATA BIAS

There are several different types of data bias in AI including sampling, measurement, labeling, temporal, demographic, and association bias.[8] Bias represents a major challenge to implementing AI in clinical radiology, and it can arise from many sources including differences in imaging protocol, biased sampling, and inaccurate labeling and annotation of training data (Fig. 3.2). Failure to identify and account for data bias could lead to misdiagnosis or unequal treatment. To date, most AI algorithms used in radiology in the United States have been trained using datasets compiled from a single institution and lack the representative sampling needed for generalizability.[9] Moreover, US and Chinese datasets are overrepresented, and nearly all the top databases in clinical AI are from high-income countries.[10] Standardization efforts in data curation and preprocessing can be taken to mitigate bias introduced by differences in imaging protocol, and efforts to systematize labeling and annotation help address bias introduced at these steps of data curation.

Model Development

The second major phase in AI development involves choosing, training, and evaluating a model suited to the desired application. This section will briefly review convolutional neural networks, summarize the major types of machine learning, discuss how a model is trained and evaluated, and identify important types and sources of model bias. Different types of algorithms and some of the key statistical methods used are covered, and a few practical examples are presented to demonstrate their use in radiologic applications. Selecting an appropriate model and learning method that aligns with the desired task, available data, and clinical requirements is important for optimizing accuracy and performance. As such, different tasks require different models best suited for the respective application at hand.

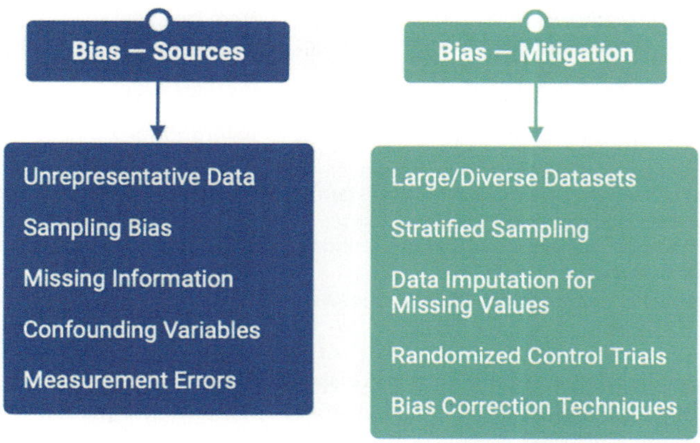

Fig. 3.2 Sources and mitigation of bias. Sources of bias in artificial intelligence (AI) development include unrepresentative data, sampling bias, missing information, confounding variables, and measurement errors. Mitigation requires evaluation and continuous monitoring for bias in clinical AI tools. Strategies range from general—curating large and diverse datasets, stratified sampling, data imputation, clinical trials—to case-specific correction techniques following bias identification. Robust countermeasures to bias mitigate equitable use and outcomes of clinical AI tools.

TABLE 3.1 ■ **Summary of Learning Methods**

Learning Method	Description	Applications	Advantages	Challenges
Supervised	Trained on labeled data to learn relationship between input and ground-truth labels	Image classification, segmentation	Well-established, accurate results	Requires labeled data that is time consuming and requires domain expertise
Unsupervised	Trained on unlabeled data to identify patterns and group by similarity	Clustering, association tasks, generative modeling	Reveals hidden patterns, less reliance on labeled data	Lack of clear ground-truth labels, complex algorithm tuning
Reinforcement	Learns by trial-and-error with positive/negative feedback, maximizing expected rewards	Image classification, segmentation, radiotherapy planning	Sequential decision-making, adaptive to changing environments	Requires careful reward design, can be computationally costly
Transfer	Uses pretrained model as a starting point, fine-tuning for a specific task	Specific medical imaging tasks with limited data	Reduced data requirements, faster model convergence	Domain gap between pretraining and specific use case
Self-Supervised	Learns from unlabeled data by creating supervisory signals (pretext tasks)	Feature extraction, attribute discovery	Utilizes unlabeled data effectively, relevant features	Design effective pretext tasks, complex model architecture
Federated	Trains a central model on local nodes with multisite internal data, preserving privacy	Collaborative model training, privacy-preserving	More (potentially diverse) data availability, privacy and data rights preserved	Infrastructure development, communication overhead

Concise overview of the various learning methods in AI development, as outlined in the text. Each method is briefly described along with sample applications in clinical radiology, advantages, and challenges. Choosing a learning method for a given application requires consideration of factors such as data availability, privacy concerns, and model performance.

Labeling images into categories is important in classification tasks, for instance classifying benign versus malignant lung nodules on a CT scan. Annotations attach information to certain parts of an image, for example whether a pixel represents functional or damaged brain tissue in stroke MRIs, and are especially important in segmentation and detection tasks. The American College of Radiology (ACR) Data Science Institute (DSI) and the RSNA have launched mass annotation efforts to improve availability and standardize the quality of training datasets for AI algorithms. The ACR-RSNA common data elements (CDEs) support integration of standardized labeling

CONVOLUTIONAL NEURAL NETWORKS

Convolutional neural networks (**CNNs**) are a type of artificial neural network especially suited for computer vision tasks due to their ability to capture both local spatial features and hierarchical representations. Typical CNN architecture consists of convolutional layers, pooling layers, and fully connected dense layers that generate output.[11] Convolution layers filter input data to extract local features such as lines and edges and output them as feature maps. Pooling layers downsample the feature maps to accelerate computation, and fully connected layers use the learned features to perform a task (e.g., classification). The U-net architecture is an example of one of the most widely used "off-the-shelf" CNNs for radiologic applications.[12] Typically, multiple models are trained and tested to determine the best for the particular task.

LEARNING METHODS

Once a network architecture is chosen, a learning method must be selected to train the model to perform a useful task. The following subsections summarize the predominant and emerging learning methods used in radiology including supervised learning, unsupervised learning, reinforcement learning, transfer learning, self-supervised learning, and federated learning (Table 3.1).

Supervised learning is by far the most employed learning method in radiologic applications with systematic review finding its use un 88% of studies.[13] In supervised learning, a model is trained on a labeled dataset that is usually preannotated by board-certified radiologists. The aim is to train the model to learn the relationship between the annotated input data and the ground-truth labels, then apply this to make predictions about unlabeled data. There are a variety of supervised learning algorithms suited for both regression problems (e.g., nonlinear regression) and classification problems (e.g., random forest).

Unsupervised learning is less common and involves training a model on an unlabeled dataset. These algorithms are often used to identify underlying features of the input data and group by similarity, making them well suited to clustering and association tasks. Another unsupervised learning task used in radiology is generative modeling, in which a model is trained on unlabeled data and asked to generate new output data similar to the input data.

Reinforcement learning algorithms train a model based on trial-and-error over time. Model agents receive positive and negative feedback from their environment and use that information to learn a sequence of actions that maximize an expected reward. A still emerging method, reinforcement learning in medical imaging has already demonstrated significant promise in image classification, image segmentation, image acquisition, and radiotherapy planning.[14]

Transfer learning involves using a model that was pretrained on a large dataset as a starting point for training it to perform an even more specific task. Several CNNs pretrained on large datasets like ImageNet[15] are publicly available and can effectively be trained further for applications specific to medical imaging.[16] This reduces the amount of data that a model may need, a key advantage in radiology where patient data is scarce and decentralized. Additionally, using models pretrained with large databases may help reduce overfitting and therefore improve generalizability.

In ***self-supervised learning***, a model learns from unlabeled data but does so by transforming the data to create supervisory signals—for example, by masking subsets of the data and asking the model to predict what has been hidden.[17] So-called "pretext tasks" in self-supervised learning are useful for finding features or attributes in the data even before providing it with explicit labeling. This allows models to incorporate features specifically relevant to the data (e.g., medical images) that may not be encoded in out-of-the-box CNNs used in transfer learning.

Federated learning, also referred to as distributed learning, is a method that trains a common central model on multiple local nodes using local private data.[18] Although not yet used on a large scale, this type of collaborative model training presents key advantages in healthcare and radiology. It provides models large amoutns of and potentially more diverse data to train on while preserving patient privacy and institutional data ownership. Federated learning is dependent on the development of infrastructure needed to host decentralized servers.

MODEL EVALUATION

Understanding which statistical measures to use and how to interpret them is critical in developing and implementing AI tools. The best way to evaluate a model depends on the specific task. In classification tasks, for example, accuracy, sensitivity, specificity, and area under the receiver operating characteristic curve (AUC) are common metrics used to evaluate model performance. Accuracy is defined as the ratio of cases on which the model was correct. Sensitivity (i.e., recall) measures the proportion of true positive cases correctly identified by an algorithm, whereas specificity measures the proportion of true negative cases correctly identified. These metrics are usually condensed into a confusion matrix, which depicts a model's performance by showing the rate of correctly and incorrectly predicted instances across different classes (e.g., true and false positive, true and false negative). AUC summarizes the overall performance of a model in discriminating positive and negative cases at different cutoff thresholds. Unlike classification tasks, segmentation tasks are best evaluated using overlap-based metrics like the Dice coefficient, mean surface distance, or Hausdorff distance.

Beyond knowing the general category of task (e.g., classification, segmentation), domain-specific knowledge is important for understanding how to interpret the evaluative metrics. Take the case of cancer screening in the general population, for instance, where the point prevalence of disease is low at any one time. A model may demonstrate high accuracy by correctly classifying the majority of patients as disease negative, but if it does so at the expense of sensitivity by incorrectly classifying most disease-positive patients as negative, then accuracy is an irrelevant metric. Understanding the goals of a model is thus critical in selecting evaluation metrics to assess its performance.

MODEL DEVELOPMENT BIAS

As in data curation, bias can occur at any step in the modeling phase of AI development. In clinical medicine, model bias is especially consequential because it may affect patient care decisions, and actively monitoring algorithms for bias is essential. The measures needed to mitigate bias are also context specific and similarly require deep domain knowledge in the clinical application of the algorithm.

Deciphering the mechanisms by which models encode bias requires access to the algorithm's training data, objective function, and prediction methodology, presenting a significant barrier to monitoring.[19] In a seminal study, US researchers with privileged access to a live widely used risk prediction algorithm demonstrated racial bias arising from prediction of healthcare cost rather than disease.[20] Because unequal access to care limits healthcare spending for African Americans in the United States, the algorithm incorrectly predicted the decrease in expenditure as a lower risk of disease. Bias by its nature goes unnoticed, and building tools to identify and correct for bias is an active area of research. In the case of deep learning, emerging methods like explainable AI (XAI) that can develop models that provide explanations for algorithm decisions present an exciting opportunity for identifying otherwise hidden bias.

Implementation

The implementation phase marks translating an algorithm into clinical practice. Successful adoption of AI tools requires thoughtful consideration of the digital infrastructure. Critically, integrating algorithms so they don't interrupt clinical workflow depends on close coordination between developers, physicians, and clinical staff. Appropriate AI governance must be formalized to oversee implementation and management of AI tools. Algorithms are also subject to oversight by the FDA that provides guidance to commercial sponsors on regulatory requirements. This section briefly summarizes these aspects of AI implementation.

Deciding what models to implement should follow objective criteria, and structured rubrics have been proposed for model evaluation in implementation decision-making.[21] Key criteria for consideration include what problem is to be solved by implementation of the AI tool, local performance metrics and ease of use, the body of scientific evidence supporting use, the degree to which encoded bias is understood, the technical readiness for implementation, the degree of monetary value a tool can contribute clinically, the impact on care providers, and the clinical impact on patients. Institutions should have in place governing bodies that assess these aspects before and after deciding to implement any given tool.

TECHNICAL INFRASTRUCTURE

A robust technical infrastructure must be in place to support the deployment of AI tools in clinical practice. This includes both hardware and software for running the algorithms, as well as the appropriate network infrastructure and AI orchestrator to transfer data between the AI host and other clinical systems. A reliable and secure data storage system is important for complying with regulatory privacy requirements and HIPAA regulations. AI algorithms must follow standards-based interoperability to integrate with other clinical information systems including electronic health records (EHRs) and the Picture Archiving and Communication System (PACS) used to manage and store patient images in radiology departments. Finally, clinical implementation requires the dedicated expertise of a full-time team of data scientists, IT professionals, and clinical experts to ensure AI algorithm reliability and performance.

AI GOVERNANCE

Establishing an AI governing body to oversee the implementation and management of AI tools in clinical practice is crucial to ensure they are used ethically, transparently, and within medical-legal and regulatory requirements. Governance committees can standardize evaluation of AI tools and direct institutional and departmental resources toward prioritizing implementation of tools poised to improve high-impact areas of clinical care. Guidelines have been proposed for organizing AI governance structures in radiology and healthcare more generally, but there remains no universal standard for institutional oversight.[20] Governance committees should engage many stakeholders and have representation from clinical and administrative leadership, ethicists, compliance and legal experts, data scientists, IT management, and end users. Although oversight mechanisms differ widely, they all establish a channel of communication between end users, the committee, leadership, and the broader organization.

FDA REGULATION

AI tools implemented in clinical practice are subject to FDA oversight to ensure patient safety and vet tool efficacy, and as the technology evolves, FDA guidance will adapt to meet the changing landscape. In 2019, the FDA published a discussion paper and request for feedback that outlined an approach for regulating machine learning software as medical devices.[22] Commensurate with the level of risk inherent to a specific application as defined by its intended use, there are three different paths (class I–III) of graded rigor for securing FDA clearance for an algorithm.[23] Additionally, the FDA has established three approval categories specifically for AI in medical imaging: CADx (computer-aided diagnosis), CADt (computer-aided triage), and CADe (computer-aided detection). CADx tools are typically considered Class III, whereas CADe software, for example, can be both Class II or Class III. In general, however, the association between a software's 'CAD' and its assigned 'Class' is determined by the intended use specified by the manufacturer. To date, there are more than 900 radiology and medical imaging–specific AI products commercially available, and the ACR-DSI maintains a current list of all FDA-cleared AI medical products.[24] The FDA provides guidance to commercial sponsors on premarket submission requirements, quality control systems, and postmarket surveillance.

Conclusion

In tracing the three main phases of AI development—data curation, modeling, and implementation—this chapter introduces key concepts and practical considerations specific to each. Particularly highlighted are the importance of properly curated and well-annotated datasets, the strategic choice of model design and learning method in the modeling phase, and the importance of ethical stewardship in clinical implementation. We also discussed some of the challenges associated with each phase, including the lack of large, diverse medical image data sets for the data curation phase, the need to monitor and correct for bias in the modeling phase, and the logistics of coordinating developers, physicians, and clinical staff during the implementation phase. Taken together, a foundational understanding of the technical principles underlying AI development in clinical radiology is essential for healthcare professionals aiming to incorporate AI into their clinical practice.

References

1. Willemink MJ, Koszek WA, Hardell C, et al. Preparing medical imaging data for machine learning. *Radiology*. 2020;295(1):4–15.
2. Aryanto KYE, Oudkerk M, Van Ooijen PMA. Free DICOM de-identification tools in clinical research: functioning and safety of patient privacy. *Eur Radiol*. 2015;25(12):3685–3695.
3. Collins SA, Wu J, Bai HX. Facial De-identification of head CT scans. *Radiology*. 2020;296(1):22.
4. Prior FW, Clark K, Commean P, et al. TCIA: an information resource to enable open science. *Conf Proc IEEE Eng Med Biol Soc*. 2013:1282–1285.
5. Yan K, Wang X, Lu L, Summers RM. DeepLesion: automated mining of large-scale lesion annotations and universal lesion detection with deep learning. *J Med Imaging (Bellingham)*. 2018;5(3):036501.
6. Rubin DL, Kahn Jr CE. Common data elements in radiology. *Radiology*. 2017;283(3):837–844.
7. Brink L, Coombs LP, Kattil Veettil D, et al. ACR's connect and AI-LAB technical framework. *JAMIA Open*. 2022;5(4):1–9.
8. Tripathi S, Gabriel K, Dheer S, et al. Dataset development review. *J Am Coll Radiol*. 2023. S1546-1440(23)00507-0.
9. Langlotz CP, Allen B, Erickson BJ, et al. A roadmap for foundational research on artificial intelligence in medical imaging: from the 2018 NIH/RSNA/ACR/The Academy workshop. *Radiology*. 2019;291(3):781–791.
10. Ardila D, Kiraly AP, Bharadwaj S, et al. End-to-end lung cancer screening with three-dimensional deep learning on low-dose chest computed tomography. *Nat Med*. 2019;25(6):954–961.
11. Mazurowski MA, Buda M, Saha A, Bashir MR. Deep learning in radiology: an overview of the concepts and a survey of the state of the art with focus on MRI. *J Magn Reson Imaging*. 2019;49(4):939–954.
12. Ronneberger O, Fischer P, Brox T. U-net: convolutional networks for biomedical image segmentation. *Lect Notes Comput Sci*. 2015;9351:234–241.
13. Kelly BS, Judge C, Bollard SM, et al. Radiology artificial intelligence: a systematic review and evaluation of methods (RAISE). *Eur Radiol*. 2022;32(11):7998–8007.
14. Zhou SK, Le HN, Luu K, V Nguyen H, Ayache N. Deep reinforcement learning in medical imaging: a literature review. *Med Image Anal*. 2021;73:102193.
15. Deng J, Dong W, Socher R, et al. ImageNet: A large-scale hierarchical image database. Proceedings of the IEEE conference on computer vision and pattern Recognition; 2009;248–255.

16. Kim HE, Cosa-Linan A, Santhanam N, Jannesari M, Maros ME, Ganslandt T. Transfer learning for medical image classification: a literature review. *BMC Med Imaging*. 2022;22(1):1–13.
17. Krishnan R, Rajpurkar P, Topol EJ. Self-supervised learning in medicine and healthcare. *Nat Biomed Eng*. 2022;6(12):1346–1352.
18. Darzidehkalani E, Ghasemi-rad M, van Ooijen PMA. Federated learning in medical imaging: part I: toward multicentral health care ecosystems. *J Am Coll Radiol*. 2022;19(8):969–974.
19. Zhang K, Khosravi B, Vahdati S, et al. Mitigating bias in radiology machine learning: 2. Model Development, *Radiol Artif Intell*. 2022;4(5):e220010.
20. Obermeyer Z, Powers B, Vogeli C, Mullainathan S. Dissecting racial bias in an algorithm used to manage the health of populations. *Science*. 2019;366(6464):447–453.
21. Daye D, Wiggins WF, Lungren MP, et al. Implementation of clinical artificial intelligence in radiology: who decides and how? *Radiology*. 2022;305(3):555–563.
22. FDA. Proposed regulatory framework for modifications to artificial intelligence/machine learning (ai/ml)-based Software as a Medical Device (SaMD). Discussion Paper and Request for Feedback. (2019). https://www.regulations.gov/document?D=FDA-2019-N-11850001.
23. Benjamens S, Dhunnoo P, Meskó B. The state of artificial intelligence-based FDA: approved medical devices and algorithms: an online database. *Npj Digit Med*. 2020;3(1):1–8 2020.
24. American College of Radiology. (n.d.). ACR AI-LAB. https://aicentral.acrdsi.org.

PART II

Interpretive Applications

PART OUTLINE

CHAPTER 4

Interpretive Applications of Artificial Intelligence in Breast Radiology

Tulasi Talluri

KEY POINTS

- Machine and deep learning techniques such as computer-aided detection and convolutional neural networks are artificial intelligence (AI) models used in breast imaging to support the radiologist in lesion detection, classification, density assessment, risk assessment, treatment response assessment, image enhancement, and decision support.
- There are currently 35 FDA-cleared applications of AI in breast imaging, of which 29 are interpretive applications, with more under development.
- Although advancements in AI have shown promise in breast imaging, its success depends on the seamless integration into existing clinical workflow, improved efficiency and demonstrated impact on patient outcomes in the real-world, larger training datasets, and worldwide equitable access to AI systems.

GLOSSARY OF TERMS AND DEFINITIONS

CADe: (computer-aided detection): A type of artificial intelligence system designed to highlight areas of potential abnormality in medical images, such as nodules, masses, or microcalcifications. CADe systems assist radiologists by drawing attention to findings that may require further evaluation, without making a diagnostic decision.

CADt: (computer-aided triage) : A type of artificial intelligence system focused on rapidly identifying potentially urgent cases, flagging them for immediate review by a clinician. It does not provide specific findings or diagnostic information but helps prioritize cases based on urgency.

CADx: (computer-aided detection): A type of artificial intelligence system that provided additional information to aid in diagnosis. This can include characterizing lesions, assessing their severity, or providing a probability of malignancy.

BI-RADS: A standardized classification system developed by the American College of Radiology to categorize breast imaging findings and guide clinical management.

Introduction

Significant advances in artificial intelligence (AI) have rapidly transformed radiology, improving interpretation of abdominal, breast, cardiac, dental, chest, musculoskeletal, and neurological imaging. Of these, breast imaging is perhaps the most widely known and researched use case for AI in radiology. Full-field digital mammography (FFDM), multiparametric magnetic resonance imaging (MRI), digital breast tomosynthesis (DBT), and automated breast ultrasound (ABUS) aid in diagnosis, prognosis, and treatment of various breast pathologies but demand increased time and expertise for image interpretation.[1] AI purports to address this challenge by automating routine tasks, reducing interpretation time, and rapidly integrating large amounts of multimodal data from electronic health records, thereby augmenting the overall efficiency and reliability of breast imaging practices.

AI can be divided into two fields: machine learning (ML) and deep learning (DL), a subset of ML. In the 1980s, mammography was one of the first imaging modalities to utilize AI, beginning with computer-aided detection (CADe), a classical form of ML that involves human-coded feature engineering to detect lesions.[2] Developments since then have resulted in computer-aided diagnosis (CADx) and computer-aided triage (CADt) for diagnosis and triaging, respectively. CAD begins with image preprocessing and segmentation to isolate regions of interest and extracts features analyzed by detection algorithms. When deviations from normal patterns are detected, these areas are marked as suspicious for further radiologist evaluation. CAD systems ideally serve as a second reader, improving sensitivity in breast imaging without replacing radiologists' expertise, but they rely on human-coded engineering and present with limited performance including a high false-positive rate. Thus many latest AI applications augment CAD with DL.

DL, a subset of ML, is based on neural networks with multiple layers, allowing it to automatically learn hierarchical representations of data without explicit feature engineering (Fig. 4.1). Unlike traditional machine learning methods, deep learning can directly process raw input data. In breast imaging, convolutional neural networks (CNNs), a type of DL architecture, have demonstrated success in tasks such as mass classification and microcalcification detection since 1994, as shown in Fig. 4.2.[1]

AI in breast imaging has diverse applications, including cancer detection, decision support, risk assessment, breast density quantitation, workflow and triage, quality evaluation, and response to neoadjuvant chemotherapy assessment.[3] As of February 2024, there were 35 FDA-cleared AI applications for breast imaging, of which 29 are interpretive applications (Table 4.1). These tools have the potential to reshape patient care by deriving greater clinical value from imaging data. Despite these advancements, there are still challenges to be addressed, such as the need for standardized data and the potential for AI to exacerbate existing healthcare disparities.

Mammography

The current gold standard in breast cancer screening is mammography, but limitations include a notable rate of missed cancers, particularly in patients with dense breasts, leading to reduced sensitivity ranging from 75% to 85% in the general screening population.[4] Despite its efficacy, DBT examinations require more time for interpretation compared to digital 2D mammography (DM) examinations, and the technique is prone to false positives, resulting in a high recall rate.[5,6] To address these challenges and optimize screening outcomes, AI algorithms emerge as a promising tool. As of February 2024, there are 22 FDA-cleared interpretive AI applications for mammography (Table 4.1). These algorithms are trained on large datasets of mammographic images and can quantify parenchymal density, detect suspicious lesions, and predict breast cancer risk with high accuracy.[7]

AI has been shown to perform consistently across different breast densities, which is crucial given that high breast density can mask tumors and is an independent risk factor for breast cancer.[8] Twelve of the interpretive AI applications for mammography are specifically for breast density assessment. Densitas, Inc. offers two applications for this purpose: DM-Density based on ML, and densityai based on DL. A study comparing densityai with expert radiologists demonstrated accuracy rates in densityai ranging from 76% for scattered fibroglandular densities, to 78% for entirely fatty breasts, to 96% for dense breasts.[9] Volpara

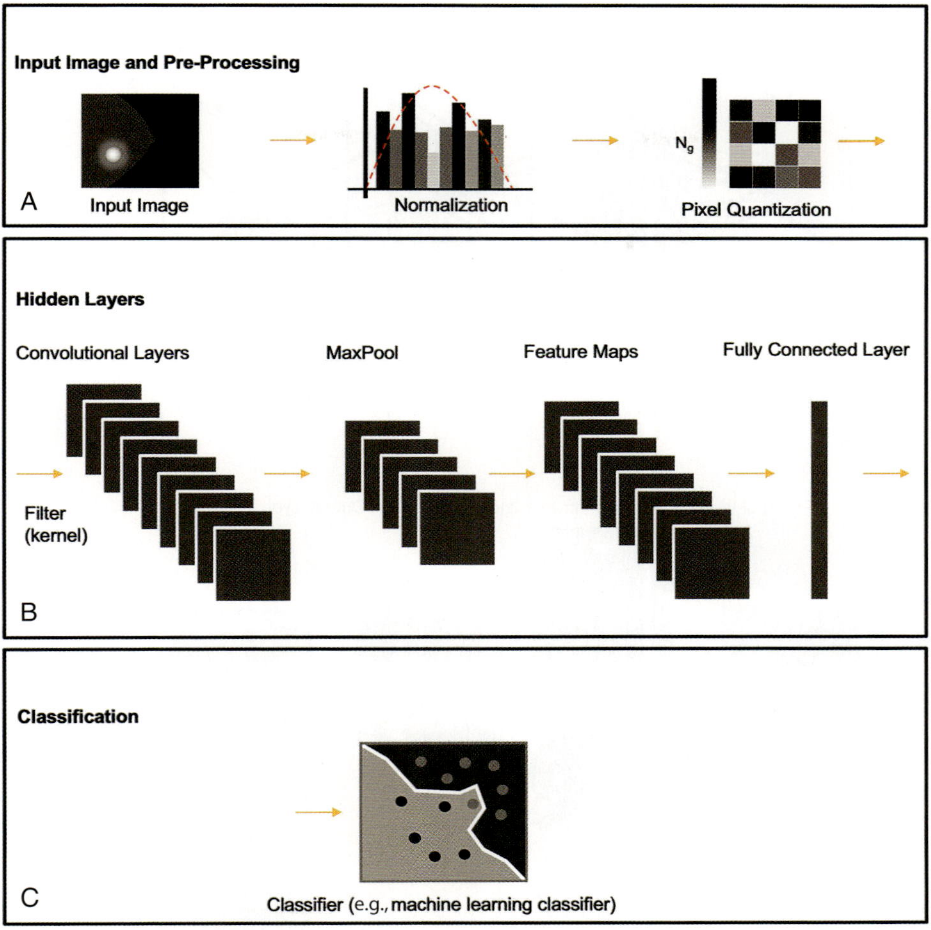

Fig. 4.1 Breast imaging for screening using artificial intelligence. (A) Image input. Breast images are acquired with standard acquisition procedures and undergo preprocessing prior to image analysis. Images are first normalized to remove variances in intensity range and brightness. Pixels (or voxels) are then quantized into a discrete gray-level scale. Whole images are often patched for better computational processing. (B) Hidden layers. Deep learning algorithms consist of several hidden layers that carry out a mathematical function. Deep convolutional neural networks (DCNN) are commonly used for image analysis. Each convolution layer of a DCNN consists of several kernels to extract feature maps, followed by an activation function. A MaxPool layer subsequently removes the insignificant parameters. The process is repeated over several layers to find the most optimal feature sets. A fully connected layer is sometimes included at the end of the hidden layers. (C) Classification of the object or pixel is carried out in the final step. Classification can be done by the DCNN itself or a separate machine learning classifier (e.g., support vector machines) that processes feature maps yielded from the hidden layers. (From Tran WT, Sadeghi-Naini A, Lu F-I, et al. Computational radiology in breast cancer screening and diagnosis using artificial intelligence. *Can Assoc Radiol J.* 2020;72(1):98–108.)

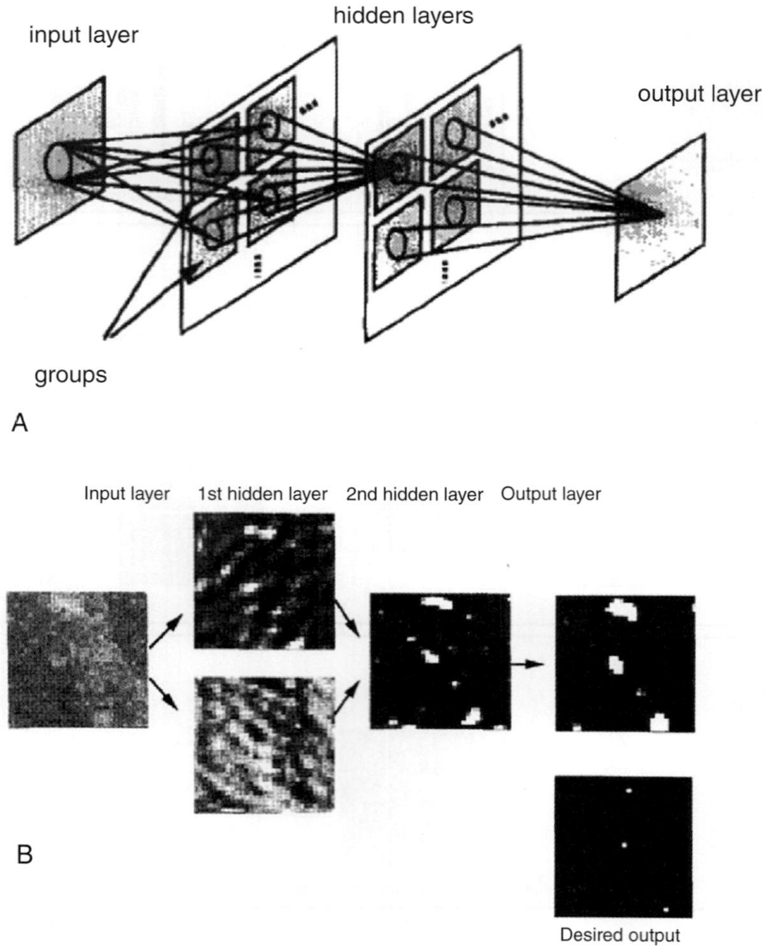

Fig. 4.2 Illustration of the first journal publication on the use of a convolutional neural network (CNN), that is, a shift-invariant neural network, in medical image analysis. The CNN was used in a computer-aided detection system to detect microcalcification on digitized mammograms and later on full-field digital mammograms. (A) A 2D shift-invariant neural network. (B) Illustration of input testing image, output image, desired output image, and responses in hidden layers. (From Zhang W, Doi K, Giger ML, Wu Y, Nishikawa RM, Schmidt RA. Computerized detection of clustered microcalcifications in digital mammograms using a shift-invariant artificial neural network. *Med Phys*. 1994;21(4):517–524.)

TABLE 4.1 ■ **Interpretive AI Applications in Breast Imaging Cleared for Use by the FDA**

Product (Manufacturer)	Category	Modality	Indication	Data Cleared
cmAngio® V1.0 (CureMetrix, Inc.)	MIMPS	MAM	Breast Arterial Calcification Identification	10/5/23
WRDensity (Whiterabbit.ai)	MIMPS	MAM	Density Assessment	10/30/20
Insight BD (Siemens Healthineers)	MIMPS	MAM	Density Assessment	2/6/18
Transpara Density 1.0.0 (ScreenPoint Medical B.V.)	MIMPS	MAM	Density Assessment	12/11/23
Visage Breast Density (Visage Imaging GmbH)	MIMPS	MAM	Density Assessment	1/29/21
PowerLook Density Assessment Software V4.0 (ICAD Inc.)	MIMPS	MAM	Density Assessment	7/12/21
Saige-Density (DeepHealth)	MIMPS	MAM	Density Assessment	12/16/22
densitas densityai (Densitas, Inc.)	MIMPS	MAM	Density Assessment	2/19/20
Volpara Imaging Software (Volpara Health Technologies Limited)	MIMPS	MAM	Density Assessment	7/27/21
DenSeeMammo (Statlife)	MIMPS	MAM	Density Assessment	6/26/18
DM-Density (Densitas, Inc.)	MIMPS	MAM	Density Assessment	2/23/18
ClariSIGMAM (Clari Pi)	MIMPS	MAM	Density Assessment	9/10/21
Quantra (Hologic, Inc.)	MIMPS	MAM	Density Assessment	10/20/17
Saige-Q (DeepHealth)	CADt	MAM	Triage	4/16/21
CogNet QmTRIAGE (MedCognetics, Inc.)	CADt	MAM	Triage	9/29/22
cmTriage (CureMetrix, Inc.)	CADt	MAM	Triage	3/8/19
HealthMammo (Nanox)	CADt	MAM	Lesion Detection	7/16/20
Transpara 1.7.2 (ScreenPoint Medical B.V.)	CADe/x	MAM	Lesion Detection and Decision Support	8/3/22
PowerLook® Tomo Detection V2 Software (ICAD Inc.)	CADe/x	MAM	Lesion Detection and Case Scores	12/6/18
MammoScreen® 2.0 (Therapixel)	CADe/x	MAM	Lesion Detection and Classification	11/26/21
ProFound AI® Software V3.0 (ICAD Inc.)	CADe/x	MAM	Lesion Detection and Classification	3/12/21
Genius AI Detection 2.0 with CC-MLO Correlation (Hologic, Inc.)	CADe/x	MAM	Lesion Detection and Classification	5/23/23
Saige-DX (DeepHealth)	CADe/x	MAM	Lesion Detection and Classification	5/12/22
Lunit INSIGHT MMG (Lunit Inc.)	CADe/x	MAM	Lesion Detection and Classification	11/17/21
Lunit INSIGHT DBT (Lunit Inc.)	CADe/x	MAM	Lesion Detection and Classification	11/6/23
BU-CAD (TaiHao Medical Inc.)	MIMPS	US	Lesion Detection and Classification	12/21/21

Continued

TABLE 4.1 ■ **Interpretive AI Applications in Breast Imaging Cleared for Use by the FDA–cont'd**

Product (Manufacturer)	Category	Modality	Indication	Data Cleared
ClearView cCAD (ClearView Diagnostics Inc.)	MIMPS	US	Lesion Classification	12/28/16
Koios DS- Breast (Koios Medical, Inc)	CADx	US	Lesion Classification	12/16/21
QuantX (Qlarity Imaging)	CADx	MR	Lesion Classification	7/19/17

CADe/x, Computer-aided detection and diagnosis; *CADt*, computer-aided triaging; *CADx*, computer-aided diagnosis; *CT*, computed tomography; *MAM*, mammography; *MIMPS*, medical image management and processing systems; *MR*, magnetic resonance; *US*, ultrasound.

Data from the FDA and American College of Radiology (ACR) website, https://aicentral.acrdsi.org/All-Ai-products#f:subspeciality=

Imaging Software (Volpara Health Technologies Limited) and Densitas' measurement of percentage density also exhibited a robust association with breast cancer risk, suggesting that AI-based breast density, when combined with clinical risk factors, can generate precise estimates of breast cancer risk.[10]

Another primary application of AI in mammography is for the detection and characterization of lesions, currently performed by six FDA-cleared applications. Fig. 4.3 depicts Transpara version 1.6.0 (ScreenPoint Medical) and Lunit INSIGHT MMG version 1.1.4.1 (Lunit Inc.) improving mammography interpretation for both novice and experienced readers, leading to increased diagnostic performance in terms of sensitivity and area under the receiver operating characteristic curve (AUC).[11] The most recent mammography AI application cleared by the FDA in May 2023, Genius AI Detection 2.0 with CC-MLO Correlation from Hologic, Inc. is a deep learning–based breast tomosynthesis cancer detection technology, demonstrating enhanced specificity compared to conventional CAD algorithms, offering accurate identification of regions of interest (ROI) with malignancy features. This allows for nuanced decision-making on complex exams, balancing patient anxiety during callbacks while minimizing false-positive markings with over a 70% reduction compared to Hologic's previous generations of 2D CAD software.[12]

Saige-Q (DeepHealth), CogNet QmTRIAGE (MedCognetics, Inc.), and cmTriage (CureMetrix, Inc.) are CADt applications used for triaging mammograms. These applications flag, notify, or assign a code to mammograms containing suspicious findings, aiding radiologists in prioritization of study interpretation and overall clinic workflow. Although not originally indicated for triaging, the Transpara 1.4.0 (ScreenPoint Medical B.V.) algorithm has been able to safely exclude normal mammograms from further radiologist evaluation, thereby reducing the workload and allowing radiologists to focus on more complex cases.[13] This reduction in workload does not come at the cost of diagnostic accuracy; in fact, AI has achieved noninferior sensitivity compared to human readings and has been suggested as a viable independent reader for breast screening.[14]

Although breast cancer screening and detection is the primary use for mammography, it captures a wealth of other valuable information in each image, yet only a fraction is typically reported. Recent advancements in AI focus on extracting more clinically relevant data, such as breast arterial calcification (BAC), a common incidental finding identified as a risk factor for cardiovascular disease in postmenopausal women.[15] The FDA cleared cmAngio® V1.0 by CureMetrix, Inc. in October 2023 to streamline the identification and reporting of BAC in mammograms, offering efficiency without additional procedures or radiation and demonstrating effectiveness across diverse breast densities.[16]

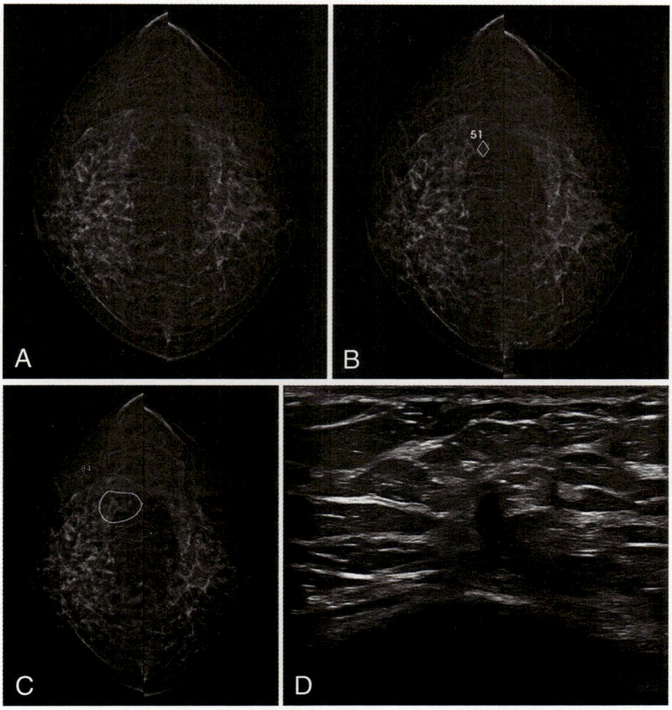

Fig. 4.3 Images from a 51-year-old woman. (a) Mammograms in CC views were rated on a LOM scale of 1 (negative) and 1 by novice readers and as 1 and 4 (low suspicion for malignancy) by experienced readers. The reports of (b) Transpara version 1.6.0 (ScreenPoint Medical) and (c) Lunit INSIGHT MMG version 1.1.4.1 (Lunit Inc.) both revealed suspicion marks in the outer portion of the right breast. When provided with the reports of Transpara version 1.6.0 (ScreenPoint Medical) and Lunit INSIGHT MMG version 1.1.4.1 (Lunit Inc.), both novice readers changed their ratings on a LOM scale of 4, but the experienced readers did not change their ratings. The area marked in both AI reports was correlated with the location of an irregular mass on (d) breast US. The mass was confirmed as a 2.4-cm, intermediate-grade, ER/PR-positive, HER2-negative invasive ductal carcinoma after breast-conserving surgery. *AI*, Artificial intelligence; *CC*, craniocaudal; *ER*, estrogen receptor; *HER2*, human epidermal growth factor receptor 2; *LOM*, likelihood of malignancy; *PR*, progesterone receptor. (From Kim HJ, Choi WJ, Gwon HY, et al. Improving mammography interpretation for both novice and experienced readers: a comparative study of two commercial artificial intelligence software. *Eur Radiol*. 2024;34(6):3924–3934.)

Breast Ultrasound

Breast ultrasound is a critical imaging modality used to differentiate between benign and malignant breast masses. However, it is not without its challenges, such as high false-positive rates and significant interobserver variability, which can lead to unnecessary biopsies and varied diagnostic outcomes.[17] There are three FDA-cleared AI systems for breast ultrasound interpretation, all for lesion detection and classification as benign or malignant. In practice, AI can serve as an adjunct tool, offering a second opinion to radiologists and suggesting whether a lesion is likely benign or malignant. This can lead to a reduction in unnecessary biopsies, as demonstrated in studies where AI systems have successfully downgraded Breast Imaging Reporting and Data System (BI-RADS) category 4A lesions to category 3, thereby avoiding biopsies without missing malignancies. Figs. 4.4 and 4.5 illustrate the performance of the BU-CAD and Koios systems for BI-RADS category assessment in breast masses detected on ultrasound. Both AI

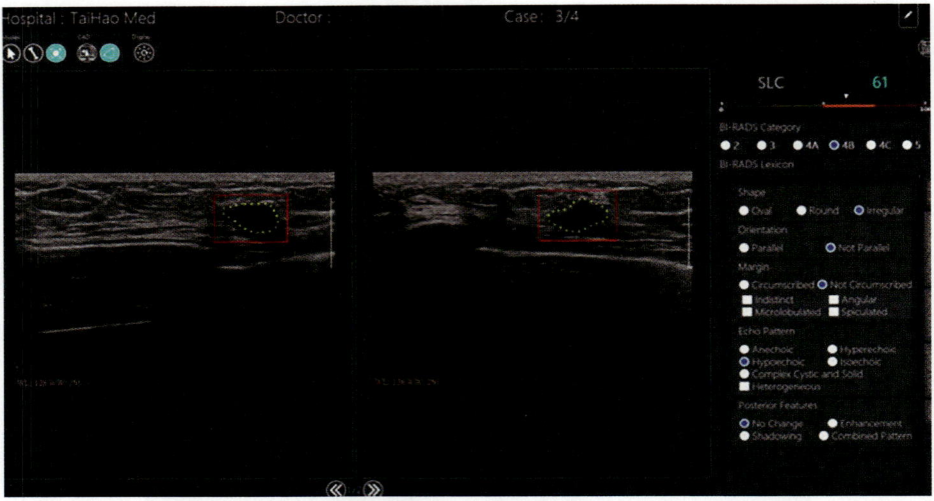

Fig. 4.4 Example of BU-CAD showing orthogonal B-mode ultrasound images of a breast mass (indicated by the red box), where the artificial intelligence decision support output (DS) displayed a high score of lesion characteristics (SLC = 61), corresponding to a Breast Imaging Reporting and Data System (BI-RADS) assessment category 4B. *Figure provided by TaiHao Medical Inc. and used with permission*. (From Brot HF, Mango VL. Artificial intelligence in breast ultrasound: application in clinical practice. *Ultrasonography*. 2023;43(1):3–14.)

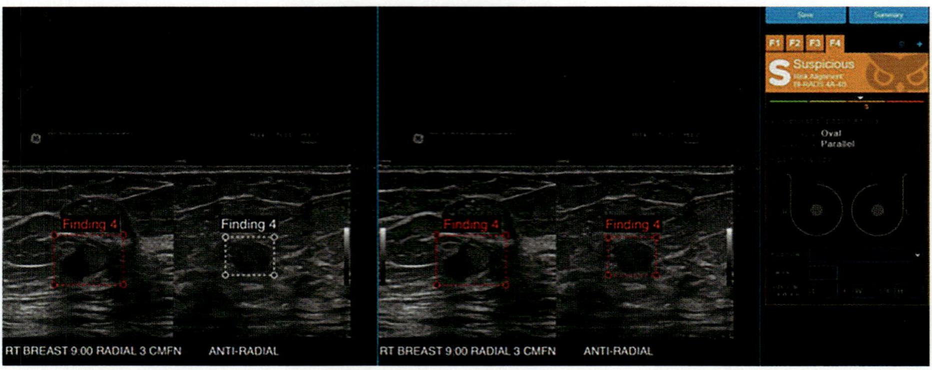

Fig. 4.5 Example of Koios decision support (DS) for breast showing the B-mode ultrasound images of invasive carcinoma with micropapillary features in a 68-year-old patient. The artificial intelligence DS output is displayed in a graphical form on the right panel, with the DS-generated output (in this case correctly classified as "suspicious") and the confidence of assessment within that category as marked by the triangular marker.

systems exhibited high sensitivity and specificity in categorizing breast masses, which could potentially reduce unnecessary biopsies and follow-ups.[18] However, it was noted that junior radiologists had an increase in sensitivity when using the AI tool, whereas experienced radiologists had decreased specificity, highlighting the importance of careful consideration before clinical implementation.[19]

Breast MRI

AI has been instrumental in enhancing the capabilities of breast MRI across various clinical scenarios, including screening accuracy and characterization of MRI lesions, risk prediction, predicting molecular subtype of breast cancer, predicting other clinical outcomes, treatment response prediction, and cancer recurrence prediction. AI can be a powerful tool for lesion segmentation in breast MRI interpretation, which involves delineating the precise boundaries of a tumor. This is crucial for accurate volume estimation, which can influence treatment planning and prognostic assessments. The only FDA-cleared application of AI in breast MRI is QuantX by Qlarity Imaging for the assessment and characterization of breast abnormalities. Notably, it is not intended for the primary interpretation of digital mammography, but rather for evaluation of patients presenting for high-risk screening, diagnostic imaging workup, or evaluation of extent of known disease.[20] QuantX utilizes a machine learning algorithm trained on segmented lesions to provide users a QI score by combining multiple lesion features, initiated by the user selecting a seed point on the image (Fig. 4.6). QI scores are added to a reference database for further image analysis.

Beyond interpretive applications such as lesion detection, AI in breast MRI is also used for prognostication and predicting treatment response. By analyzing the imaging characteristics of breast tumors, AI models can extract quantitative imaging biomarkers that are indicative of the tumor's genetic makeup and behavior. This information can be used to tailor personalized

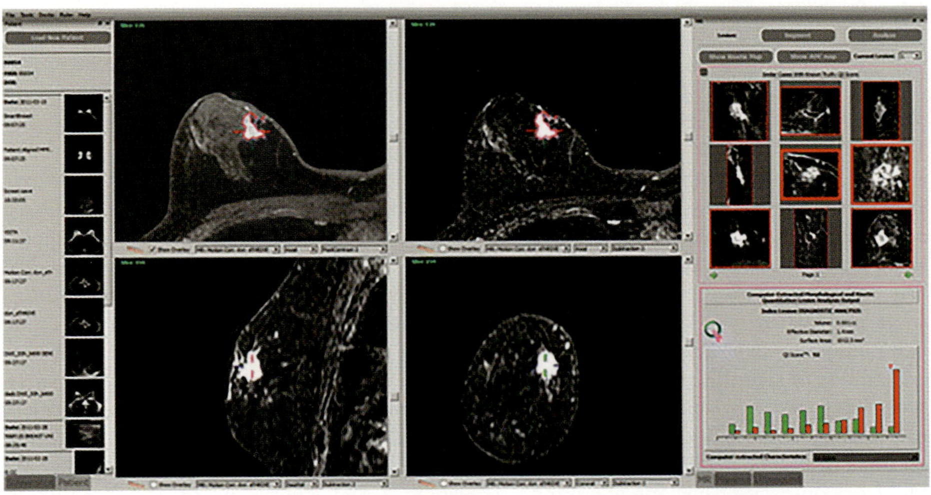

Fig. 4.6 Screenshot of artificial intelligence system user interface. Enhancing mass was segmented with software using seed point input from the reader as described in text. (From Jiang Y, Edwards AV, Newstead GM. Artificial intelligence applied to breast MRI for improved diagnosis. *Radiology*. 2020;298(1):38–46.)

treatment plans and predict how a patient might respond to a particular therapy, thus paving the way for precision medicine in breast cancer care.[17] Additionally, AI-augmented clinical decision strategies are being developed to integrate imaging findings with genomic, pathologic, and clinical data.[21]

Other Applications

In addition to the aforementioned FDA-cleared commercial applications for interpretive AI in breast imaging, there are also several investigational and open access AI algorithms under development. Jiang, Edwards, and Newstead report on an integrated AI system within computer-aided diagnosis software that significantly improved radiologists' ability to distinguish between malignant and benign lesions on breast MRI scans.[22] Another application, driven by deep learning, has shown promise in refining breast cancer risk assessment and enabling personalized screening strategies.[23] Fig. 4.7 shows the output of one such AI algorithm developed using a large-scale dataset, demonstrating superior diagnostic performance compared to radiologists, with significant improvements in sensitivity for detecting cancers with specific characteristics such as mass, distortion, or asymmetry. In one retrospective study, the strategic use of an AI system employing maximum intensity projection (MIP) of postcontrast subtracted breast MRI images achieved diagnostic performance comparable to senior radiologists and outperformed junior counterparts in classifying non-mass enhancement (NME) lesions.[24] Compelling data from an AI system assisting radiologists in assessing indeterminate BI-RADS 0 mammograms demonstrated effective reduction in unnecessary follow-ups and benign biopsy rates without compromising detection of highly malignant tumors.[25] Similar results were observed in an AI support system that enhanced the accuracy of breast radiologists in interpreting wide-angle DBT images, reducing reading time and demonstrating noninferior performance in malignancy detection.[26]

Limitations

As the potential of AI in breast imaging gains recognition, caution must be exercised in clinical implementation. Several barriers to conception and implementation of breast AI applications in clinical practice have been identified, with model training dataset size and quality emerging as a predominant concern.[27] There is substantial variation in data accessibility, with DM and DBT studies typically featuring extensive datasets acquired from numerous centers, whereas MRI studies tend to lack data diversity.[28] This discrepancy is further exacerbated by imbalances in clinical data due to disease prevalence, data availability, and population characteristics. Lack of model transparency is a recurring barrier due to the "black box" nature of AI algorithms that may conceal bias, necessitating efforts toward increasing clinician and patient trust in imaging findings. Meanwhile, the implementation of AI in clinical practice remains limited, with challenges including the lack of prospective clinical studies and the necessity for multicenter evaluations to establish generalizability of algorithms. The need for robust external validation studies also becomes apparent to showcase the adaptability of AI algorithms across diverse screening populations and settings, considering factors like race, ethnicity, risk factors, and imaging modalities. Ethical barriers to AI implementation in breast imaging encompass concerns about liability, emphasizing the need for clarity on decision-making and error responsibility. Legal, ethical, and economic challenges further include issues related to patient privacy, fair AI practices, cybersecurity, and economic considerations, necessitating careful navigation for responsible and effective integration of AI technologies.[29]

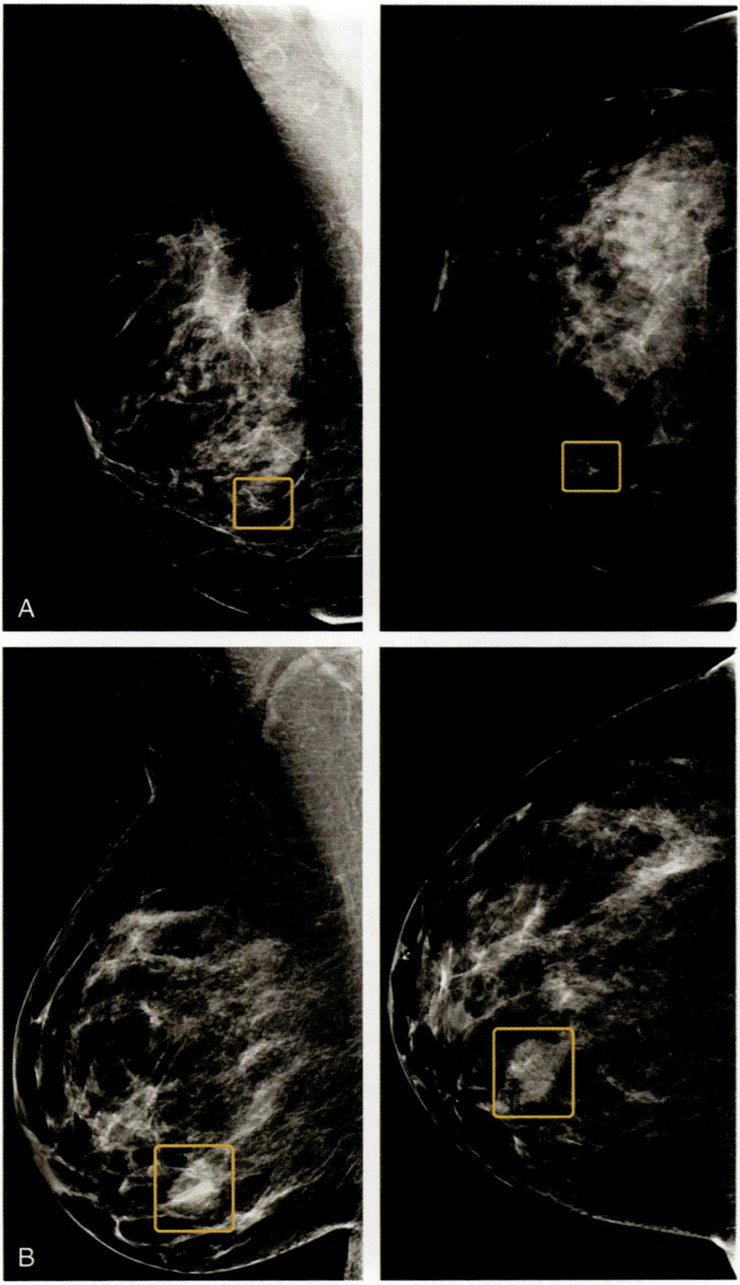

Fig. 4.7 (A) A sample cancer case that was missed by all six readers in the US reader study but correctly identified by the AI system. The malignancy, outlined in *yellow*, is a small, irregular mass with associated microcalcifications in the lower inner right breast. (B) A sample cancer case that was caught by all six readers in the U.S. reader study but missed by the AI system. The malignancy is a dense mass in the lower inner right breast. *Left*, mediolateral oblique view; *right*, craniocaudal view. (From McKinney SM, Sieniek M, Godbole V, et al. International evaluation of an AI system for breast cancer screening. *Nature*. 2020;577:89–94.)

References

1. Hu Q, Giger ML. Clinical artificial intelligence applications: breast imaging. *Radiol Clin North Am.* 2021;59(6):1027–1043. http://doi.org/10.1016/j.rcl.2021.07.010.
2. Bitencourt A, Daimiel Naranjo I, Lo Gullo R, Rossi Saccarelli C, Pinker K. AI-enhanced breast imaging: where are we and where are we heading? *Eur J Radiol.* 2021;142:109882. http://doi.org/10.1016/j.ejrad.2021.109882.
3. Taylor CR, Monga N, Johnson C, Hawley JR, Patel M. Artificial intelligence applications in breast imaging: current status and future directions. *Diagnostics (Basel).* 2023;13(12):2041, doi:10.3390/diagnostics13122041.
4. Batchu S, Liu F, Amireh A, Waller J, Umair M. A review of applications of machine learning in mammography and future challenges. *Oncology.* 2021;99:483–490. https://doi.org/10.1159/000515698.
5. Kim H, Kim H, Han B, et al. Changes in cancer detection and false-positive recall in mammography using artificial intelligence: a retrospective, multireader study. *Lancet Digit Health.* 2020;2(3):e138–e148. https://doi.org/10.1016/s2589-7500(20)30003-0.
6. Sechopoulos I, Teuwen J, Mann R. Artificial intelligence for breast cancer detection in mammography and digital breast tomosynthesis: state of the art. *Semin Cancer Biol.* 2021;72:214–225. https://doi.org/10.1016/j.semcancer.2020.06.002.
7. Yoon JH, Kim E-K. Deep learning-based artificial intelligence for mammography. *Korean J Radiol.* 2021;22(8):1225–1239. https://doi.org/10.3348/kjr.2020.1210.
8. Freer PE. Mammographic breast density: impact on breast cancer risk and implications for screening. *Radiographics.* 2015;35(2):302–315. http://doi.org/10.1148/rg.352140106.
9. Food and Drug Administration. *Densityai.* 2020. https://www.accessdata.fda.gov/cdrh_docs/pdf19/K192973.pdf.
10. Astley SM, Harkness EF, Sergeant JC, et al. A comparison of five methods of measuring mammographic density: a case-control study. *Breast Cancer Res.* 2018;20:10. https://doi.org/10.1186/s13058-018-0932-z.
11. Kim HJ, Choi WJ, Gwon HY, et al. Improving mammography interpretation for both novice and experienced readers: a comparative study of two commercial artificial intelligence software. *Eur Radiol.* 2024;34(6):3924–3934.
12. Hologic. *Addressing Reading Distractions.* 2023. https://www.hologic.com/sites/default/files/Genius%20AI%20Detection%20Point-of-Care%20Triaging%20Case%20Study.pdf.
13. Rodriguez-Ruiz A, Lång K, Gubern-Merida A, et al. Can we reduce the workload of mammographic screening by automatic identification of normal exams with artificial intelligence? A feasibility study. *Eur Radiol.* 2019;29(9):4825–4832. http://doi.org/10.1007/s00330-019-06186-9.
14. Lauritzen AD, Rodríguez-Ruiz A, von Euler-Chelpin MC, et al. An artificial intelligence-based mammography screening protocol for breast cancer: outcome and radiologist workload. *Radiology.* 2022;304(1):41–49. http://doi.org/10.1148/radiol.210948.
15. Iribarren C, Chandra M, Lee C, et al. Breast arterial calcification: a novel cardiovascular risk enhancer among postmenopausal women. *Circ Cardiovasc Imaging.* 2022;15(3):e013526.
16. CureMetrix. CureMetrix Receives FDA Clearance for cmAngio®, First-of-Its-Kind Solution for Detecting Breast Arterial Calcification. *EIN Presswire.* 2023.
17. Sheth D, Giger M. Artificial intelligence in the interpretation of breast cancer on MRI. *J Magn Reson Imaging.* 2019;51(5):1310–1324. https://doi.org/10.1002/jmri.26878.
18. Brot HF, Mango VL. Artificial intelligence in breast ultrasound: application in clinical practice. *Ultrasonography.* 2023;43(1):3–14. https://www.ncbi.nlm.nih.gov/pmc/articles/PMC10766882/.
19. Wu G, Zhou L, Xu J, et al. Artificial intelligence in breast ultrasound. *World J Radiol.* 2019;11:19–26. https://doi.org/10.4329/wjr.v11.i2.19.
20. 510(k) premarket notification. accessdata.fda.gov. 2019. Accessed 22, 2025.https://www.accessdata.fda.gov/scripts/cdrh/cfdocs/cfPMN/pmn.cfm?ID=K191959.
21. Meyer-Bäse A, Morra L, Meyer-Bäse U, Pinker K. Current status and future perspectives of artificial intelligence in magnetic resonance breast imaging. *Contrast Media Mol Imaging.* 2020;2020:6805710. https://doi.org/10.1155/2020/6805710.
22. Jiang Y, Edwards AV. Newstead GM. Artificial intelligence applied to breast MRI for improved diagnosis. *Radiology.* 2021;298(1):38–46. https://doi.org/10.1148/radiol.2020200292.

23. Gastounioti A, Desai S, Ahluwalia VS, Conant EF, Kontos D. Artificial intelligence in mammographic phenotyping of breast cancer risk: a narrative review. *Breast Cancer Res.* 2022;24(1):14. https://doi.org/10.1186/s13058-022-01509-z.
24. Wang L, Chang L, Luo R, et al. An artificial intelligence system using maximum intensity projection MR images facilitates classification of non-mass enhancement breast lesions. *Eur Radiol.* 2022;32(7):4857–4867. https://doi.org/10.1007/s00330-022-08553-5.
25. Yi C, Tang Y, Ouyang R, et al. The added value of an artificial intelligence system in assisting radiologists on indeterminate BI-RADS 0 mammograms. *Eur Radiol.* 2022;32(3):1528–1537. https://doi.org/10.1007/s00330-021-08275-0.
26. Rodríguez-Ruiz A, Krupinski E, Mordang JJ, et al. Detection of breast cancer with mammography: effect of an artificial intelligence support system. *Radiology.* 2019;290(2):305–314. https://doi.org/10.1148/radiol.2018181371.
27. Lokaj B, Pugliese MT, Kinkel K, Lovis C, Schmid J. Barriers and facilitators of artificial intelligence conception and implementation for breast imaging diagnosis in clinical practice: a scoping review. *Eur Radiol.* 2024;34(3):2096–2109. https://doi.org/10.1007/s00330-023-10181-6.
28. Zhang X, Zhang Y, Zhang G, et al. Deep learning with radiomics for disease diagnosis and treatment: challenges and potential. *Front Oncol.* 2022;12:773840. https://doi.org/10.3389/fonc.2022.773840.
29. Bi WL, Hosny A, Schabath MB, et al. Artificial intelligence in cancer imaging: clinical challenges and applications. *CA Cancer J Clin.* 2019;69(2):127–157. https://doi.org/10.3322/caac.21552.

CHAPTER 5

Artificial Intelligence in Cardiovascular Imaging

Marvee Espiritu ■ Rajat Chand

KEY POINTS

- Artificial intelligence (AI)-based algorithms have shown promising results in increasing diagnostic accuracy and efficiency in interpreting a variety of cardiac imaging modalities including echocardiography, CT, MRI, and nuclear imaging.
- Several AI-based models have FDA approval for clinical use in cardiovascular imaging.
- Ethical and regulatory limitations still exist that limit widespread adoption of AI in the clinical setting.

GLOSSARY OF TERMS AND DEFINITIONS

Single Photon Emission Computed Tomography (SPECT): A medical imaging modality based on nuclear medical imaging and tomographic reconstruction models that convey functional information.

Fractional Flow Reserve–Computed Tomography (FFR-CT): A noninvasive imaging modality based on computational fluid dynamics to calculate coronary atheroma burden using data obtained from computed tomography coronary angiography.

Coronary Artery Calcium Score: Measurement of calcified plaque in the coronary arteries based on CT scan.

Angiography: Radiographic visualization of blood vessels after injection of radiopaque substance

Introduction

According to the most recent data from the World Health Organization (WHO), cardiovascular diseases are the leading causes of death worldwide with approximately 18 million deaths in 2019, secondary to cardiovascular-related causes.[1] The utilization of artificial intelligence (AI) in cardiovascular radiology has gained significant attention due to its ability to yield more accurate and efficient image interpretation. Recent studies have demonstrated the promising role of AI in various cardiac imaging modalities such as echocardiography, computed tomography (CT), magnetic resonance imaging (MRI), nuclear cardiology, and angiography.[2,3,4] This chapter highlights the most recent advances and uses of AI within cardiac imaging as well current limitations of the technology.

ECHOCARDIOGRAPHY

Echocardiography is one the most widely utilized imaging modalities in cardiology. Echocardiography is noninvasive ultrasound used to assess various biomechanics of the heart such as structural abnormalities, valvular function, and myocardial contractility. However, one of the major limitations of echocardiography is the subjective and technologist/operator-dependent nature of the image interpretation, which often leads to interobserver variability. AI addresses this limitation by producing accurate, consistent, and automated interpretations of echocardiograms. A study by Zhang et al.[5] utilized 14,035 echocardiograms to train convolutional neural network (CNN) models across varying tasks such as automated identification of 23 viewpoints and segmentation of cardiac chambers (Fig. 5.1). The performance of the AI was compared with manual segmentation and measurements from 8666 echocardiograms during routine clinical workflow. Their CNN model was able to accurately identify 96% of parasternal long-axis imaging views, and the study showed comparable or superior output by the automated measurements compared to manual measurements.[5] Madani et al.[6] trained a convolutional neural network to recognize 15 different echocardiographic views using 267 real-world echocardiograms with over 200,000 images. Using this CNN algorithm, the AI correctly classified 15 echocardiographic views with 97.8% accuracy compared with 70.2% to 84.0% accuracy among board-certified echocardiographers when charged with the same task.[6] Several companies including Zebra Medical Vision (Nanox.AI Petah Tikva, Israel) and Arterys (Tempus Radiology, San Francisco, CA) are currently developing AI-based echocardiography software.

COMPUTED TOMOGRAPHY

CT is another imaging modality used to analyze various pathologies in cardiovascular imaging. In particular, coronary artery calcium (CAC) score on cardiac CT has been well regarded as an independent predictor of cardiac events and mortality risk. However, the manual measurement of CAC score on cardiac CT can be time consuming, and its accuracy may be limited by motion artifacts. In a study by Al'Aref et al.,[7] the authors utilized a machine learning model to predict coronary artery disease in 35,281 patients using the combination of coronary artery calcium score and clinical factors. Machine learning in conjunction with coronary artery calcium score resulted in a more accurate assessment of obstructive coronary artery disease (CAD) with area under the curve (AUC) of 0.881 compared with machine learning alone (AUC 0.773) or coronary artery calcium score (AUC 0.866).[7]

CT ANGIOGRAPHY

CT angiography (CTA) is widely utilized for the evaluation of cardiovascular diseases serving as the first-line diagnostic imaging modality for pulmonary embolism and aortic dissection. CTA is also being increasingly used for standard clinical assessment of patients with low-intermediate pretest probability of CAD. However, the radiation dose associated with CTA has been a main concern. Wolterink et al.[2] showed the feasibility of deriving CAC score from coronary CT angiography. A CNN model was trained on 250 patients who underwent both CT angiography and nonenhanced cardiac CT scans. The model quantified CAC scores on CT angiography comparable to CAC quantification derived from nonenhanced cardiac CT in 83% of the patients.[2] The findings of this study showed that patients may undergo CAC quantification while undergoing CT angiography without undergoing additional cardiac CT scans, thereby reducing radiation dose exposure.

In 2021, the FDA approved Zebra Coronary Artery Calcium Solution, an AI-based software that aids in the quantification of coronary artery calcium on CT scans. The software stratifies the CT image into three categories (low, medium, high) depending on the extent of coronary artery calcium deposit with the goal of identifying at-risk patients and providing them with appropriate preventative care to mitigate their risk of future cardiovascular events.[8]

FRACTIONAL FLOW RESERVE–COMPUTED TOMOGRAPHY

Another use of AI in cardiac imaging is in fractional flow reserve–computed tomography (FFR-CT) in the diagnosis of CAD. FFR-CT is an alternative imaging technique used to detect

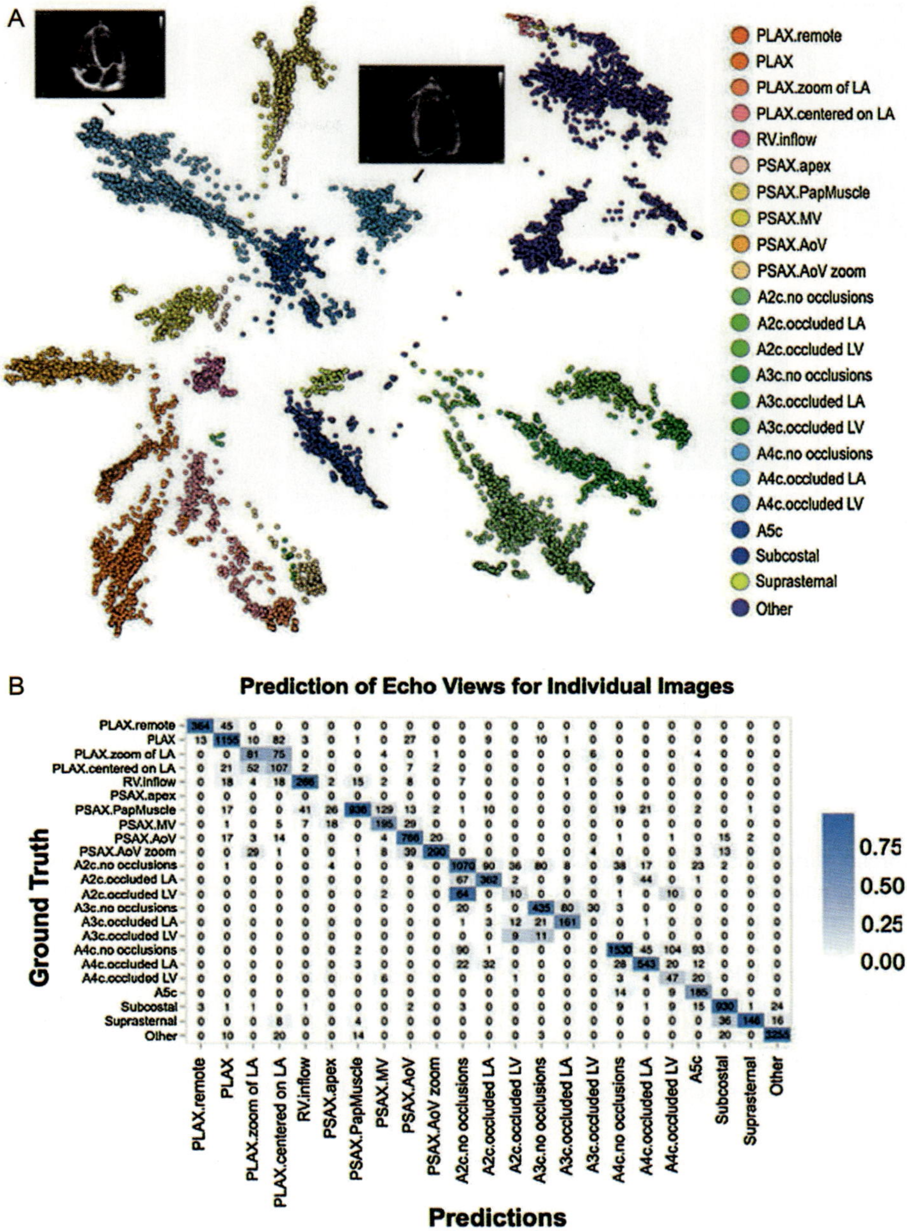

Fig. 5.1 Discrimination of echocardiographic views through the use of convolutional neural networks. (A) Groups of test images that corresponds to 23 different echocardiographic views, including views with or without occlusion. (B) Successful (numbers along diagonal) and unsuccessful (off-diagonal) view classifications within the test data set. *A2c*, Apical 2-chamber; *A3c*, apical 3-chamber; *A4c*, apical 4-chamber; *echo*, echocardiogram; *LV*, left ventricular; *PLAX*, parasternal long axis. (Image adapted from Zhang J, Gajjala S, Agrawal P, et al. Fully automated echocardiogram interpretation in clinical practice. *Circulation*. 2018;138(16):1623–1635.)

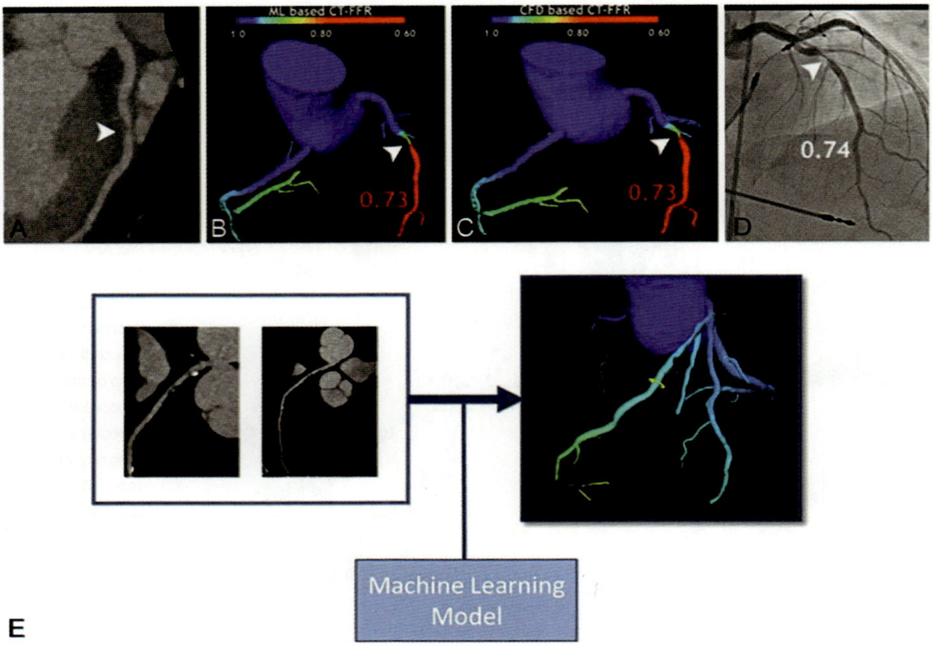

Fig. 5.2 (A) Coronary computed tomography showing coronary artery stenosis (*arrowhead*). (B) Machine-learning based calculation of CT-FFR (*arrowhead* represents degree of stenosis). (C) Computational fluid dynamics (CFD)-based calculation of CT-FFR (*arrowhead* represents degree of stenosis). (D) Coronary angiography measuring degree of stenosis (*arrowhead*). (E) The process of reconstructing a three-dimensional image from a coronary CT after utilization of machine learning model. (Image reproduced from Siegersma KR, Leiner T, Chew DP, Appelman Y, Hofstra L, Verjans JW. Artificial intelligence in cardiovascular imaging: state of the art and implications for the imaging cardiologist. *Neth Heart J.* 2019;27(9):403–413.)

coronary artery stenosis based on CTA images. FFR measurement is defined as the ratio between the maximum blood flow feasible in a diseased or stenosed coronary artery and the maximum blood flow in a nondiseased coronary artery. Jian et al.[9] compared the performance of a machine-learning (ML)-based coronary CT angiography (cCTA)-derived fractional flow reserve (CT-FFR) against FFR as the reference for the detection of coronary calcification severity. When tested on 442 patients in a multicenter study, ML-based cCTA-derived FFR yielded an accuracy of 0.90, sensitivity of 0.84, and specificity of 0.94. ML-based cCTA-derived FFR also showed improved detection of ischemia compared with cCTA alone in lesions with moderate calcification.[9] Fig. 5.2 is a schematic diagram showing the use of AI in FFR-CT (Fig. 5.2).[3]

MAGNETIC RESONANCE IMAGING

Cardiac MRI is another diagnostic modality widely used in cardiology that provides detailed structural and functional images of the heart. The high-resolution images obtained through MRI make it the gold standard for the evaluation and quantification of left ventricular function, mass, and volume. However, cardiac MR imaging is particularly challenging because it may be limited by physiologic constraints, in particular cardiac and respiratory motion. In addition, manual segmentation of the right and left ventricles is currently the standard of practice for cardiac MR (CMR), which is often time consuming and subject to intra- and interobserver variability. Use of AI in cardiac MRI has gained traction due to its potential to enhance diagnostic accuracy and optimize workflow.

Winther et al.[10] utilized a deep learning algorithm, *vnet*, to facilitate automated segmentation of the right and left ventricular endocardium and epicardium in order to estimate cardiac volume and mass. The algorithm performed equally or superior to human experts when presented with the same task.[10] Similarly, Fahmy et al.[11] created a deep fully convolutional neural network (FCN) to achieve segmentation of the myocardium in T1-weighted images of patients with hypertrophic cardiomyopathy. The algorithm was trained and tested by using manually segmented images of 210 patients plus additional images from 455 patients segmented by an expert using a semiautomatic tool. The FCN algorithm offered automated and accelerated segmentation compared to the manual segmentation of two expert readers. The automated T1 calculations from the FCN algorithm were within good agreement with the manual calculations (Pearson correlation coefficient, $r = 0.82$; $slope = 1.01$; $P < .0001$), showing the potential of AI to automate the tedious and time-consuming manual segmentation of cardiac MR.[11]

NUCLEAR IMAGING

Nuclear cardiology, specifically the use of single photon emission computed tomography (SPECT) and positron emission tomography (PET) myocardial perfusion imaging (MPI), has also been a clinically valuable tool in the diagnosis and management of coronary artery diseases. These imaging modalities provide critical information with regards to cardiac perfusion and function. Recent studies have explored the role of AI in nuclear cardiology, specifically in tasks related to improving image quality, automated image quantification and segmentation, disease diagnosis, and prognosis. Juarez-Orozco et al.[12] evaluated the performance of a deep learning model in 1185 patients for identifying myocardial ischemia or increased risk of major adverse cardiovascular events (MACE) using PET myocardial perfusion imaging. The integration of deep learning in PET myocardial perfusion significantly outperformed all comparator models with an area under the receiver operating curve (AUC) of 0.90, accuracy of 0.82, sensitivity of 87%, and specificity of 77%.[12] These findings are supported by another study that showed improved accuracy of deep learning in predicting myocardial perfusion and degree of myocardial ischemia in patients without known CAD.[4] Furthermore, machine learning algorithms have been implemented to predict early coronary revascularization (ECR) within 90 days after SPECT imaging yielding an AUC higher than standard quantitative analysis and outperforming expert interpretation by nuclear cardiologists.[13]

Although SPECT is a clinically valuable imaging modality to assess cardiovascular disease, concerns about radiation risks associated with this imaging technique has been raised. In order to obtain high-quality images, sufficient radiopharmaceutical dose must be used to avoid yielding poor signal-to-noise ratio (SNR). Recent studies have explored strategies to decrease the injected radiopharmaceutical dose without compromising diagnostic performance. With the integration of deep learning, noise suppression in the image was achieved at low radiation, and the predicted standard-dose images were comparable to reference standard-dose images at half- and at quarter-dose levels.[14]

LIMITATIONS

The recent advancements in research have shown tremendous promise regarding the use of AI in cardiovascular imaging. Several AI-based applications have already been approved by the FDA for use in echocardiography and CT scan with the goal of streamlining workflow and improving diagnostic accuracy. However, limitations still exist that limit adoption of AI in cardiovascular healthcare. AI-based software must undergo a comprehensive evaluation and approval by the FDA, which delays introduction of the technology to the consumer market. In addition, further studies are warranted to determine whether the use of such technologies leads to improved patient outcomes and lower healthcare costs. Furthermore, the performance of AI algorithms is dependent on the data cohort on which the model is trained. Ethnic, age, gender, and medical diversity must be utilized to create unbiased algorithms, which requires large diverse datasets in the training and validation of the algorithm.

Conclusion

AI is a tool that may be utilized to improve diagnostic accuracy and streamline workflow in cardiovascular imaging. However, human input and expertise is still vital in the overall patient assessment and management.

Resources

U.S. Food & Drug Administration: Artificial Intelligence and Machine Learning (AI/ML)-Enabled Medical Devices.

References

1. Organization WH. Cardiovascular Diseases. https://www.who.int/news-room/fact-sheets/detail/cardiovascular-diseases-(cvds)#:~:text=Cardiovascular%20diseases%20(CVDs)%20are%20the,%2D%20and%20middle%2Dincome%20countries.
2. Wolterink JM, Leiner T, de Vos BD, van Hamersvelt RW, Viergever MA, Išgum I. Automatic coronary artery calcium scoring in cardiac CT angiography using paired convolutional neural networks. *Med Image Anal.* 2016;34:123–136. http://doi.org/10.1016/j.media.2016.04.004.
3. Administration UF& D. *Section 510 K Premarket Notification of Intent.* Accessed February 10, 2023. https://www.accessdata.fda.gov/cdrh_docs/pdf21/K210085.pdf.
4. Di Jiang M, Zhang XL, Liu H, et al. The effect of coronary calcification on diagnostic performance of machine learning-based CT-FFR: a Chinese multicenter study. *Eur Radiol.* 2021;31(3):1482–1493. http://doi.org/10.1007/s00330-020-07261-2.
5. Zhang J, Gajjala S, Agrawal P, et al. Fully automated echocardiogram interpretation in clinical practice. *Circulation.* 2018;138(16):1623–1635. http://doi.org/10.1161/CIRCULATIONAHA.118.034338.
6. Siegersma KR, Leiner T, Chew DP, Appelman Y, Hofstra L, Verjans JW. Artificial intelligence in cardiovascular imaging: state of the art and implications for the imaging cardiologist. *Neth Heart J.* 2019;27(9):403–413. https://doi.org/10.1007/s12471-019-01311-1.
7. Winther HB, Hundt C, Schmidt B, et al. ν-net: deep learning for generalized biventricular mass and function parameters using multicenter cardiac MRI data. *JACC Cardiovasc Imaging.* 2018;11(7):1036–1038. http://doi.org/10.1016/j.jcmg.2017.11.013.
8. Madani A, Arnaout R, Mofrad M, Arnaout R. Fast and accurate view classification of echocardiograms using deep learning. *NPJ Digit Med.* 2018;1:6. http://doi.org/10.1038/s41746-017-0013-1.
9. Fahmy AS, El-Rewaidy H, Nezafat M, Nakamori S, Nezafat R. Automated analysis of cardiovascular magnetic resonance myocardial native T(1) mapping images using fully convolutional neural networks. *J Cardiovasc Magn Reson Off J Soc Cardiovasc Magn Reson.* 2019;21(1):7. http://doi.org/10.1186/s12968-018-0516-1.
10. Juarez-Orozco LE, Martinez-Manzanera O, van der Zant FM, Knol RJJ, Knuuti J. Deep learning in quantitative PET myocardial perfusion imaging: a study on cardiovascular event prediction. *JACC Cardiovasc Imaging.* 2020;13(1 Pt 1):180–182. http://doi.org/10.1016/j.jcmg.2019.08.009.
11. Betancur J, Commandeur F, Motlagh M, et al. Deep learning for prediction of obstructive disease from fast myocardial perfusion SPECT: a multicenter study. *JACC Cardiovasc Imaging.* 2018;11(11):1654–1663. http://doi.org/10.1016/j.jcmg.2018.01.020.
12. Al'Aref SJ, Maliakal G, Singh G, et al. Machine learning of clinical variables and coronary artery calcium scoring for the prediction of obstructive coronary artery disease on coronary computed tomography angiography: analysis from the CONFIRM registry. *Eur Heart J.* 2020;41(3):359–367. http://doi.org/10.1093/eurheartj/ehz565.
13. Hu L-H, Betancur J, Sharir T, et al. Machine learning predicts per-vessel early coronary revascularization after fast myocardial perfusion SPECT: results from multicentre REFINE SPECT registry. *Eur Hear journal Cardiovasc Imaging.* 2020;21(5):549–559. http://doi.org/10.1093/ehjci/jez177.
14. Aghakhan Olia N, Kamali-Asl A, Hariri Tabrizi S, et al. Deep learning-based denoising of low-dose SPECT myocardial perfusion images: quantitative assessment and clinical performance. *Eur J Nucl Med Mol Imaging.* 2022;49(5):1508–1522. http://doi.org/10.1007/s00259-021-05614-7.

CHAPTER 6

Interpretive Applications: Chest

Rasheed Abdullah ■ Mustafa Azam

KEY POINTS

- Artificial intelligence (AI) enhances early detection and personalized treatment of lung diseases such as cancer and chronic obstructive pulmonary disease (COPD).
- AI's quantitative analysis improves the accuracy and objectivity of chest imaging assessments.
- FDA-approved AI products and emerging technologies are revolutionizing diagnosis and treatment in chest imaging.

GLOSSARY OF TERMS AND DEFINITIONS

Early Detection and Diagnosis: The application of AI algorithms to identify signs of diseases such as lung cancer in their initial stages, enabling timely medical interventions.

Deep Learning: A subset of machine learning that involves algorithms inspired by the structure and function of the brain called artificial or convolutional neural networks; used extensively in AI applications for chest imaging to analyze complex patterns in data.

Quantitative Analysis: The application of AI algorithms to provide exact measurements related to lung function, airway dimensions, and other critical features, aiding in diagnosis and treatment planning.

Computer-Aided Detection (CADe): A type of AI application designed to assist radiologists by identifying and highlighting regions of interest in medical images, such as pulmonary nodules in chest CT scans.

CT DICOM Data: Digital Imaging and Communications in Medicine (DICOM) data from computed tomography (CT) scans, often used as input for AI algorithms in chest imaging.

Feature Extraction: The process of transforming input data into a set of features that can be mathematically analyzed; often a crucial step in AI algorithms for tasks like image recognition and classification in chest imaging.

Transfer Learning (TL): A machine learning technique in which a pretrained model is adapted as a starting point for a new but related task, often used in AI applications for chest imaging to adapt existing models for specific medical applications.

Introduction

Artificial intelligence has likely had its biggest impact thus far in the realm of chest imaging. AI algorithms are revolutionizing the early detection and diagnosis of lung diseases, particularly lung cancer. By analyzing radiological images with high speed and accuracy, AI can identify subtle signs of cancer and other pulmonary diseases that may be missed by human radiologists. This

TABLE 6.1 ■ **Overview of Current FDA-Approved AI Products in Chest Imaging**

Product Name	Developer	Primary Function	Special Features
syngo.CT Lung CAD VD20	Siemens Healthcare	Detection of pulmonary nodules on chest CT	Can be used as a first or second reader
AI-Rad Companion (Pulmonary)	Siemens Medical Solutions	Assessment of thoracic diseases on chest CT	Lung segmentation, lobe measurement
LungVision System	Body Vision Medical	Enhancing pulmonary procedures on chest CT	Integrates 3D CT datasets with real-time fluoroscopic X-ray images
CINA CHEST	Avicenna.AI	Early detection of critical conditions like PE and AD on chest CT	Rapid notifications, high sensitivity and specificity
syngo.CT CaScoring SOMARIS/8 VB70	Siemens Medical Solutions	Evaluation of calcified coronary lesions on chest CT	Calculates various scores like Agatston-equivalent score
iNtuition-Structural Heart Module	TeraRecon	Structural heart assessment on chest CT	Advanced visualization techniques and reporting capabilities

early detection enables timely interventions, leading to better treatment outcomes. AI also aids in characterizing and monitoring various pulmonary diseases like chronic obstructive pulmonary disease (COPD) and idiopathic pulmonary fibrosis (IPF), allowing for personalized treatment plans based on precise quantification of disease severity.

AI's strength in quantitative analysis is particularly beneficial in chest imaging. Algorithms can automate tedious and time-consuming manual measurements and provide precise measurements related to lung function, airway dimensions, and other critical features. This quantitative approach enhances the accuracy of diagnosis, prognosis, and treatment planning. It also allows for more objective follow-up evaluations, helping clinicians make data-driven decisions.

Several FDA-approved AI products are already in use (Table 6.1), enhancing the accuracy and efficiency of chest imaging. These include tools for detecting pulmonary nodules, assessing thoracic diseases, and aiding in pulmonary procedures. Additionally, there are promising applications under development, particularly for the detection and monitoring of COVID-19 and other infectious diseases, as well as chronic conditions like idiopathic pulmonary fibrosis, tuberculosis (TB), and COPD. These emerging technologies are expected to further advance the field, offering high accuracy and efficiency in diagnosis and treatment planning.

This chapter gives an overview of the current state of AI in chest imaging, its practical applications, and the promising future developments in this field.

Current Needs

EARLY DETECTION AND DIAGNOSIS

One of the most promising applications of AI in chest imaging is the early detection and diagnosis of lung cancer. AI algorithms can analyze radiological images with unprecedented speed and accuracy, identifying subtle signs of cancer that might escape human detection. By detecting lung cancer at its incipient stages, AI enables timely interventions, leading to better treatment outcomes and improved survival rates. Several studies have shown that AI can enhance the sensitivity of lung cancer detection, ultimately saving lives.[1] These algorithms, trained on extensive datasets of chest images, can recognize even the faintest shadows or anomalies that may indicate malignancy. Several commercial products, discussed further in this chapter, are being utilized to detect lung nodules (Fig. 6.1).

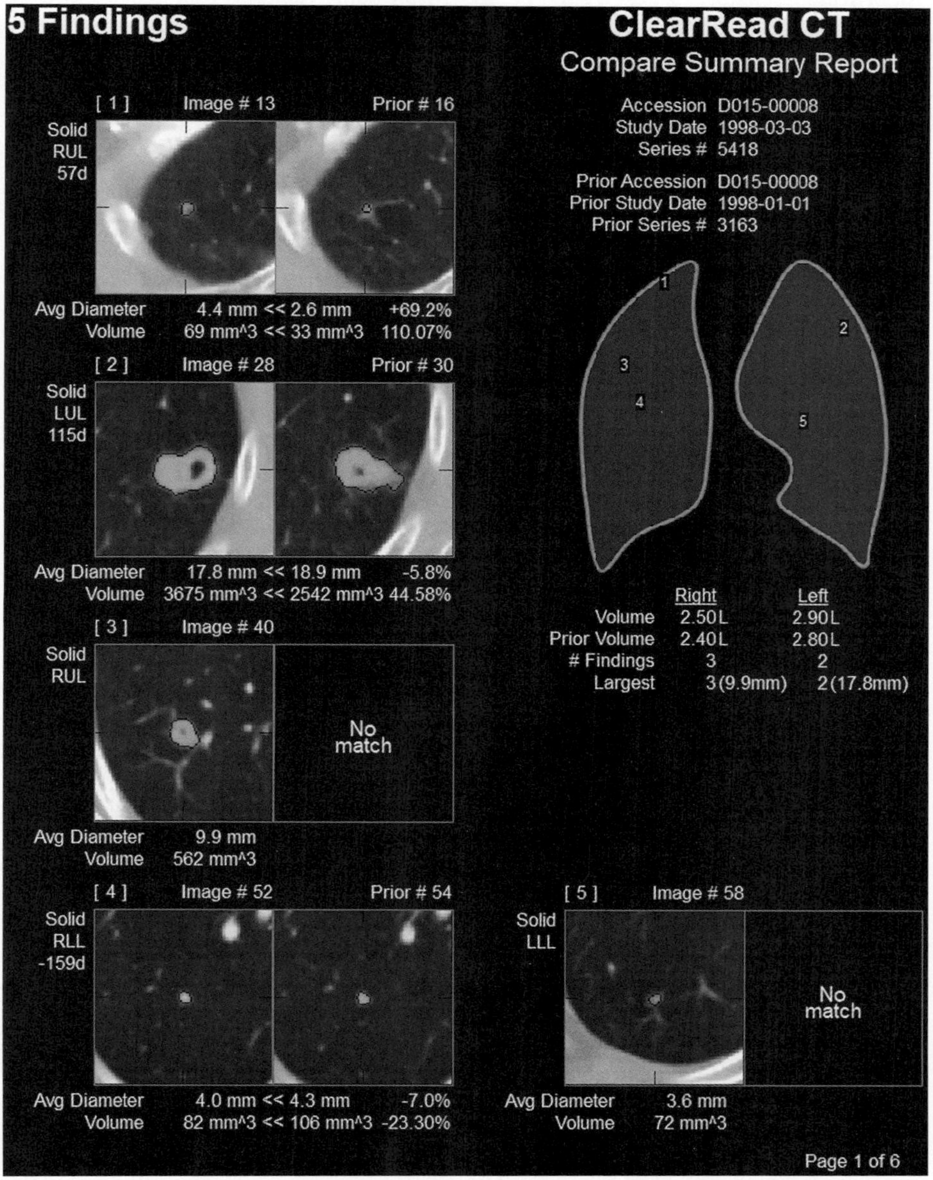

Fig. 6.1 Report from commercial product using computer-aided detection (CAD) software to detect lung nodules and compare with previous studies. (From ClearRead CT – Riverain; n.d. https://www.riveraintech.com/clearread-ai-solutions/clearread-ct/.)

CHARACTERIZATION AND MONITORING OF PULMONARY DISEASES

Beyond lung cancer, AI algorithms are invaluable for characterizing and monitoring a range of pulmonary diseases, such as COPD and IPF. These algorithms can precisely quantify disease severity, identify subtle changes in lung structure, and predict disease trajectories. One study employed a deep-learning application to characterize COPD severity in smokers and predict risk of acute respiratory distress (ARD) events.[2] By providing clinicians with detailed insights, AI facilitates the development of personalized treatment plans, ensuring that patients receive the most appropriate interventions tailored to their specific needs. This personalized approach is vital for managing chronic conditions and optimizing patient outcomes.

QUANTITATIVE ANALYSIS

AI's quantitative prowess extends to chest imaging by enabling advanced analysis of lung function, airway dimensions, and other relevant features. Through quantitative metrics, AI can offer precise measurements that aid in diagnosis, prognosis, and treatment planning. For instance, AI can assess lung function by measuring airway obstruction in COPD, helping clinicians gauge disease severity and guiding therapeutic decisions. This quantitative approach not only enhances the accuracy of assessments but also allows for more objective follow-up evaluations.

Current FDA-Approved Products

SYNGO.CT LUNG CAD VD20

The syngo.CT Lung CAD VD20, developed by Siemens Healthcare, is an AI application designed to enhance the accuracy and efficiency of chest imaging, particularly in the detection of pulmonary nodules on CT. This computer-aided detection (CADe) tool serves as an invaluable assistant to radiologists when reviewing multidetector computed tomography (MDCT) scans of the chest. Its purpose is to identify solid and subsolid (part-solid and ground glass) pulmonary nodules that might be overlooked by human review alone. The AI algorithm processes images from various MDCT scanners and highlights regions of interest (ROIs) for radiologists to investigate further. Notably, the syngo.CT Lung CAD can be employed in two different ways: as a concurrent first reader or as a second reader after the initial review by a radiologist. This AI application provides radiologists with a powerful tool to improve nodule detection, ultimately leading to more accurate diagnoses and better patient outcomes.[3]

AI-RAD COMPANION

The AI-Rad Companion (Pulmonary), designed by Siemens Medical Solutions, serves as a tool for assessment of thoracic disease. Leveraging CT Digital Imaging and Communications in Medicine (DICOM) data, the AI-Rad Companion (Pulmonary) utilizes machine learning and deep learning algorithms to deliver both quantitative and qualitative analyses of lung conditions. It offers a variety of functions such as lung segmentation, lung lobe measurement, detection of areas with abnormal Hounsfield values, and the ability to categorize and measure lung lesions. Furthermore, this AI application can interface with external devices such as syngo.CT Lung CAD, which enhances its diagnostic capabilities. With the recent introduction of features like pulmonary density and bidirectional lesion diameter, it provides even more comprehensive assessments. This innovative technology assists healthcare providers in swiftly and accurately evaluating lung diseases, which is especially crucial in the realm of chest imaging, aiding in the early detection and management of thoracic conditions.[3]

LUNGVISION SYSTEM

The LungVision System, developed by Body Vision Medical, utilizes the power of AI to enhance pulmonary procedures. This AI application allows users to integrate previously acquired 3D CT datasets with real-time fluoroscopic x-ray images of the same anatomical region. This integration enables precise navigation of catheters and devices during pulmonary procedures, providing invaluable support to physicians. By overlaying segmented 3D CT data onto live fluoroscopic images, LungVision aids in guiding endobronchial tools to the precise target locations within the patient's lungs. This system complies with stringent medical device standards and has undergone comprehensive performance testing, ensuring its reliability in clinical settings.[3]

CINA CHEST

The CINA CHEST (Computer-Aided Triage and Notification Software for Chest Imaging), developed by Avicenna.AI, utilizes AI for the early detection and prioritization of critical conditions such as pulmonary embolism (PE) and aortic dissection (AD) in chest and thoraco-abdominal CT angiography. This AI application operates in parallel with standard image interpretation, analyzing DICOM images to flag and communicate suspected positive findings of PE and AD to radiologists and clinicians. CINA CHEST provides rapid notifications, accompanied by compressed preview images for informational purposes, facilitating early triage and timely patient care. Notably, the application doesn't alter the original medical images and is not intended for primary diagnosis but serves as a valuable tool to aid radiologists in quickly identifying critical cases. The performance data show that CINA CHEST performs with high sensitivity and specificity, making it a valuable addition to chest imaging workflows, enhancing diagnostic speed and ultimately improving patient outcomes.[3]

SYNGO.CT CASCORING SOMARIS/8 VB70

The syngo.CT CaScoring SOMARIS/8 VB70 is a post-processing application developed by Siemens Medical Solutions designed to evaluate calcified coronary lesions using chest imaging data from CT scans. This AI application takes noncontrast cardiac CT images and allows radiologists to interactively identify and classify calcified lesions within the coronary arteries. It calculates various scores, including the Agatston-equivalent score, mass score, and volume score for each coronary artery, providing a comprehensive assessment of coronary calcium burden. Furthermore, it enables users to create detailed reports that include calcium scoring data, images, cited literature, and other relevant information. This AI application aids in the early detection and monitoring of coronary artery calcifications, which is crucial for assessing cardiovascular health and guiding patient care.[3]

INTUITION-STRUCTURAL HEART MODULE

The iNtuition-Structural Heart Module, developed by TeraRecon, is an AI application that has significantly advanced the field of chest imaging, particularly in the context of structural heart assessment. This module allows clinicians to visualize and measure various structures within the heart and blood vessels. By employing automatic and manual centerline detection, segmentation of cardiovascular structures, and precise measurement tools for dimensions (such as diameters, lengths, areas, and volumes), the module enhances preoperative planning and sizing for cardiovascular interventions. Additionally, it aids in postoperative evaluations, providing valuable insights into patient outcomes. The software also enables calcium quantification and scoring to assess for and monitor calcifications within the heart and vessels. With its advanced visualization techniques and reporting capabilities, this AI application is playing a pivotal role in improving diagnostic accuracy, treatment planning, and overall patient care in the field of chest imaging.[3]

Applications Under Development

There are several applications of artificial intelligence (AI) in radiology as they apply to chest imaging that are currently under development. This section highlights only some of these developments but focuses on some of the unique algorithmic approaches being honed for future applications.

Among these, researchers have been exploring the use of AI-based algorithms for the detection and monitoring of COVID-19 on chest imaging modalities. Panahi et al. (2022) proposed an accurate and automatic technique based on a deep residual network to analyze chest x-ray images for COVID-19 diagnosis. Their model achieved an accuracy of 92.1%.[4]

El-Shafai et al. (2022) proposed an automated diagnosis framework that includes image acquisition, preprocessing, and classification using transfer learning (TL) models. They focused on leveraging deep convolutional neural networks (DCNNs) to create an automated diagnosis system for COVID-19. Their framework incorporates image acquisition, preprocessing, and classification stages, utilizing TL to adapt preexisting models for this specific medical application. Two types of TL—fine tuning and deep tuning—were employed on a variety of neural network architectures such as DenseNet, ResNet, and VGG. The models were tested on datasets comprising 9270 chest x-rays and 2762 chest CT images, with varying training-to-testing ratios. Remarkably, their approach achieved an average accuracy rate of 98.49% for multiclass classification and 97.64% for binary classification. These findings underscore the potential of AI-based algorithms in providing highly accurate and efficient diagnostic solutions for COVID-19 using chest imaging modalities.[5]

Ragab et al. (2023) similarly aimed to develop a Deep Transfer Learning Based COVID-19 monitoring system. They introduced the Intelligent Firefly Algorithm Deep Transfer Learning Based COVID-19 Monitoring System (IFFA-DTLMS), a sophisticated AI-based framework for COVID-19 diagnosis using chest radiographs. The system primarily employs the DenseNet121 architecture for feature extraction, optimized by the Firefly Algorithm (FFA) for hyperparameter tuning. Additionally, an Autoencoder-Long Short Term Memory (AE-LSTM) model is utilized for the final diagnosis and classification of COVID-19. The model was experimentally validated using a CXR image dataset containing 32,224 samples under the COVID class and 6448 samples under the healthy class. Although the paper did not explicitly mention the accuracy rates, it emphasized the model's enhanced performance and wide-ranging experimental validation. This work adds to the growing body of evidence supporting the efficacy of AI-based algorithms in the rapid and accurate diagnosis of COVID-19 through chest imaging.[6]

AI algorithms are also being leveraged to develop applications that can quantify the severity of lung diseases, including but not limited to idiopathic pulmonary fibrosis (IPF), TB, and COPD on chest imaging.

Pakzad et al. (2021) developed a model that focused on IPF, a lung disease characterized by excessive fibrosis. They introduced AirQuant, an automated computational pipeline designed to quantify airway abnormalities in IPF using volumetric CT imaging. Unlike the other models that focus on infectious diseases like COVID-19, AirQuant aims to provide estimates of IPF disease extent and severity. The pipeline uses deep learning–based airway segmentation to parcellate the airway tree into its lobes and generational branches, deriving structural measures from chest CT scans. Notably, AirQuant computes airway "inter-tapering" and airway tortuosity, measures that were found to be significantly altered in IPF patients compared to healthy controls. The system is open source and has the potential to serve as a novel imaging biomarker for IPF severity and disease extent.[7]

Fati et al. (2022) focused on the early detection of TB using chest x-ray images. They proposed two distinct approaches that employ a combination of artificial intelligence techniques for diagnosis. The first approach hybridizes two convolutional neural networks (CNN) models, namely Res-Net-50 and GoogLeNet, and uses principal component analysis (PCA) for feature reduction. The support vector machine (SVM) algorithm is then used for classification. The second approach utilizes artificial neural networks (ANN) based on fused features extracted by ResNet-50 and GoogleNet models. These features are then combined with those extracted by the gray-level co-occurrence matrix (GLCM), discrete wavelet transform (DWT), and local binary pattern (LBP) algorithms. Remarkably, the ANN approach achieved an accuracy of 99.2% on the first dataset and 99.8% on the second dataset for diagnosing TB. These methods aim to assist healthcare professionals in diagnosing TB at an early stage, thereby increasing the chances of patient survival.[8]

Siebert et al. (2023) outlined a clinical protocol for an observational case-control study that aims to develop deep learning algorithms for the diagnosis and severity stratification of interstitial lung disease (ILD) and COPD. Unlike the other studies that are already in the implementation or validation phase, Siebert et al. are in the planning stage, focusing on digitally acquired lung sounds and lung ultrasound (LUS) images. Their algorithm, named DeepBreath, will be trained to differentiate ILD from non-ILD sounds and images, predict ILD clinical severity, and differentiate ILD from COPD. The study also aims to categorize subtypes of ILD, such as IPF versus nonspecific interstitial pneumonia (NSIP). This adds another layer to the growing body of work that leverages AI for the diagnosis and monitoring of lung diseases, extending beyond infectious diseases like COVID-19 to chronic conditions like ILD and COPD.[9]

Rapid advancements are transpiring within the applications utilizing AI algorithms in chest imaging. These algorithms are not only demonstrating high accuracy in recognizing infectious diseases such as COVID-19 but are also showing promise in quantifying the severity of chronic lung diseases like IPF, TB, and COPD. Ongoing research and development are expected to lead to new and innovative uses of this technology in the future.

References

1. Ardila D, Kiraly AP, Bharadwaj S, et al. End-to-end lung cancer screening with three-dimensional deep learning on low-dose chest computed tomography. *Nat Med.* 2019;25(6):954–961. https://doi.org/10.1038/s41591-019-0447-x.
2. González G, Ash SY, Vegas-Sánchez-Ferrero G, et al. Disease staging and prognosis in smokers using deep learning in chest computed tomography. *Am J Respir Crit Care Med.* 2018;197(2):193–203. https://doi.org/10.1164/rccm.201705-0860OC.
3. FDA. Artificial Intelligence and Machine Learning (AI/ML)-Enabled Medical Devices. *US Food & Drug Administration.* 2022. https://www.fda.gov/medical-devices/software-medical-device-samd/artificial-intelligence-and-machine-learning-aiml-enabled-medical-devices.
4. Panahi A, Askari Moghadam R, Akrami M, Madani K. Deep residual neural network for COVID-19 detection from chest X-ray images. *SN Comput Sci.* 2022;3(2):169.
5. El-Shafai W, Algarni AD, El Banby GM, El-Samie A, Fathi E, Soliman NF. Classification framework for COVID-19 diagnosis based on deep CNN models. *Intell Autom Soft Comput.* 2022;31(3):1561–1575. https://www.techscience.com/iasc/v31n3/44842.
6. Ragab M, Al-Rabia MW, Binyamin SS, Aldarmahi AA. Intelligent firefly algorithm deep transfer learning based COVID-19 monitoring system. *Comput Mater Contin.* 2023;74(2):2889–2903. https://www.techscience.com/cmc/v74n2/50240.

7. Pakzad A, Cheung WK, Quan K, et al. Evaluation of automated airway morphological quantification for assessing fibrosing lung disease. *arXiv preprint arXiv:2111.10443*. 2021. https://arxiv.org/pdf/2111.10443.pdf.
8. Fati SM, Senan EM, ElHakim N. Deep and hybrid learning technique for early detection of tuberculosis based on X-ray images using feature fusion. *Appl Sci*. 2022;12(14):7092. https://www.mdpi.com/2076-3417/12/14/7092.
9. Siebert JN, Hartley MA, Courvoisier DS, et al. Deep learning diagnostic and severity-stratification for interstitial lung diseases and chronic obstructive pulmonary disease in digital lung auscultations and ultrasonography: clinical protocol for an observational case–control study. *BMC Pulm Med*. 2023;23(1):1–16. https://www.ncbi.nlm.nih.gov/pmc/articles/PMC10234685/.

CHAPTER 7

Artificial Intelligence in Emergency Radiology

Nadeen Aladham ■ Rajat Chand

KEY POINTS

- AI Advancements in Emergency Radiology
  - AI is significantly enhancing workflow efficiency and improving diagnostic accuracy of findings requiring urgent management in emergency radiology through applications for finding detection, order entry, imaging protocols, and report generation, helping reduce radiologist burnout.
- Example Companies With FDA-Approved Products
  - FDA-approved AI tools such as Viz.AI's Contact, Qure.ai, and Zebra Medical Vision leverage deep learning to rapidly identify critical conditions in emergency department settings (e.g., large-vessel occlusion in stroke, intracranial hemorrhage, cervical spine fractures), improving diagnostic accuracy, accelerating triage, and enhancing overall patient outcomes.
- Implementation Challenges and Future Potential
  - While the integration of AI presents opportunities for improved patient outcomes, challenges remain regarding capital investment, reimbursement, and the need for ongoing monitoring and governance to ensure effective deployment.

GLOSSARY OF TERMS AND DEFINITIONS

AI: Artificial intelligence; the simulation of human intelligence processes by machines, particularly computer systems, to perform tasks that typically require human cognition.

Diagnostic Accuracy: The degree to which a test correctly identifies (sensitivity) or excludes (specificity) a condition, reflecting the reliability of the diagnostic process.

Emergency Radiology: A subspecialty of radiology focused on the diagnosis and management of acute medical conditions through imaging techniques in emergency settings.

FDA Approval: The process by which the U.S. Food and Drug Administration evaluates and authorizes the safety and effectiveness of medical products, including software applications in healthcare.

Imaging Protocols: Standardized procedures and guidelines used to obtain and interpret medical images to ensure consistency, accuracy, and quality in radiological evaluations.

Radiologist Burnout: A state of physical, emotional, and mental exhaustion experienced by radiologists, often resulting from excessive workload, stress, and lack of work-life balance.

Reimbursement: The process by which healthcare providers receive payment for services rendered, including the coverage of costs for specific treatments or technologies by insurance companies or government programs.

Workflow Efficiency: The effectiveness of a process in achieving its objectives with minimal waste, time, or resources, often enhanced by streamlined procedures and technology.

Artificial intelligence (AI) is rapidly evolving within radiology, particularly in emergency settings, offering significant advantages for both radiologists and patients.[1,4] By optimizing imaging workflows, enhancing diagnostic accuracy, and alleviating radiologist burnout, AI is proving to be a valuable asset in emergency radiology. It aids in various tasks such as order entry, study protocol management, scan scheduling, image acquisition, and report generation, ultimately improving steps throughout the imaging lifecycle.

However, selecting and implementing AI tools in emergency radiology can be complex and requires substantial financial investment. Radiologists need to understand how to screen, select, implement, and monitor AI software effectively.[2] It's essential for them to evaluate their practices and pinpoint areas that could benefit from AI integration, engaging in discussions with fellow radiologists and referring clinicians to address specific needs. Once a potential AI opportunity is identified, solutions can be assessed using guidelines like ÉCLAIR (Evaluate Commercial AI Solutions in Radiology).[3]

Numerous companies have developed applications to aid radiologists in diagnostics and workflow management within emergency departments. The FDA has approved several AI applications tailored for emergency radiology a sample of which is listed in Table 7.1.[1,3]

The Viz.AI product Contact uses deep learning to identify large-vessel occlusion (LVO) in acute stroke patients—an urgent condition requiring immediate intervention.[5] This algorithm analyzes CT angiography images and can detect LVO in under 5 minutes, significantly accelerating diagnosis. One study that compared Viz.ai detection of an internal carotid artery (ICA) or middle cerebral artery first segment (MCA-M1) occlusion to the gold-standard computed tomography angiogram (CTA) of 220 patients. AI tool performance demonstrated sensitivity and specificity were 78.2% and 97%, respectively.[6]

In September 2020, the Centers for Medicare and Medicaid Services (CMS) introduced a New Technology Add-On Payment (NTAP) for detecting LVO in acute stroke patients, offering up to $1300 reimbursement per use for qualifying Medicare patients. This marked the first instance of a reimbursable AI product in radiology, although the actual reimbursement value varies based on patient care and institutional volume.[7]

Qure.ai has developed FDA-approved software that utilizes deep learning to automatically detect and analyze head CT scans for signs of intracranial hemorrhage, significantly aiding radiologists in prioritizing critical cases and enhancing patient outcomes.[8] Similarly, Zebra Medical Vision has designed AI applications that can identify findings indicative of a variety of conditions, including acute chest pain, stroke, and trauma.[9]

AI applications are also under development to improve areas like cervical spine fracture detection and emergency ultrasound diagnostics, with companies like Zebra Medical Vision and Butterfly Network leading the charge. These innovations aim to increase diagnostic accuracy and improve patient outcomes while reducing healthcare costs.[10,11]

Workflow integration is crucial during implementation, addressing both technical aspects and user experience. Prioritizing software that requires minimal manual input from radiologists is advisable. Most vendors typically offer trial periods at little or no cost, allowing institutions to assess the software's compatibility with their patient population. Smooth deployment often involves collaboration with existing vendors and informatics staff, often facilitated by performing a pilot project with specific outcomes metrics. Continuous performance monitoring is vital, as even FDA-approved applications can show significant variability across different patient populations and equipment.

TABLE 7.1 ■ **List of FDA-Approved AI Applications in Radiology**

Service	Company	Description
V8/XV8/XH8, V7/XV7/XH7, V6/XV6/XH6 Diagnostic Ultrasound System	Samsung Medison Co., Ltd.	High-resolution diagnostic ultrasound systems optimized for general and specialized imaging needs, including obstetric, gynecological, and cardiovascular applications
Clarius OB AI	Clarius Mobile Health Corp.	A portable, AI-enhanced ultrasound system focused on obstetric imaging, facilitating real-time fetal assessments
Radiography 7300 C	Philips Medical Systems DMC GmbH	Digital radiography system that offers high-quality imaging for various radiographic applications, emphasizing reduced radiation dose
Relu Creator	Relu BV	Imaging software that automates the process of medical image segmentation for various anatomical regions, enhancing workflow efficiency
RS85 Diagnostic Ultrasound System	Samsung Medison Co., Ltd.	High-end diagnostic ultrasound system with AI features for advanced imaging in cardiology, obstetrics, and musculoskeletal assessments
Cardiac CT Function Software Application	Circle Cardiovascular Imaging	Software that provides advanced cardiac CT analysis, including automated segmentation and quantification of cardiac functions
CINA-VCF	Avicenna.AI	AI tool for vertebral compression fracture detection and assessment on CT scans, designed to support diagnosis and treatment planning
uPMR 790	Shanghai United Imaging Healthcare Co., Ltd.	Advanced MRI system with high-field imaging capabilities, suited for various clinical applications including neurology and oncology
LVivo IQS	DiA Imaging Analysis Ltd.	AI-powered echocardiography tool that assesses cardiac function through real-time quantification and automated measurements
Syngo Carbon Enterprise Access (VA40A)	Siemens Healthcare GmbH	A unified platform for enterprise-wide access to medical images and reports, enhancing cross-departmental collaboration
YSIO X.pree	Siemens Medical Solutions	Digital radiography system with intelligent workflow features, aimed at improving radiographic efficiency and image quality
uOmnispace.CT	Shanghai United Imaging Healthcare Co., Ltd.	Comprehensive CT imaging system with AI capabilities, designed for whole-body imaging and quick diagnostic assessments
Heuron ICH	Heuron Co., Ltd.	AI software for intracranial hemorrhage detection, utilizing CT imaging for rapid identification of potential bleeding sites
BriefCase-Quantification	Aidoc Medical, Ltd.	AI platform for prioritizing and quantifying medical imaging studies, helping radiologists focus on urgent cases

The potential applications of AI in emergency radiology are many, with several software solutions already FDA approved and others currently in development. Although there's much work to do to harness this technology fully, the increasing number of FDA-approved AI applications and growing awareness of AI's benefits in healthcare suggest a promising future for AI in emergency radiology.

In summary, AI applications in emergency radiology are expanding rapidly, with the potential to enhance patient outcomes and streamline workflows. Companies such as Enlitic, Zebra Medical Vision, and Aidoc are already providing FDA-approved AI solutions for critical issues like pneumothorax, intracranial hemorrhages, and acute stroke. Ongoing development aims to address specific needs like pulmonary embolism detection, cervical spine fractures, and pediatric head trauma.[12] Although the evolution of AI and deep learning holds great promise for supporting radiologists in emergency settings, careful implementation, monitoring, and governance structures are crucial to avoid redundancy and ensure efficiency. Additionally, reimbursement challenges remain a significant hurdle to large-scale AI adoption in healthcare. Despite these obstacles, the benefits of AI in emergency radiology highlight the importance of staying informed about advancements in this dynamic field.[13]

Acknowledgment

During the preparation of this work the authors used ChatGPT, a generative AI technology, for assistance with chapter layout and content specific to the referenced articles. After using this tool, the authors reviewed and edited the content. These authors take full responsibility for what is written.

References

1. Jalal S, Parker W, Ferguson D, Nicolaou S. Exploring the role of artificial intelligence in an emergency and trauma radiology department. *Can Assoc Radiol J*. 2020;72(1):167–174. SAGE Publications. https://doi.org/10.1177/0846537120918338.
2. Becker CD, Kotter E, Fournier L, Martí-Bonmatí L. Current practical experience with artificial intelligence in clinical radiology: a survey of the European Society of Radiology. *Insights Imaging*. 2022;13(1):107. Springer Science and Business Media LLC. https://doi.org/10.1186/s13244-022-01247-y.
3. Omoumi P, Ducarouge A, Tournier A, et al. To buy or not to buy-evaluating commercial AI solutions in radiology (the ECLAIR guidelines). *Eur Radiol*. 2021;31(6):3786–3796. https://doi.org/10.1007/s00330-020-07684-x.
4. Moulik SK, Kotter N, Fishman EK. Applications of artificial intelligence in the emergency department. *Emerg Radiol*. 2020;27(4):355–358. Springer Science and Business Media LLC. https://doi.org/10.1007/s10140-020-01794-1.
5. Viz.ai. *Viz LVO: AI-Powered Stroke Detection*; 2023. https://www.viz.ai/publications.
6. Karamchandani RR, Helms AM, Satyanarayana S, et al. Automated detection of intracranial large vessel occlusions using Viz. ai software: experience in a large, integrated stroke network. *Brain Behav*. 2023;13(1):e2808.
7. Centers for Medicare & Medicaid Services (CMS). New Medical Services and New Technologies. *CMS.gov*. 2020.
8. Qure.ai. *qER: AI-Powered Head CT Scan Analysis*; 2023. https://www.qure.ai.
9. Zebra Medical Vision. *AI1 for Acute Chest Pain*; n.d. https://whatsnext.nuance.com/healthcare-ai/zebra-medical-vision-ai1-transforms-patient-care/.
10. Zebra Medical Vision. Zebra medical vision secures its 5th FDA clearance, making its vertebral compression fractures AI solution available in the U.S. *Business Wire*. 2020. https://www.businesswire.com/news/home/20200518005487/en/Zebra-Medical-Vision-Secures-its-5th-FDA-Clearance-Making-Its-Vertebral-Compression-Fractures-AI-Solution-Available-in-the-U.S.
11. Butterfly Network. *Butterfly Blueprint*; n.d. https://www.butterflynetwork.com/blueprint.
12. Cheikh AB, Gorincour G, Nivet H, et al. How artificial intelligence improves radiological interpretation in suspected pulmonary embolism. *Eur Radiol*. 2022;32(9):5831–5842. Springer Science and Business Media LLC. https://doi.org/10.1007/s00330-022-08645-2.
13. Liew C. The future of radiology augmented with artificial intelligence: a strategy for success. *Eur J Radiol*. 2018;102:152–156. Elsevier BV. https://doi.org/10.1016/j.ejrad.2018.03.019.

CHAPTER 8

Artificial Intelligence in Gastrointestinal Imaging

Marvee Espiritu ■ Rajat Chand

KEY POINTS

- Artificial intelligence (AI) is advancing gastrointestinal imaging particularly in colonoscopy and CT colonography.
- The US FDA has approved the use of AI-based technology to aid in colon cancer screening and polyp detection.
- Several studies have shown the clinical utility of AI in improving efficiency and providing high diagnostic accuracy in various gastrointestinal diseases.

GLOSSARY OF TERMS AND DEFINITIONS

Endoscopy: A medical procedure that uses an endoscope, an instrument composed of an optical lens, light sources, and image sensor, to evaluate the interior of a hollow body cavity such as the esophagus or stomach.

CT Colonography: Also known as virtual colonoscopy, a minimally invasive imaging modality that uses computed tomography to evaluate the colon and rectum.

Pneumoperitoneum: The abnormal presence of air or gas in the peritoneal cavity.

Hemoperitoneum: The abnormal presence of blood in the peritoneal cavity.

Intussusception: A medical condition in which a part of the intestine invaginates into an adjacent intestinal segment, often leading to bowel obstruction.

Hemothorax: The presence of blood in the pleural space.

Introduction

Artificial intelligence (AI) has been demonstrated to improve clinical accuracy and efficiency in the medical field. AI has particularly revolutionized the field of gastrointestinal radiology in diagnosing and managing gastrointestinal pathologies. In the last few decades, considerable research has been conducted in the development of technology-assisted applications that could potentially be utilized in gastrointestinal imaging to improve diagnosis, management, and prognosis of gastrointestinal diseases. This chapter will explore the current advances and applications of AI in both upper and lower gastrointestinal diseases.

Applications of AI in Gastrointestinal Imaging

Endoscopy is a widely utilized imaging modality in diagnosing numerous gastrointestinal pathologies such as gastric ulcers and esophageal cancer. Therefore a high level of accuracy is critical to decrease the likelihood of missing potentially cancerous lesions. AI algorithms can be utilized to analyze endoscopic images with the potential to identify abnormal lesions or areas of abnormal growth. The algorithms can be trained to recognize specific patterns, such as those associated with cancer, thereby potentially increasing diagnostic accuracy. Several studies have shown promising results in the integration of AI in endoscopy to diagnose and treat upper gastrointestinal diseases. A recent study by Zhang et al.[1] analyzed the diagnostic accuracy of AI in characterizing protruding lesions in the esophagus. The study developed convolutional neural network (CNN)-based models to identify and differentiate subtypes of esophageal protruded lesions (Fig. 8.1). AI outperformed expert endoscopists in the diagnostic accuracy of image interpretation. Furthermore, combining AI and endoscopist predictions improved diagnostic accuracy of esophageal lesions compared to endoscopists alone.[1] AI has also shown promise in detecting esophageal cancer from CT images. A retrospective study that examined VGG16, an image recognition model of CNN, for detection of esophageal cancer showed 84.2% diagnostic accuracy.[2]

A growing number of companies and research studies are exploring AI's potential for application to gastrointestinal imaging. In 2021, the FDA approved the AI tool GI Genius (Medtronic GI Genius, Minneapolis, MN) that aids in the detection of lesions suspicious for colon cancer during colonoscopy. The approval was issued after assessment of the safety and efficacy of the software in a multicenter, randomized-controlled trial that examined a total of 230 subjects assigned to either AI-assisted colonoscopy or non-AI colonoscopy.[3] During colonoscopy, the GI Genius system generates a marker superimposed on the colonoscopy images in the event that it detects a potentially cancerous lesion, which may then prompt the endoscopist to further investigate the lesion. Results of the randomized-controlled trial showed lower adenoma miss rate (AMR), 15.5% in AI-assisted colonoscopy compared to 32.4% non-AI colonoscopy, suggesting higher diagnostic accuracy in AI colonoscopy compared to standard colonoscopy.[3] Another AI-assisted device approved by the FDA is SKOUT (SKOUT, Iterative Health, Cambridge, MA), a computer-aided detection device that aids in polyp detection for colorectal cancer screening during colonoscopy. The device, developed by Iterative Scopes, was evaluated in a US. multicenter randomized controlled trial involving 1359 patients randomized to either standard colonoscopy or computer-aided detection colonoscopy (CADe) (Fig. 8.2). Results of the trial showed improved adenoma detection compared to standard colonoscopy as measured by adenomas per colonoscopy (APC) of 0.83 versus 1.05 (P = .002) for standard and CADe, respectively.[4] Although the use of AI in gastrointestinal radiology is still in its infancy, colonoscopy is still considered the gold standard in the diagnosis and management of colonic lesions.

Further application of AI in gastrointestinal radiology is its utilization in virtual colonoscopy or CT colonography in the detection of colonic polyps. AI algorithms in CT colonography permit the use of this minimally invasive technique in detecting polyps by constructing a three-dimensional image of the colon and rectum via CT images.[5]

Applications of AI in Gastrointestinal Diseases

AI has also shown promise in assessing inflammatory bowel disease (IBD) such as ulcerative colitis (UC) and Crohn's disease (CD). UC and CD are debilitating diseases that, combined, affect approximately 6.8 million individuals worldwide.[6] In ulcerative colitis, disease severity during endoscopic evaluation is one factor that determines therapeutic response. A retrospective study compared the ability of deep learning models in grading endoscopic severity of UC with that of experienced human endoscopists. In this study, AI was programmed to categorize UC disease severity into remission (Mayo 0 or 1) or moderate/severe disease (Mayo 2 or 3). AI performance was found to be comparable human endoscopists with area under the curve (AUC) of 0.96 (95% CI, 0.967–0.972), positive predictive value (PPV) of 0.87 (95% CI, 0.85–0.88), sensitivity of 83% (95% CI, 0.808–0.854), and specificity of 96% (95% CI, 0.951–0.971).[7]

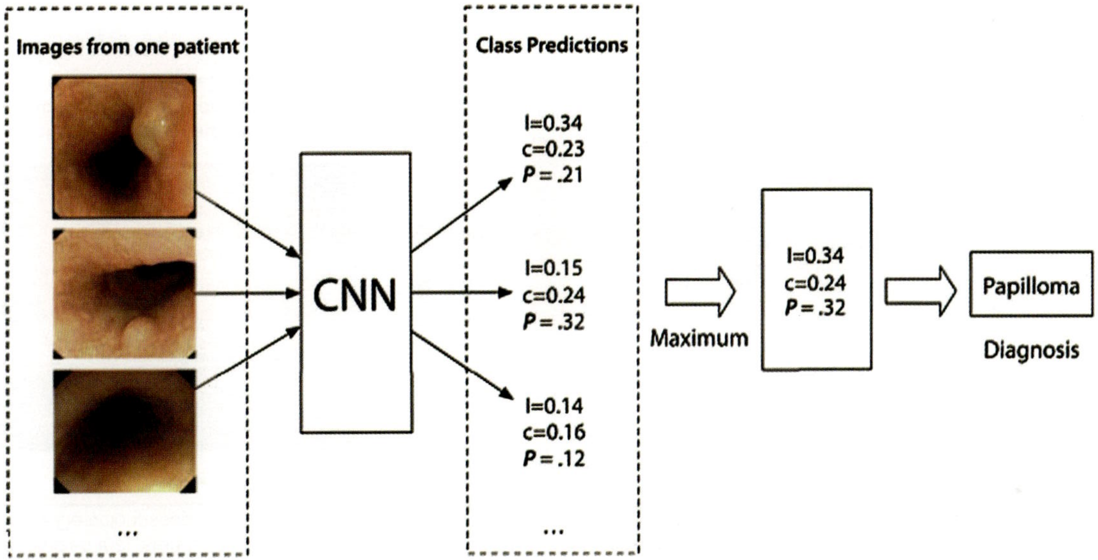

Fig. 8.1 The utilization of convolutional neural network algorithm to predict disease diagnosis. (Image adapted from Zhang M, Zhu C, Wang Y, et al. Differential diagnosis for esophageal protruded lesions using a deep convolution neural network in endoscopic images. *Gastrointest Endosc*. 2021;93(6):1261–1272.e2).

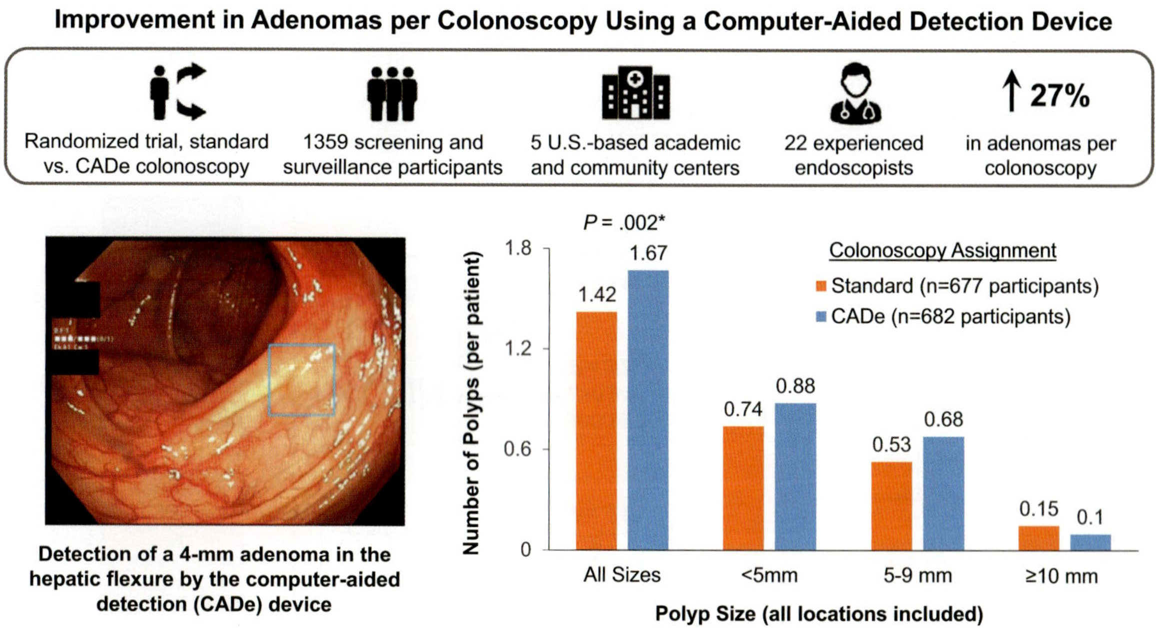

Fig. 8.2 Key findings of the randomized controlled trial that evaluated the performance of SKOUT, an FDA-approved computer-assisted device used in the detection of polyps during colorectal cancer screening via colonoscopy. (Image adapted from Shaukat A, Lichtenstein DR, Somers SC, et al. Computer-aided detection improves adenomas per colonoscopy for screening and surveillance colonoscopy: a randomized trial. *Gastroenterology*. 2022;163(3):732–741.)

Another study designed a deep neural network algorithm for the evaluation of UC (DNUC). The AI was initially trained using 40,758 images of colonoscopies and 6885 biopsies from 2012 patients with UC. The accuracy of the DNUC algorithm was tested on 875 patients achieving an accuracy of 90.1% (95% CI, 0.892–0.909) in identifying endoscopic remission and 92.9% accuracy (95% CI, 0.921–0.937) in identifying histologic remission.[8] AI has also shown promise in detecting small bowel ulcers in patients with CD. A study assessed the diagnostic accuracy of a deep learning algorithm in detecting small bowel ulcers on capsule endoscopy (CE). The algorithm was assessed on 17,640 small bowel capsule endoscopy images from 49 patients, achieving an accuracy of 96.7%.[9]

Artificial intelligence has also made significant strides in the field of emergency gastrointestinal radiology, particularly in the diagnosis of bowel obstruction, intussusception, appendicitis, hemoperitoneum, pneumoperitoneum, trauma, and abdominal aortic aneurysms. Interpretation of radiological images in the emergency setting can be particularly demanding with large volumes of images and the need for rapid turnaround times. The use of AI in the emergency setting may assist radiologists in both accuracy and speed of image interpretation, which in turn can enable the clinician to provide diagnosis and treatment planning in a timely manner. Studies have demonstrated promising results in the application of AI in detecting bowel obstructions on CT scans. The algorithms can also predict the likelihood of the patient requiring surgery, thereby potentially aiding in the clinical decision-making process. A study examined the diagnostic accuracy of a deep convolutional neural network in detecting high-grade small bowel obstruction patterns on abdominal radiographs after training with 7768 supine abdominal radiographs classified as either obstructive or nonobstructive. Following training, the neural network achieved area under the receiver operator curve (AUC) of 0.97, sensitivity of 91%, and specificity of 92%, showing high accuracy in the detection of high-grade small bowel obstruction with AI.[10] Another study examined the role of AI in detecting small bowel obstruction using a model trained on 990 plain abdominal radiographs divided into either normal findings or small bowel obstruction (Fig. 8.3). The images were also characterized based on radiology reports and subsequent CT scans. Model diagnostic accuracy achieved an AUC of 0.961, sensitivity of 91%, and specificity of 93%.[11]

AI has also been utilized in the detection of pneumoperitoneum on CT scans of patients presenting with acute abdominal pain. A retrospective study assessed the accuracy of an AI algorithm in detecting pneumoperitoneum in 331 patients where 31 patients had pneumoperitoneum (either large, moderate, or small). Test of accuracy showed AUC of 0.77 (95% CI, 0.66–0.87), sensitivity of 52%, and specificity of 99%. When patients with small peritoneum (<0.25 mL of free air) were excluded, AUC increased to 0.96 (95% CI, 0.89–1.0) with sensitivity of 81%, specificity of 99%, and positive likelihood ratio was 82 (95% CI, 0.27–0.254). The study suggests a role for AI in ruling in pneumoperitoneum.[12]

With regards to trauma, AI has also shown promise in assisting the detection of hemoperitoneum. Focused assessment with sonography for trauma (FAST) or extended FAST (eFAST) exams are considered the gold standard for detection of peritoneal/pleural free fluid, hemothorax, hemoperitoneum, and pericardial effusion. Findings of the FAST or eFAST examination determines whether a patient requires surgical management. There is a constant need for accurate and rapid interpretation of FAST/eFAST examinations, thereby leading to studies determining the role of AI in this setting. In a pilot study by Sjogren et al.,[13] the authors tested the feasibility of automating abdominal free fluid detection with FAST exam in the setting of trauma. The authors of the study developed an algorithm to detect hypoechoic regions of interests based on specific criteria and threshold values. These hypoechoic regions are then defined as either "free fluid" or "not free fluid" based on the analysis of features related to geometric properties of the shape (linearity, curvilinearity, radius angle covariance, roundness, position, and area) as well as features related to the grayscale color properties of the shape (echogenicity, echo variability). The sensitivity and specificity of the AI algorithm in detecting free fluid on FAST exam were 100% and

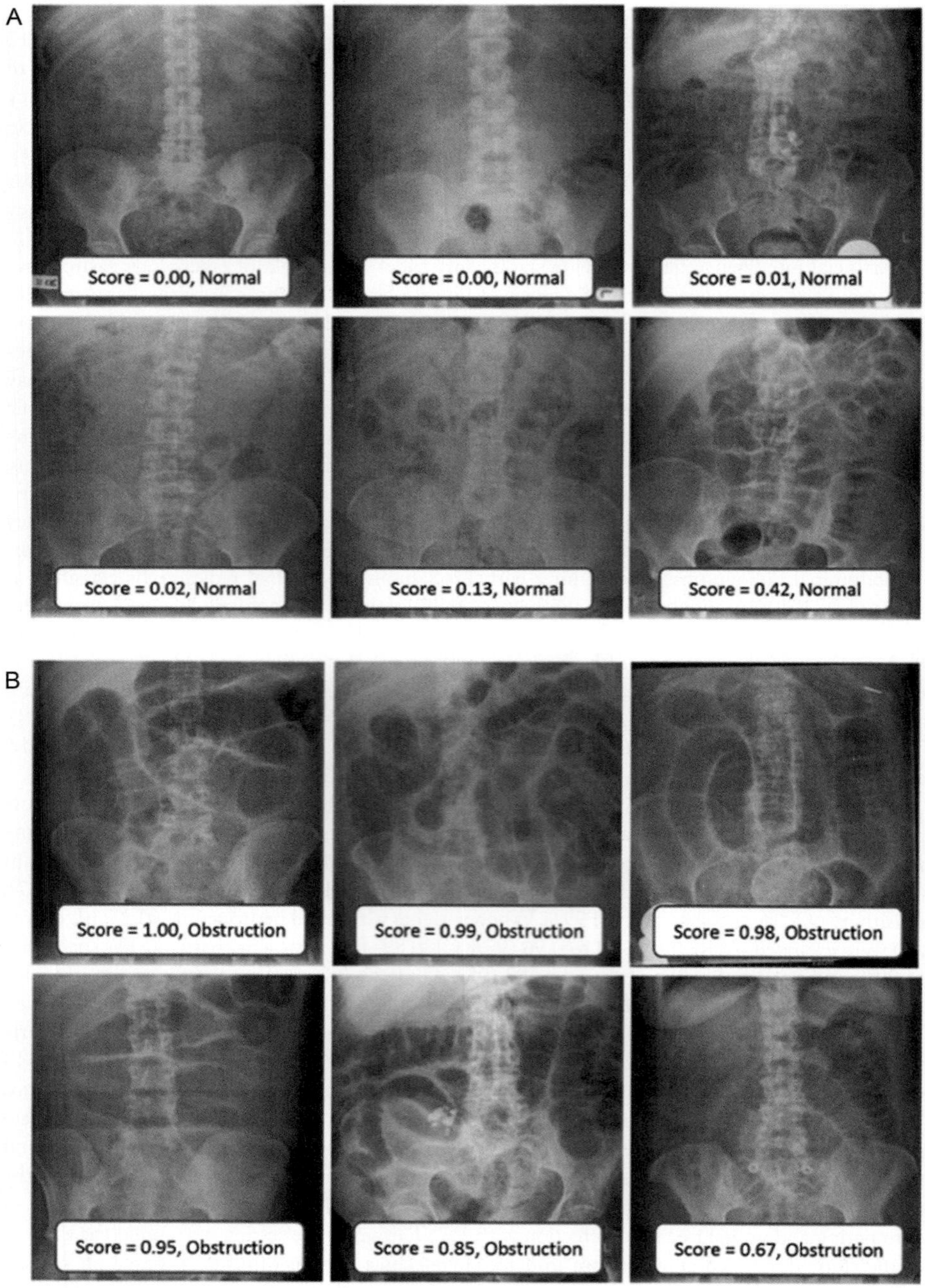

Fig. 8.3 Plan abdominal radiographic images correctly identified as normal or obstruction using a deep learning model. (Image adapted from Kim DH, Wit H, Thurston M, et al. An artificial intelligence deep learning model for identification of small bowel obstruction on plain abdominal radiographs. *Br J Radiol*. 2021;94(1122):20201407.)

90%, respectively, which were comparable to the human interpretation of FAST exams.[13] These results suggest the utility of AI in rapid detection of free fluid in the abdomen. Further studies are warranted to determine the clinical utility of AI in the analysis of other components of the FAST exam. Nevertheless, the utilization of automated detection systems in imaging interpretation in the setting of trauma may lead to expedited clinical assessment and efficient use of hospital resources.

Limitations

The aforementioned studies highlight the recent advances of AI in the field of gastrointestinal radiology. It is important to note that there remain barriers that preclude the widespread adoption of AI in the clinical setting. One such barrier includes the ethical considerations when standardizing the AI algorithm to the general population. The training models utilized in the AI algorithm must represent data from a diverse population to avoid potential bias, which could lead to adverse consequences for patients. In addition, it is difficult to adapt AI technologies and algorithms developed at one institution to the generalized clinical practice as systems and workflows vary. In order to obtain the US FDA approval, these algorithms must yield reproducible results that satisfy the framework set forth by the FDA.

Conclusion

Several AI applications have been integrated into clinical practice within the last decade, proving to be valuable tools for physicians in disease diagnosis and management. Nevertheless, further studies, including clinical validation via prospective tests and randomized-controlled trials, are warranted to determine the clinical utility of this technology in improving patient outcomes and decreasing healthcare costs.

Resources

US Food & Drug Administration: Artificial Intelligence and Machine Learning (AI/ML)-Enabled Medical Devices.

References

1. Zhang M, Zhu C, Wang Y, et al. Differential diagnosis for esophageal protruded lesions using a deep convolution neural network in endoscopic images. *Gastrointest Endosc*. 2021;93(6):1261–1272. e2. http://doi.org/10.1016/j.gie.2020.10.005.
2. Takeuchi M, Seto T, Hashimoto M, et al. Performance of a deep learning-based identification system for esophageal cancer from CT images. *Esophagus*. 2021;18(3):612–620. http://doi.org/10.1007/s10388-021-00826-0.
3. Wallace MB, Sharma P, Bhandari P, et al. Impact of artificial intelligence on miss rate of colorectal neoplasia. *Gastroenterology*. 2022;163(1):295–304. e5. http://doi.org/10.1053/j.gastro.2022.03.007.
4. Shaukat A, Lichtenstein DR, Somers SC, et al. Computer-aided detection improves adenomas per colonoscopy for screening and surveillance colonoscopy: a randomized trial. *Gastroenterology*. 2022;163(3):732–741. http://doi.org/10.1053/j.gastro.2022.05.028.
5. Bielen D, Kiss G. Computer-aided detection for CT colonography: update 2007. *Abdom Imaging*. 2007;32(5):571–581. http://doi.org/10.1007/s00261-007-9293-2.
6. GBD 2017 Inflammatory Bowel Disease Collaborators. The global, regional, and national burden of inflammatory bowel disease in 195 countries and territories, 1990–2017: a systematic analysis for the Global Burden of Disease Study 2017. *Lancet Gastroenterol Hepatol*. 2020;5(1):17–30. http://doi.org/10.1016/S2468-1253(19)30333-4.

7. Stidham RW, Liu W, Bishu S, et al. Performance of a deep learning model vs human reviewers in grading endoscopic disease severity of patients with ulcerative colitis. *JAMA Netw Open*. 2019;2(5):e193963. http://doi.org/10.1001/jamanetworkopen.2019.3963.
8. Takenaka K, Ohtsuka K, Fujii T, et al. Development and validation of a deep neural network for accurate evaluation of endoscopic images from patients with ulcerative colitis. *Gastroenterology*. 2020;158(8):2150–2157. http://doi.org/10.1053/j.gastro.2020.02.012.
9. Klang E, Barash Y, Margalit RY, et al. Deep learning algorithms for automated detection of Crohn's disease ulcers by video capsule endoscopy. *Gastrointest Endosc*. 2020;91(3):606–613.e2. http://doi.org/10.1016/j.gie.2019.11.012.
10. Cheng PM, Tran KN, Whang G, Tejura TK. Refining convolutional neural network detection of small-bowel obstruction in conventional radiography. *AJR Am J Roentgenol*. 2019;212(2):342–350. http://doi.org/10.2214/AJR.18.20362.
11. Kim DH, Wit H, Thurston M, et al. An artificial intelligence deep learning model for identification of small bowel obstruction on plain abdominal radiographs. *Br J Radiol*. 2021;94(1122):20201407. http://doi.org/10.1259/bjr.20201407.
12. Brejnebøl MW, Nielsen YW, Taubmann O, Eibenberger E, Müller FC. Artificial intelligence based detection of pneumoperitoneum on CT scans in patients presenting with acute abdominal pain: a clinical diagnostic test accuracy study. *Eur J Radiol*. 2022;150:110216. http://doi.org/10.1016/j.ejrad.2022.110216.
13. Sjogren AR, Leo MM, Feldman J, Gwin JT. Image segmentation and machine learning for detection of abdominal free fluid in focused assessment with sonography for trauma examinations: a pilot study. *J Ultrasound Med*. 2016;35(11):2501–2509. http://doi.org/10.7863/ultra.15.11017.

CHAPTER 9

Genitourinary

Alice Hou

KEY POINTS

- A background of clinically relevant AI concepts, presented in the context of GU imaging
- Four comprehensive tables of federally approved AI products for prostate cancer, bladder volume, kidney stones, and ovarian cancer
- Challenges of current practices in GU diagnostics, and an overview of ongoing research in the field

GLOSSARY OF TERMS AND DEFINITIONS

Artificial Intelligence: A branch of computer science that involves the simulation of human intelligence processes by machines, including learning, reasoning, and self-correction.

Machine Learning: A subset of artificial intelligence that involves the development of algorithms that enable computers to learn without being explicitly programmed to do so.

Deep Learning: A subset of machine learning that focuses on the development and training of artificial neural networks designed to emulate the structure and function of the human brain.

Convolutional Neural Network Models: A class of deep learning algorithms used in effectively capturing spatial hierarchies of patterns in data.

Computer-Aided Detection Systems: Software algorithms that utilize artificial intelligence and pattern recognition to analyze medical images and highlight areas of abnormalities that may warrant further attention.

Cancer Antigen-125: A protein biomarker that is often used as a tumor marker to aid in the diagnosis, monitoring, and management of ovarian cancer.

Introduction

Once an esoteric concept, artificial intelligence (AI) has now become a commonplace tool in everyday life as well as many areas of medicine. Specifically, it has brought us deep learning, which is a subset of AI and machine learning that trains neural networks designed to emulate the structure and function of the human brain. It allows for automaticity in analyzing large datasets, identifying patterns, image recognition, feature quantitation, and anomaly detection. Additionally, it provides a consistency and objectivity to the variability and subjectivity that exists in imaging interpretation across different readers and institutions.

In genitourinary (GU) medicine, AI's radiological applications have enabled groundbreaking advancements in the visualization and treatment planning of the prostate, bladder, kidneys, and female reproductive organs. With a market forecasted to top $19 billion by 2032[1] and 25% of articles in major radiology journals now studying AI in radiology,[2] the technology is on its way to reshape the healthcare industry and is here to stay. This chapter provides an overview of the research landscape and approved AI technology for genitourinary radiology.

Prostate

Perhaps the best example of AI in GU medicine is its application in prostate cancer. Prostate cancer is the second leading cause of death in biological males in the United States, accounting for 18.8 per 100,000 men annually.[3] Currently, multiparametric magnetic resonance imaging (mpMRI) is the main diagnostic imaging modality for prostate cancer and is used for its early detection, staging, and active surveillance.[4] It assesses lesions through the standardized Prostate Imaging Reporting and Data System (PI-RADS) score, but its usefulness is limited due to its inherently subjective scoring system and high inter-reader variability.[5] Although expert radiologists may miss 2.6% of clinically significant prostate cancers, a less experienced reader may miss almost 30% of cancers.[6] Furthermore, current methods of manual segmentation of the prostate gland are time consuming, tedious, and subjective. AI, and specifically automated segmentation algorithms and computer-aided detection (CAD) systems, can increase efficiency, reduce subjectivity and errors, and achieve outcomes with minimal manual input from radiologists. Currently, 12 AI products have been approved for clinical use and are commercially available for prostate cancer imaging (Table 9.1).[7–9]

Bladder

Bladder cancer is the most common malignancy of the urinary tract,[10] and due to its high recurrent rate and necessary follow-up and surveillance, it is now one of the most expensive cancers to manage.[11] Although there are no currently approved AI tools for bladder cancer imaging, much research has been applied to cystoscopy imaging to improve its efficacy in cancer detection. Current research uses convolutional neural network (CNN) models, which are a type of deep learning algorithm that uses three-dimensional data for image classification and object recognition tasks.[12] Like prostate cancer detection, CAD systems have also been explored for segmentation, as wide range of variations in bladder shapes and sizes exist, impacting tumor detection.[10]

One area in which AI has found success in managing bladder health is in postvoid residual bladder volume (PVR) measurement. Instead of going through the tedious steps of manually calculating bladder volume, AI-integrated portable ultrasound machines can automatically measure bladder volume in seconds, offering convenient evaluation of urinary retention, neurogenic bladder, or urinary tract obstruction. This allows healthcare providers to quickly determine catheterization needs, potentially avoiding inappropriate use of catheters.[13]

Currently, five AI products have been approved for clinical use and are commercially available for PVR measurement (Table 9.2).[7–9] Although the devices are currently only FDA cleared for use by healthcare providers, there is ongoing research evaluating the efficacy and reliability of self-monitoring in voiding dysfunction patients.[14]

Kidneys

Renal cell carcinoma (RCC) is the 6th most common malignancy in men and 10th in women.[15] Its current diagnostic imaging workup is hampered by a suboptimal ability to correctly distinguish RCC from benign lesions,[16] and although percutaneous renal lesion biopsies have high diagnostic accuracy, it is invasive and sometimes difficult to perform.[17] Although no AI models designated for RCC imaging have yet been approved for clinical use, there has been extensive research in using deep learning to effectively characterize renal masses. In addition to using AI to distinguish

TABLE 9.1 ■ **Prostate AI Products**

Company	Product Name	FDA Approval Class (510(k) Number)	CE Approval Class	Available Since	Main Features
Advantis Medical Imaging Single Member P.C. (Eindhoven, North Brabant, Netherlands)	Advantis Platform	Class II (K222975)	N/A	03/2023	Organ segmentation and lesion detection
Avenda Health, Inc. (Culver City, CA, USA)	Avenda Health AI Prostate Cancer Planning Software	Class II (K221624)	N/A	11/2022	Organ segmentation and lesion detection
GE Healthcare (Chicago, IL, USA)	PROView DL	Class II (K193306)	N/A	11/2020	Organ segmentation and lesion detection
HealthLytix (San Diego, CA, USA)	RSI-MRI+	Class II (K191278)	N/A	11/2019	Organ segmentation and lesion detection
JLK (Seoul, South Korea)	JPC-01K	N/A	Class I - MDD	04/2019	Lesion detection
Lucida Medical (Cambridge, United Kingdom)	Prostate Intelligence	N/A	Class IIb - MDR	05/2021	Organ segmentation and lesion detection
Merge CAD Inc (Ann Arbor, MI, USA)	CADstream	Class II (K092954)	N/A	11/2009	Organ segmentation and lesion detection
Mediaire (Berlin, Germany)	mdprostate	N/A	Class IIb - MDR	08/2023	Organ segmentation and lesion detection
Quantib BV/ DeepHealth (Rotterdam, South Holland, Netherlands)	Quantib Prostate (Saige Prostate)	Class II (K202501)	Class IIb - MDR	10/2020	Organ segmentation and lesion detection
Quibim S.L. (Valencia, Spain)	qp-Prostate	Class II (K203582)	Class IIb - MDR	02/2021	Organ segmentation
ScanMed/Bot Image (Omaha, NE, USA)	ProstatID	Class II (K212783)	N/A	07/2022	Organ segmentation and lesion detection
Siemens healthineers (Forchheim, Bavaria, Germany)	AI-Rad Companion Prostate MR Syngo.MR	Class II (K193283)	Class IIb - MDR	07/2020	Organ segmentation and lesion detection

TABLE 9.2 ■ **Bladder AI Products**

Company	Product Name	FDA Approval Class (510(k) Number)	CE Approval Class	Available Since	Main Features
Butterfly Network, Inc. (Burlington, MA, USA)	Auto 3D Bladder Volume Tool	Class II (K200980)	N/A	06/2020	Bladder volume measurement
Clarius Mobile Health Corp. (Vancouver, British Columbia, Canada)	Clarius Bladder AI	Class II (K232257)	N/A	11/2023	Bladder volume measurement
DiA Imaging Analysis Ltd (Be'er-Sheva, Israel)	LVivo platform (includes LVivo Bladder)	Class II (K200232)	Class IIa - MDD	06/2020	Bladder volume measurement
Exo Inc (Santa Clara, CA, USA)	Bladder AI (AIBV01)	Class II (K230497)	N/A	06/2023	Bladder volume measurement
Verathon (Bothell, WA, USA)	BladderScan Prime PLUS	Class II (K172356)	N/A	09/2017	Bladder volume measurement

TABLE 9.3 ■ **Kidney AI Product**

Company	Product Name	FDA Approval Class (510(k) Number)	CE Approval Class	Available Since	Main Features
Imaging Biometrics, LLC (Elm Grove, WI, USA)	StoneChecker	Class II (K191530)	Class I - MDD	09/2019	CT post-processing for kidney stones

between benign and malignant solid and cystic masses, it has also proven helpful in identifying benign oncocytomas versus malignant chromophobe RCC.[15]

AI technology has, however, been successful and approved for use in kidney stone management (Table 9.3).[7–9] As the prevalence of kidney stones has continued to increase in recent decades,[18] there have been concerted efforts to improve detection and treatment. The most crucial diagnostic step is accurate analysis of stone composition, which is done through techniques such as infrared spectroscopy, x-ray diffraction, and chemical analysis.[19] AI technology can aid clinical decision-making by using CT texture analysis to examine stone characteristics including volume, density, skin-to-stone distance, among others. This helps identify patients most suited for lithotripsy.

Gynecology—Ovary, Cervix, Uterus

Gynecological AI research studying cervical and endometrial cancers has included evaluating colposcopy, hysteroscopy, and MR images in verifying the diagnostic accuracy of deep learning

TABLE 9.4 ■ **Ovarian AI Product**

Company	Product Name	FDA Approval Class (510(k) Number)	CE Approval Class	Available Since	Main Features
DeepTrace Technologies Srl (Milan, Lombardy, Italy)	TRACE4OC	N/A	Class I - MDD	05/2021	Ovarian cancer classification

algorithms.[20] AI has also been used in creating prediction models for lymph node metastasis.[21] Ovarian cancer remains the most researched gynecological malignancy due to its high mortality rate, with 300,000 cases diagnosed worldwide in 2018 and 180,000 associated deaths.[22] Lack of accurate screening tools remain a barrier, as biological markers like Cancer Antigen-125 (CA-125) have been shown to be sensitive but not specific, and ultrasound imaging lacks the ability to detect ovarian cancer at its early stages. Although not yet FDA approved, there is AI technology available in Europe for predicting malignancy risks of ovarian masses based on transvaginal ultrasound imaging and serum CA-125 levels (Table 9.4).[7–9]

Conclusion

AI tools are revolutionizing many aspects of modern medical fields, and radiology is no exception. Understanding the power of these applications in genitourinary medicine will require an appreciation of its science as well as an awareness of its possible shortcomings and ethical pitfalls. For the technology to reach its full potential, it will also require thoughtful integration of diverse inputs and imaging that match our global population, as well as collaboration with physicians and patients alike.

References

1. AI in Medical Imaging Market Trends, Analysis Report, 2032. Global Market Insights Inc., Accessed February 29, 2024. www.gminsights.com/industry-analysis/artificial-intelligence-in-medical-imaging-market.
2. Bluemke DA, Moy L, Bredella MA, et al. Assessing radiology research on artificial intelligence: a brief guide for authors, reviewers, and readers—from the Radiology editorial board. *Radiology.* 2020;294:487–489.
3. Giona S. *The Epidemiology of Prostate Cancer.* Exon Publications; 2021:1-5.
4. Turkbey B, Brown AM, Sankineni S, Wood BJ, Pinto PA, Choyke PL. Multiparametric prostate magnetic resonance imaging in the evaluation of prostate cancer. *CA Cancer J Clin.* 2016;66(4):326–336.
5. Smith CP, Harmon SA, Barrett T, et al. Intra- and interreader reproducibility of PI-RADSv2: a multireader study. *J Magn Reson Imag.* 2019;49(6):1694–1703.
6. Hietikko R, Kilpeläinen TP, Kenttämies A, et al. Expected impact of MRI-related interreader variability on ProScreen prostate cancer screening trial: a pre-trial validation study. *Cancer Imaging.* 2020;20(1):72.
7. AI for Radiology – Products. https://grand-challenge.org/aiforradiology/.
8. ACR Data Science Institute AI Central – FDA Cleared AI Medical Products. https://aicentral.acrdsi.org/
9. Center for Devices and Radiological Health. *Artificial Intelligence and Machine Learning (AI/ML)-Enabled Medical D.* U.S. Food and Drug Administration, FDA. www.fda.gov/medical-devices/software-medical-device-samd/artificial-intelligence-and-machine-learning-aiml-enabled-medical-devices.
10. Borhani S, Borhani R, Kajdacsy-Balla A. Artificial intelligence: a promising frontier in bladder cancer diagnosis and outcome prediction. *Crit Rev Oncol Hematol.* 2022;171:103601.
11. Kassouf W, Traboulsi SL, Schmitz-Drager B, et al. Follow-up in non-muscle-invasive bladder cancer-International bladder cancer network recommendations. *Urol Oncol.* 2016;34(10):460–468.

12. Ikeda A, Nosato H, Kochi Y, et al. Support system of cystoscopic diagnosis for bladder cancer based on artificial intelligence. *J Endourol.* 2020;34(3):352–358.
13. Stephens K. FDA clears clarius mobile health bladder AI scanner. *AXIS Imaging News.* 2024.
14. Jalfon M, Gardezi M, Heckscher D, et al. Agreement and reliability of patient-measured postvoid residual bladder volumes. *Urology.* 2024;184:62–68.
15. Yilmaz EC, Belue MJ, Turkbey B, Reinhold C, Choyke PL. A brief review of artificial intelligence in genitourinary oncological imaging. *Can Assoc Radiol J.* 2023;74(3):534–547.
16. Kim JH, Li S, Khandwala Y, et al. National trends of preoperative imaging modalities before partial nephrectomy for renal masses in the U.S. from 2007–2015. *Can Urol Assoc J.* 2019;13:89–94.
17. Roussel E, Capitanio U, Kutikov A, et al. Novel imaging methods for renal mass characterization: a collaborative review. *Eur Urol.* 2022;81:476–488.
18. Scales CD, Smith AC, Hanley JM, Saigal CS. Urologic diseases of America project prevalence of kidney stones in the United States. *Eur Urol.* 2012;62:160–165. https://doi.org/10.1016/j.eururo.2012.03.052.
19. Hameed BMZ, Shah M, Naik N, et al. The ascent of artificial intelligence in endourology: a systematic review over the last 2 decades. *Curr Urol Rep.* 2021;22:53. https://doi.org/10.1007/s11934-021-01069-3.
20. Tian X, Sun C, Liu Z, et al. Prediction of response to preoperative neoadjuvant chemotherapy in locally advanced cervical cancer using multicenter CTbased radiomic analysis. *Front Oncol.* 2020;10:77.
21. Xu X, Li H, Wang S, et al. Multiplanar MRI-based predictive model for preoperative assessment of lymph node metastasis in endometrial cancer. *Front Oncol.* 2019;9:1007.
22. Okunade KS, Dawodu O, Adenekan M, et al. Prognostic impact of pretreatment thrombocytosis in epithelial ovarian cancer. *Niger J Clin Pract.* 2020;23(8):1141–1147.

CHAPTER 10

Artificial Intelligence In Head and Neck Radiology: Current Innovations, Challenges, and Future Directions

Srikanth Mahankali

KEY POINTS

- AI achieves 94% sensitivity in detecting early-stage malignancies, improving 5-year survival rates by 15% through timely interventions.
- FDA-approved tools reduce vascular reconstruction time from 2 hours to 8 minutes, enhancing stroke management.
- Ethical challenges, including GDPR (General Data Protection Regulation) compliance and algorithmic bias, necessitate global regulatory harmonization for equitable AI deployment.

GLOSSARY OF TERMS AND DEFINITIONS

Artificial Intelligence (AI): Computational systems that analyze medical imaging data through machine learning (e.g., convolutional neural networks for tumor detection).

Radiomics: Quantitative extraction of imaging features (e.g., texture heterogeneity in MRI) to predict treatment responses.

Convolutional Neural Networks (CNNs): Deep learning models using convolutional layers to detect spatial patterns in imaging data (e.g., nasopharyngeal carcinoma on MRI).

Multimodal Integration: Fusion of CT, PET, and genomic data to stratify head and neck cancer subtypes.

Algorithmic Bias: Disparities in AI performance due to underrepresentation of minority groups in training datasets.

DICOM: Standard protocol ensuring interoperability of imaging data across PACS and AI platforms.

Computer-Aided Detection (CAD): AI tools that highlight suspicious regions (e.g., lymph node metastases on CT).

Introduction

The integration of artificial intelligence (AI) into head and neck imaging represents a transformative leap in radiology, addressing long-standing challenges in early diagnosis, workflow efficiency, and personalized care.[1] Since the advent of deep learning in the 2010s, AI has evolved from basic pattern recognition to sophisticated systems capable of analyzing complex imaging datasets with pixel-level precision.[2] For example, convolutional neural networks (CNNs) now detect subtle malignancies like human papillovirus (HPV)-associated oropharyngeal carcinomas, which are frequently missed in conventional imaging due to their submucosal location and lack of contrast enhancement.[3,4] A landmark 2024 multicenter trial validated an AI model that identifies extranodal extension in head and neck squamous cell carcinoma (HNSCC) with 94% accuracy, outperforming human radiologists by 18%.[5]

FDA-approved platforms leverage automated segmentation and radiomics to standardize diagnostic workflows.[6] These tools quantify tumor volumes in under 5 minutes, compared to 30+ minutes for manual methods, while reducing inter-reader variability by 40%.[7] Beyond diagnostics, AI optimizes treatment planning—predictive models enhance radiation therapy targeting by 28%, minimizing collateral damage to critical structures like the parotid glands.[8] However, challenges persist, including data silos, ethical dilemmas, and interoperability issues. For instance, a 2025 survey revealed that 62% of radiology departments struggle to integrate AI tools with legacy PACS systems.[9] This chapter explores these advancements and barriers, offering actionable strategies for sustainable AI adoption (Fig. 10.1).

Current Applications and Clinical Impact

1. **Early Detection and Diagnosis**
   AI excels in identifying early-stage malignancies through advanced pattern recognition in CT, MRI, and PET scans.[10] For example:
   - **CNN-Based Nasopharyngeal Carcinoma Detection:** A 2023 study trained a ResNet-50 model on 12,000 contrast-enhanced MRI scans, achieving 92% sensitivity and 88% specificity in distinguishing malignant lesions from benign hyperplasia.[11] The model's attention maps highlight subtle asymmetries in the nasopharyngeal mucosa, enabling radiologists to prioritize high-risk cases.
   - **HPV-Associated Oropharyngeal Cancer:** AI algorithms detect submucosal tumors by analyzing textural heterogeneity in T2-weighted MRI sequences, achieving 89% specificity.[12] A 2024 retrospective analysis at MD Anderson Cancer Center (Houston, TX, USA) demonstrated that AI reduced diagnostic delays by 40%, correlating with a 15% improvement in 5-year survival rates.[13]
2. **Disease Characterization and Monitoring**
   AI has been shown to standardize assessments of thyroid nodules, lymphadenopathy, and salivary gland diseases:
   - **Thyroid Nodule Classification:** A U-Net-based AI model, trained on a diverse dataset of 15,000 ultrasound images, demonstrated exceptional performance in differentiating benign from malignant thyroid nodules, achieving 95% diagnostic accuracy.[14] This model analyzes key sonographic features, including microcalcifications, hypoechoic regions, and irregular margins, which are critical for malignancy risk stratification. By quantifying these features with pixel-level precision, the AI outperformed conventional Thyroid Imaging Reporting and Data System (TI-RADS) criteria, reducing unnecessary biopsies by 30% in a multicenter validation cohort.[15] The system provides probabilistic malignancy scores, enabling clinicians to prioritize high-risk nodules for biopsy while safely deferring intervention in low-risk cases. This approach not only streamlines workflows but also minimizes patient anxiety and healthcare costs associated with overtreatment.[14]
   - **Tumor Regression Analysis:** Longitudinal AI monitoring tracks tumor volumes in HNSCC patients during chemoradiotherapy, enabling dynamic adjustments to treatment regimens.[16] A 2025 study at Memorial Sloan Kettering Cancer Center (New York City, NY, USA) reported a 22% reduction in treatment-related toxicity using AI-guided adaptive radiotherapy.[17]

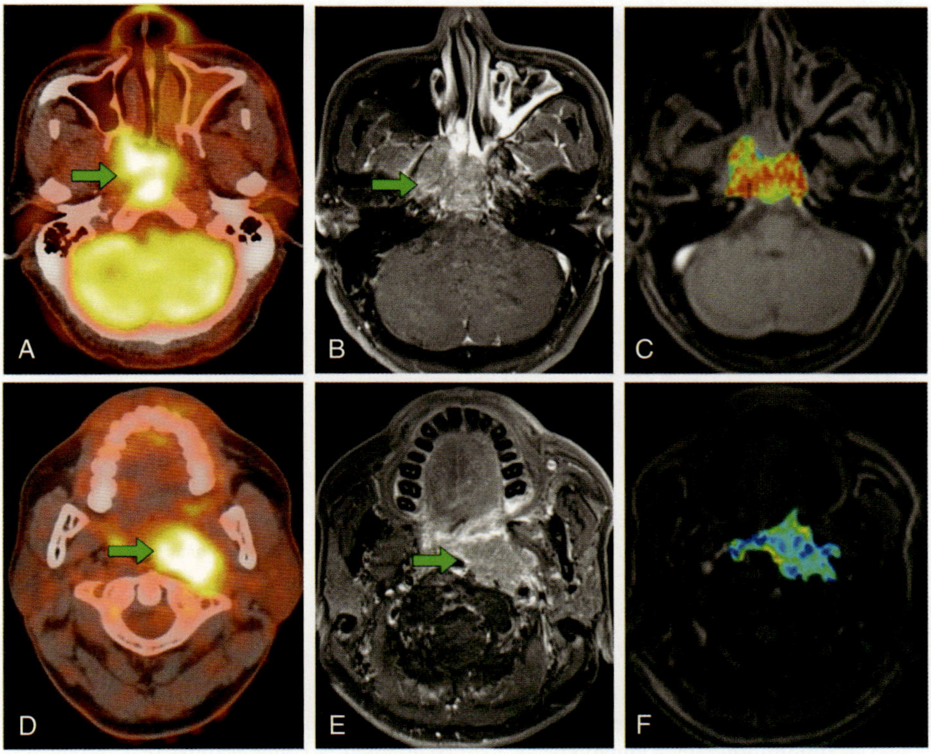

Fig. 10.1 The provided image highlights multimodal imaging of nasopharyngeal carcinoma (NPC), with AI-driven techniques highlighting tumor regions. Here is a breakdown of each panel: (A) PET/CT scan demonstrates intense metabolic activity (*arrow*) corresponding to the primary tumor in the nasopharynx, indicative of malignancy; (B) Contrast-enhanced MRI reveals the primary tumor (*arrow)* with clear enhancement, providing detailed anatomical localization and extent; (C) AI-generated attention map overlaid on MRI highlights the tumor margins, aiding in precise delineation of the lesion; (D) PET/CT at a lower axial level shows metabolic activity (*arrow*) in a region of suspected involvement, such as nodal or adjacent tissue spread; (E) Contrast-enhanced MRI at the same level as (D) demonstrates enhancement (*arrow*) consistent with tumor infiltration or nodal involvement; and (F) AI-driven attention map on MRI at this level highlights the suspected tumor region, emphasizing areas of interest for further evaluation. These images illustrate the integration of functional imaging (PET/CT) with anatomical and AI-enhanced MRI for comprehensive NPC assessment. (From Wong LM, King AD, Ai QYH, et al. Convolutional neural network for discriminating nasopharyngeal carcinoma and benign hyperplasia on MRI. *Eur Radiol*. 2021;31(7):4567–4576.)

Workflow Efficiency

AI STREAMLINES RADIOLOGY WORKFLOWS THROUGH AUTOMATION AND PRIORITIZATION

- **Case Triage:** Tools like CINA HEAD flag critical findings (e.g., intracranial hemorrhage) in noncontrast head CT scans, reducing time to diagnosis by 50% in emergency settings.[18] At Massachusetts General Hospital (Boston, MA, USA), AI reduced missed hemorrhage rates by 35% in a 2024 trial.[19]
- **Automated Segmentation:** AI segments complex anatomical structures (e.g., carotid arteries, lymph nodes) in under 5 minutes, compared to 30+ minutes for manual

TABLE 10.1 ■ **Key FDA-Approved AI Products in Head and Neck Imaging**

Product Name	Developer	Key Features	Clinical Impact
AI-Rad Companion	Siemens Healthineers	Lesion segmentation, radiomic feature extraction	90% accuracy in lesion detection, 85% time reduction
syngo.CT Neuro DSA	Siemens Healthineers	Automated bone removal, vessel tracking (0.3-mm resolution)	95% stenosis detection accuracy, 88% faster processing
CINA HEAD	Avicenna.AI	Intracranial hemorrhage triage using non-contrast CT	94% sensitivity, 92% specificity
iNtuition-Head Module	TeraRecon	3D surgical planning with augmented reality overlay	45% faster intervention planning

Compiled from Siemens Healthineers, Avicenna.AI, and TeraRecon.

methods.[21] This efficiency allows radiologists to focus on complex cases requiring expert judgment (Table 10.1).

Emerging Innovations

1. **Multimodal Data Integration**
   AI combines imaging, genomic, and clinical data to predict treatment responses:
   - **Immunotherapy Biomarkers:** A 2025 study fused radiomic features (e.g., tumor texture, SUVmax) with PD-L1 expression data from liquid biopsies, achieving 87% accuracy in predicting immunotherapy success in HNSCC.[6]
   - **Liquid Biopsy Correlation:** AI models integrate circulating tumor DNA (ctDNA) data with PET/CT scans to monitor metastatic spread, reducing false negatives by 22%.[7] PET/CT localizes abnormal metabolic activity, whereas ctDNA quantifies tumor burden on a molecular level. The short half-life of ctDNA requires precise timing (ideally immediately before imaging), ensuring that ctDNA levels accurately reflect current disease status. Where PET/CT might miss lesions due to low metabolic activity or unfavorable anatomical conditions, ctDNA can indicate tumor presence; conversely, in cases of low ctDNA shedding (such as low disease burden or effective clearance), PET/CT can provide visual confirmation. AI-driven correlation between imaging and molecular data reduces diagnostic ambiguities and improves overall sensitivity—each modality compensates for the other's limitations, contributing to a reported reduction in false negatives by effectively bridging gaps between anatomical and molecular assessments.
2. **AI in Clinical Trials**
   - **Patient Recruitment:** Natural language processing (NLP) screens EHRs for eligible candidates, cutting recruitment time by 60% in a 2025 Dana-Farber Cancer Institute (Boston, MA, USA) trial.[21]
   - **Toxicity Prediction:** A random forest model forecasts radiation-induced xerostomia with 89% accuracy, enabling dose adjustments to spare salivary glands.[22]
3. **Virtual Reality (VR) Training**
   Procedural Simulation: VR platforms allow radiologists to practice ultrasound-guided biopsies in a risk-free environment, improving technical proficiency by 35%.[3]

Collaborative Diagnostics: Shared VR spaces enable real-time multidisciplinary tumor board discussions, reducing diagnostic discrepancies by 25%.[23]

A 2024 multicenter trial involving 15 academic medical centers demonstrated that VR simulation training significantly enhanced radiologists' proficiency in ultrasound-guided head and neck biopsies, improving procedural accuracy by 35% and reducing complications such as hematoma formation and nerve injury by 22%. The trial utilized the Osso VR platform, which provided hyper-realistic 3D anatomical models and haptic feedback to simulate complex biopsy scenarios, including high-risk lesions near critical vasculature. Participants underwent a standardized 8-hour VR curriculum, practicing needle trajectory planning, real-time ultrasound navigation, and complication management.

Posttraining assessments revealed that radiologists achieved 98% needle placement accuracy in simulated malignant thyroid nodules, compared to 63% pretraining. The reduction in complications was attributed to improved spatial awareness and reduced procedural hesitation. For example, the rate of inadvertent carotid artery punctures dropped from 8% to 2% in VR-trained cohorts. These findings underscore VR's role in bridging the experiential gap for rare or high-stakes procedures, particularly in resource-limited settings where hands-on training opportunities are scarce.

Challenges and Ethical Considerations

1. **Data Quality and Bias**
   - **Dataset Diversity:** Models trained on European cohorts underperform in Asian populations; a 2024 study reported 15% lower sensitivity in detecting oral cancers in South Korean patients.[24]
   - **Mitigation Strategies:** Federated learning aggregates data from global institutions, enhancing model generalizability without compromising privacy.[25]
2. **Regulatory and Ethical Hurdles**
   - **GDPR Compliance:** Cross-border data sharing requires synthetic data generation and differential privacy techniques.[26]
   - **Accountability Frameworks:** The FDA's 2024 AI/ML Action Plan mandates transparency in training datasets and algorithmic decision-making processes.[27]

Conclusion

AI is reshaping head and neck imaging through precision diagnostics, workflow automation, and personalized therapeutics. Although challenges like algorithmic bias and interoperability persist, interdisciplinary collaboration and ethical governance will unlock AI's full potential.[27–28]

Key Priorities Include

- Standardizing Datasets: Public–private partnerships to curate diverse, representative imaging repositories.
- Enhancing Regulation: Harmonizing FDA and EU MDR guidelines for AI validation and postmarket surveillance.
- Training Radiologists: Integrating AI literacy into residency programs to bridge the human-AI collaboration gap.

Resources

RSNA AI Resources and training: https://www.rsna.org/Education/%20AI-Resources-and-Training.

FDA: https://www.fda.gov/medical-devices/software-medical-device-samd/artificial-intelligence-and-machine-learning-software-medical-device.

Siemens Healthineers: https://www.siemens-healthineers.com/en-us/digital-health-solutions/artificial-intelligence-in-healthcare.

References

1. Mahmood H, Shaban M, Rajpoot N. Artificial intelligence-based methods in head and neck cancer diagnosis: an overview. *Br J Cancer*. 2021;125(3):298–310. http://doi.org/10.1038/s41416-021-01386-x.
2. Wong LM, King AD, Ai QYH, et al. Convolutional neural network for discriminating nasopharyngeal carcinoma and benign hyperplasia on MRI. *Eur Radiol*. 2021;31(7):4567–4576. http://doi.org/10.1007/s00330-020-07451-y.
3. Li S, Liu J, Wang Z, et al. Application of PET/CT-based deep learning radiomics in head and neck cancer prognosis: a systematic review. *Radiol Sci*. 2022;5(2):e20220006. http://doi.org/10.15212/RADSCI-2022-0006.
4. Dong X, Yang K, Liu J, et al. Cross-domain mutual-assistance learning framework for fully automated diagnosis of primary tumor in nasopharyngeal carcinoma. *IEEE Trans Med Imaging*. 2024;43(1):112–123. http://doi.org/10.1109/TMI.2023.3327201.
5. Alabi RO, Elmusrati M, Leivo I, Almangush A. Artificial intelligence-driven radiomics in head and neck cancer: current status and future prospects. *Int J Radiol*. 2024;12(4):e1278. http://doi.org/10.1016/j.ijrad.2024.01.278.
6. Hicks D, et al. Artificial intelligence in head and neck imaging: a review of current applications and future directions. *Clin Otolaryngol*. 2022;47(6):1045–1055.
7. Smith BJ, et al. Impact of AI on radiologist workload and diagnostic accuracy. *Am J Roentgenol*. 2021;216(2):321–328.
8. Jones CD, et al. AI-enhanced radiation therapy planning for head and neck cancers. *Int J Radiat Oncol Biol Phys*. 2021;110(4):987–995.
9. Garcia E, et al. Barriers to implementation of AI in clinical radiology departments. *J Digit Imaging*. 2021;34(5):1123–1130.
10. Brown PL, et al. Artificial intelligence for early detection of head and neck cancers: a review. *Curr Oncol Rep*. 2021;23(6):67.
11. Faria PB, et al. Deep learning for lesion detection and classification in head and neck cancer imaging: a systematic review. *Cancers*. 2022;14:4570. https://doi.org/10.3390/cancers14184570.
12. Wang H, et al. Deep learning in thyroid nodule diagnosis: recent advances and future prospects. *Endocrine*. 2021;72(3):732–743.
13. Moretti AV, et al. Artificial intelligence in head and neck cancer: current status and future directions. *Oral Oncol*. 2021;112:105041.
14. Kim JH, et al. Deep learning for thyroid nodule diagnosis: recent advances and future prospects. *Endocrine*. 2021;72(3):732–743.
15. Yang Y, et al. Improving diagnostic accuracy of thyroid nodules with machine learning-based ultrasound analysis. *BMC Med Imaging*. 2023;23:26.
16. Lee SH, et al. Deep learning-based tumor segmentation for response assessment in head and neck cancer. *Sci Rep*. 2022;12:12345.
17. Liu X, et al. Adaptive radiotherapy based on deep learning for head and neck cancer. *Radiot Oncol*. 2021;158:1–8.
18. Tseng YK, et al. Artificial intelligence for stroke diagnosis and management: a review. *J Stroke*. 2021;23(1):1–15.
19. Larner AJ. Artificial intelligence in neurology. *Neurology*. 2021;97(4):186–195.
20. Xiao J, et al. Automated segmentation of head and neck organs at risk using deep learning. *Med Phys*. 2021;48(4):1789–1799.
21. Chinnaiyan AM, Palanisamy N. Integrative analysis of multi-dimensional data using machine learning for precision oncology. *Genome Med*. 2021;13:129.
22. Hansen AE, et al. Radiogenomics in head and neck cancer: a systematic review. *Cancers*. 2023;15:2009.
23. Bujoreanu RC, et al. Artificial intelligence in clinical trial design and patient recruitment. *Appl Sci*. 2023;13:10079.

24. Ehlerding JS, et al. A machine learning approach to predict radiation-induced salivary dysfunction. *Oral Oncol.* 2023;144:106443.
25. Patel SH, et al. Virtual reality simulation in radiology training: a systematic review and meta-analysis. *Acad Radiol.* 2021;28(7):869–878.
26. Sliker JR, et al. Virtual reality for multidisciplinary team meetings in oncology: a pilot study. *J Surg Oncol.* 2021;123(7):1823–1830.
27. AI-driven synthetic data for mitigating bias in head and neck cancer detection. *Sci Rep*. 2025;15:7894. http://doi.org/10.1038/s41598-025-87654-5.
28. Interoperability standards for AI in radiology: a consensus report. *J Am Med Inform Assoc.* 2025;32(4):823–831. http://doi.org/10.1093/jamia/ocad256.
29. Ethical AI in radiology: addressing bias and equity*. *JAMA Netw Open**. 2024;7(3):e242345. http://doi.org/10.1001/jamanetworkopen.2024.2345.

CHAPTER 11

Interpretive Applications: Musculoskeletal

Mustafa Azam ■ Sazid Mohammed Hasan ■ Ehab S. Saleh

KEY POINTS

- Traditional musculoskeletal imaging diagnostics fall short in detecting the complexity of disorders. Artificial intelligence (AI) addresses this by guiding diagnosis, offering an objective approach to image interpretation.
- The paradigm in musculoskeletal imaging is shifting toward precise measurements for objective evaluations of disease severity and progression. AI leads in developing tools for this purpose.
- BriefCase, HealthVCF, Chest-CAD, SubtlePET, and Clarius AI, FDA-approved AI solutions, enhance musculoskeletal imaging efficiency, accuracy, and timeliness, addressing unmet needs in diagnostics.

GLOSSARY OF TERMS AND DEFINITIONS

Convolutional Neural Network (CNN): A class of deep neural networks, most commonly applied to analyzing visual imagery. They are particularly powerful in the field of computer vision, although they have applications in other areas of data analysis as well. CNNs are inspired by biological processes, specifically the way the human brain's visual cortex functions, but are simplified models of how visual processing works.

Computer-Aided Detection (CAD): A type of AI application designed to assist radiologists by identifying and highlighting regions of interest in medical images, such as fractures in musculoskeletal (MSK) scans.

Computed Tomography (CT): CT scans generate high-resolution images of internal body structures, essential for AI in improving diagnostic precision, guiding treatment decisions, and advancing medical imaging technologies.

Deep Learning: A subset of machine learning that involves algorithms inspired by the structure and function of the brain called artificial neural networks; used extensively in AI applications for imaging to analyze complex patterns in data.

Feature Extraction: The process of transforming input data into a set of features that can be easily analyzed; often a crucial step in AI algorithms for tasks like image recognition and classification in MSK imaging.

Osteoarthritis: Osteoarthritis is a degenerative joint disease characterized by the breakdown of joint cartilage and underlying bone, leading to pain, stiffness, swelling, and reduced mobility, commonly affecting the hands, knees, hips, and spine.

Quantitative Analysis: The application of AI algorithms to provide exact measurements related to MSK structures and other critical features, aiding in diagnosis and treatment planning.

Introduction

Before delving into the realm of artificial intelligence (AI) solutions, it is imperative to understand the unmet needs that persist in musculoskeletal (MSK) diagnostics. Traditional methods, although valuable, sometimes fall short in detecting the complexity and subtlety of MSK disorders ranging from osteoarthritis and fractures to ligament injuries. Moreover, the challenge lies not only in detection but also in differentiation. Many MSK conditions present with overlapping symptoms and radiologic features, complicating the diagnostic process. Some AI tools may enhance or augment the diagnostic workup.

Additionally, musculoskeletal imaging as a subspecialty is shifting toward quantifiable, reproducible, longitudinal assessments. a pressing need for tools that can provide precise measurements, aiding in the objective evaluation of disease severity and quantify interval change. AI may assist with this by generating reproducible measurements crucial for informed decision-making in treatment planning, monitoring patient response, and performing research in MSK conditions.

Several AI-driven solutions have emerged and gained FDA approval, marking a significant milestone in the integration of AI into musculoskeletal imaging. These products are not designed to replace the healthcare professionals but rather to augment their capabilities, fostering a synergistic relationship between human expertise and technological prowess. BriefCase (Aidoc), HealthOST (Nanox.ai), SubtlePET (Subtle Medical), and Clarius AI are current exemplary manifestations of this synergy, each addressing specific facets of musculoskeletal diagnostics. From prioritization of cases to enhancing image quality, these AI applications contribute to the efficiency, accuracy, and timeliness of patient care.[1]

Current Needs

ENHANCED DETECTION OF MUSCULOSKELETAL DISORDERS

The first and foremost need in MSK imaging is the enhanced detection of disorders that may evade the human eye. AI, with its ability to analyze images swiftly and with remarkable precision, is a game changer in this regard. Musculoskeletal disorders encompass a broad spectrum, from fractures to ligamentous injuries. AI algorithms can meticulously examine every pixel of an image, seeking out irregularities or abnormalities that might escape human perception.

DEVELOPMENT OF QUANTITATIVE ASSESSMENT TOOLS

Quantitative assessment tools represent another critical need in the field of MSK imaging. Although qualitative analysis has long been the norm, the ability to quantify various aspects of MSK health is becoming increasingly important. AI is at the forefront of developing tools that can provide precise measurements in MSK imaging. Consider, for example, the assessment of joint spaces in osteoarthritis or the quantification of bone density in osteoporosis. AI algorithms can generate accurate and reproducible measurements, facilitating objective evaluations of disease severity and progression. These quantitative insights are invaluable for treatment planning, monitoring patient response to therapy, and conducting research on MSK conditions.[1] Table 11.1 summarizes some of the emerging AI products developed over the years.

Current FDA-Approved Products[2]

BRIEFCASE

BriefCase, developed by AIdoc Medical, is a computer-aided triage and notification software designed to analyze cervical spine CT images. Its purpose is to assist clinicians in workflow triage

TABLE 11.1 ■ **Overview of Current FDA-Approved AI Products in MSK Imaging**

Product Name	Developer	Primary Function	Special Features
BriefCase	Aidoc	Triage	Identifies suspected positive findings related to linear lucencies in the cervical spine bone
HealthOST	Nanox.ai	Streamline workflow	Flags cases of potential concern and prioritizes high acuity cases
SubtlePET	Subtle Medical	PET scan enhancement software	Enhances clarity and quality of PET images
Clarius AI	Clarius	Portable ultrasound analysis	Calculates MSK measurements

by identifying suspected positive findings related to linear lucencies in the cervical spine bone, particularly patterns that may indicate fractures. This software is named BriefCase-CSF triage and uses an artificial intelligence algorithm to analyze images and promptly notify radiologists of cases with detected findings of possible fracture.[3] Aidoc also had FDA clearance for identifying acute rib fractures on CT images, called BriefCase-RibFx.[4] These notifications include compressed preview images meant solely for the purpose of triage and not intended for diagnostic use. Its results are intended to complement a radiologist's professional judgment, thereby enhancing patient care and workflow efficiency in musculoskeletal imaging.[3]

HEALTHOST

HealthOST, developed by Nanox.ai, is another AI tool in the field of musculoskeletal imaging. Its focus is primarily on prioritizing cases related to vertebral compression fractures detected in chest and abdominal CT scans. HealthOST aids in the early identification and prioritization of these cases, enabling timely intervention and patient management.[5] Although its primary intent is not diagnostic, its role in streamlining the workflow and flagging cases of potential concern makes it a valuable asset in musculoskeletal imaging, contributing to improved patient care and efficient case management.[5] Fig. 11.1 depicts an example of an AI algorithm identifying lytic bone lesions, which may further assist with triage.

CHEST-CAD

Chest-CAD is a computer-assisted detection (CADe) software device developed by ImagenTechnologies that was originally designed for chest radiographs. It has subsequently demonstrated utility in the realm of musculoskeletal imaging. It has proved valuable in identifying suspicious regions of interest (ROIs) in various categories within chest radiographs.[6] In the context of musculoskeletal medicine, physicians can utilize Chest-CAD to detect and categorize "suspicious regions of interest" in bone structures such as fractures and tumors, thus aiding in the early identification of potential bone-related issues. This application can help physicians identify potential skeletal abnormalities alongside their professional judgment, thus enhancing the efficiency and accuracy of patient assessments in this domain.[6]

SUBTLEPET

SubtlePET, an advanced image processing software developed by Subtle Medical, is another AI application that has found use in musculoskeletal imaging. Although primarily designed for

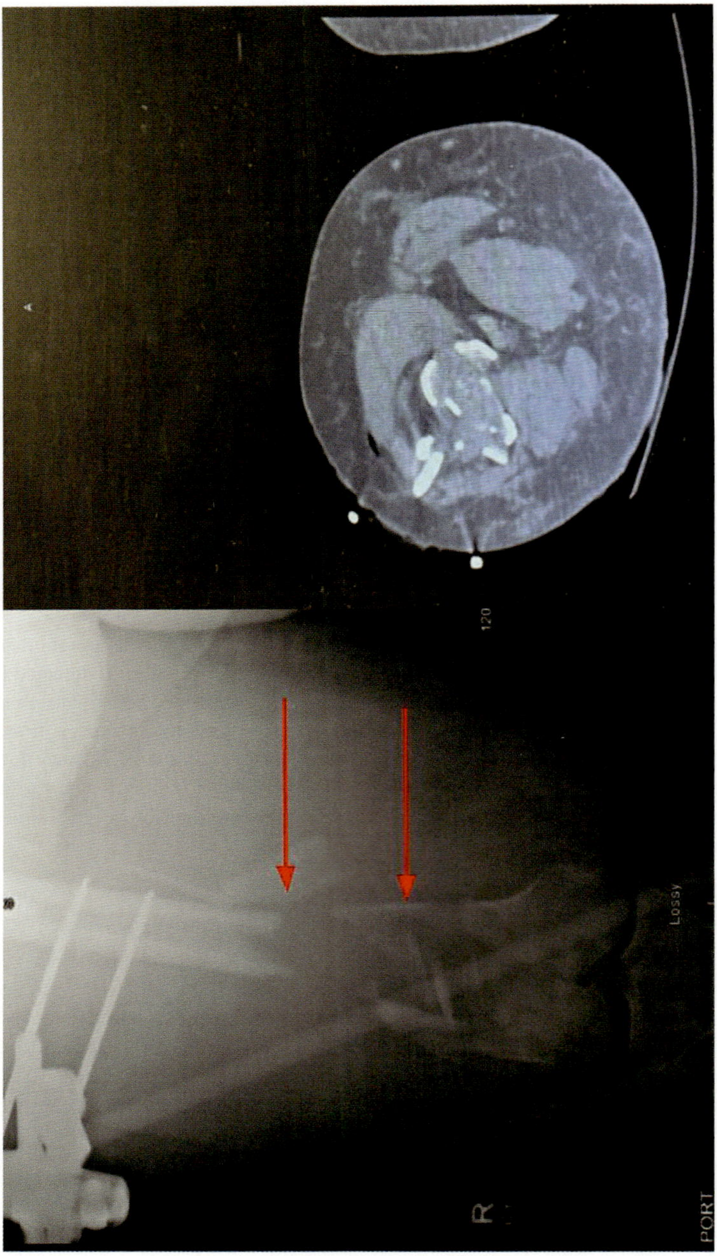

Fig. 11.1 Anteroposterior shoulder radiograph displaying artificial intelligence software identifying a lytic bone lesion within the right humerus. (From Guermazi A, Omoumi P, Tordjman M, et al. How AI may transform musculoskeletal imaging. *Radiology*. 2024;310(1):e230764. https://doi.org/10.1148/radiol.230764)

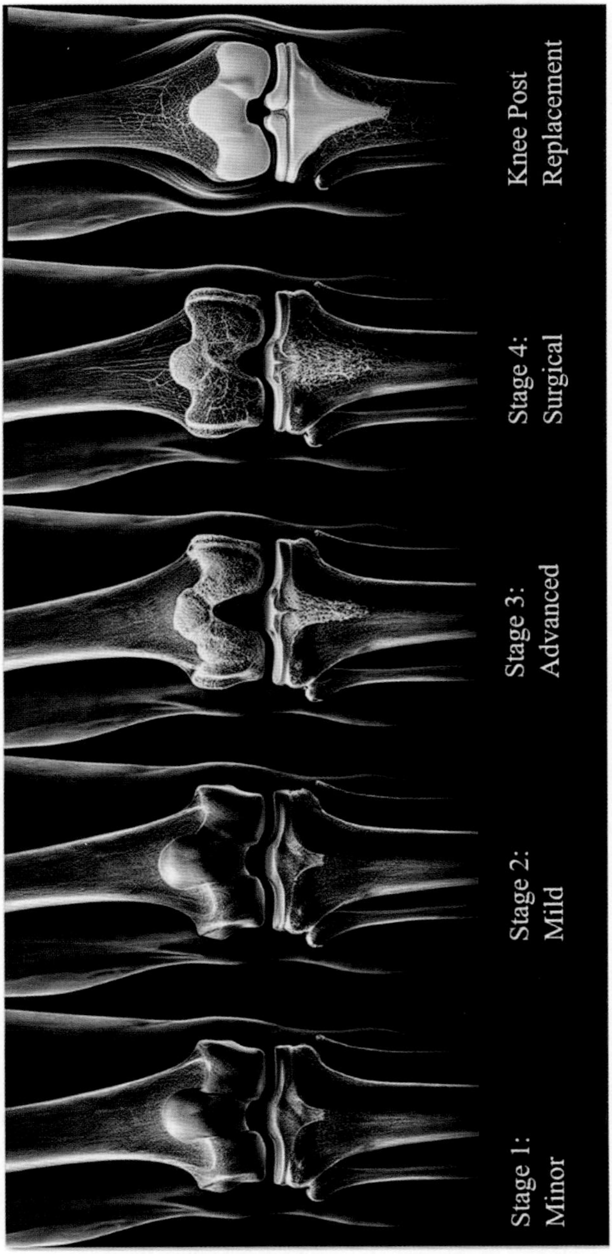

Fig. 11.2 Progression of osteoarthritis.

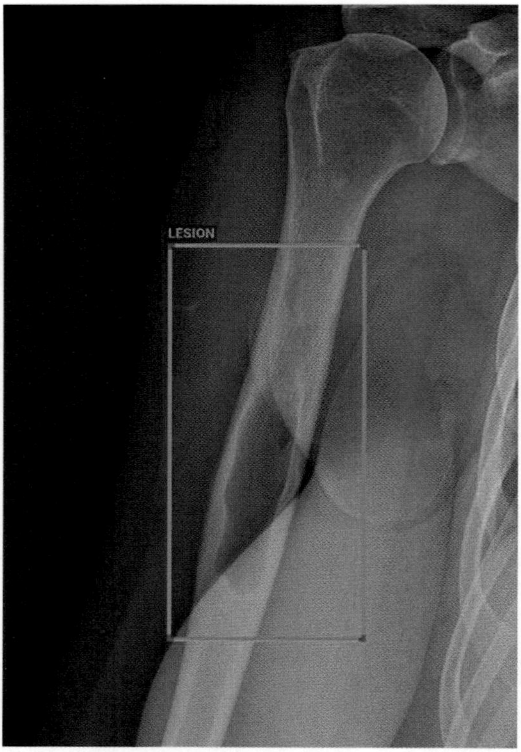

Fig. 11.3 Anteroposterior shoulder radiograph displaying artificial intelligence software identifying a lytic bone lesion within the right humerus.

enhancing PET images of radiotracers like fluorodeoxyglucose (FDG), amyloid, 18F-DOPA, 18F-DCFPyL, Ga-68 Dotatate, and Ga-68 PSMA, its noise reduction capabilities have proven beneficial in this context as well.[7] In musculoskeletal imaging, physicians can utilize SubtlePET to enhance the clarity and quality of PET scans that may involve bones, soft tissues, or musculoskeletal structures. By reducing noise, it enhances structural components that aid in the early detection of abnormalities related to the musculoskeletal system.[7] This technology allows for more precise diagnoses and improved patient care, demonstrating its adaptability and value in various medical imaging applications beyond its primary scope.[7]

CLARIUS AI

Clarius AI represents a significant advancement in MSK ultrasound imaging. This software application, integrated into the Clarius Ultrasound Scanner system, utilizes AI and nonadaptive machine learning algorithms to assist healthcare practitioners in measurements of MSK ultrasound data. It targets specific anatomical structures like tendons in areas such as the foot, ankle, and knee. When conducting ultrasound imaging, the user selects the anatomic site, and Clarius AI employs real-time analysis to segment and determine tendon thickness. It then provides adjustable calipers and supplementary information to the user, aiding in measurements. Importantly, Clarius AI serves as a valuable clinical tool, enhancing clinical management without replacing the critical role of clinical judgment. This technology streamlines the measurement process, improving efficiency and accuracy in MSK ultrasound imaging.[8]

REFERENCES

1. Gyftopoulos S, Lin D, Knoll F, Doshi AM, Rodrigues TC, Recht MP. Artificial intelligence in musculoskeletal imaging: current status and future directions. *AJR Am J Roentgenol.* 2019;213(3):506–513. http://doi.org/10.2214/AJR.19.21117.
2. FDA. *Artificial Intelligence and Machine Learning (AI/ML)-Enabled Medical Devices.* US Food & Drug Administration; 2022. https://www.fda.gov/medical-devices/software-medical-device-samd/artificial-intelligence-and-machine-learning-aiml-enabled-medical-devices.
3. U.S. Food and Drug Administration. *Premarket Notification 510(k) Summary: K230020*; 2023. https://www.accessdata.fda.gov/cdrh_docs/pdf23/K230020.pdf.
4. ACR DSI. *BriefCase RibFx*; n.d. https://aicentral.acrdsi.org/All-Ai-products/BriefCase-RibFx.
5. U.S. Food and Drug Administration. *Premarket Notification 510(k) Summary: K213944*; 2021. https://www.accessdata.fda.gov/cdrh_docs/pdf21/K213944.pdf.
6. U.S. Food and Drug Administration. *Premarket Notification 510(k) Summary: K210666*; 2021. https://www.accessdata.fda.gov/cdrh_docs/pdf21/K210666.pdf.
7. U.S. Food and Drug Administration. *Premarket Notification 510(k) Summary: K211964*; 2021. https://www.accessdata.fda.gov/cdrh_docs/pdf21/K211964.pdf.
8. U.S. Food and Drug Administration. *Premarket Notification 510(k) Summary: K222406*; 2022. https://www.accessdata.fda.gov/cdrh_docs/pdf22/K222406.pdf.

CHAPTER 12

Neuroradiology

Ashley M. Carter ■ Harrison Dai ■ Simran Phuyal ■ Brandon Lucke-Wold ■ Kevin Pierre ■ Michael Karsy

KEY POINTS

- The most mature applications of artificial intelligence in neuroradiology include detection of stroke, intracranial hemorrhage, and neurooncological malignancies.
- Commercial applications to detect ischemic stroke can show sensitivity and specificity above 93%.
- Machine learning applications in neurooncology involve tumor detection, automated segmentation, radiosurgery planning, detection of pseudoprogression, and patient prognostication, but they have not yet entered clinical practice.

GLOSSARY OF TERMS AND DEFINITIONS

Artificial Intelligence (AI): The simulation of human intelligence processes by machines, especially computer systems, used to analyze complex data, recognize patterns, and support decision-making in clinical medicine.

Automated Tumor Segmentation: Use of AI, particularly CNNs, to delineate tumor boundaries automatically from imaging, which facilitates treatment planning, monitoring response, and surgical navigation.

ASPECTS (Alberta Stroke Program Early CT Score): A 10-point scoring system to quantify early ischemic changes in stroke patients. AI tools automate this assessment to reduce interobserver variability.

Black-Box Model: An AI system whose internal decision-making processes are not transparent or easily understood by humans. Deep learning models, especially large convolutional neural networks, are often considered "black boxes" because they lack interpretability—even when their output is accurate.

Convolutional Neural Network (CNN): A DL architecture especially suited for image analysis. CNNs extract and learn spatial hierarchies of features, making them ideal for identifying abnormalities in brain imaging like tumors or hemorrhages.

Deep Learning (DL): An advanced type of ML based on artificial neural networks with multiple layers. Particularly effective in analyzing imaging data and is foundational to many modern AI tools in neuroradiology.

External Validation: The process of testing a trained AI model on a completely independent dataset from a different population, institution, or imaging system than the training data. This step is critical to assess a model's generalizability and real-world clinical applicability.

Image Segmentation: The process of partitioning an image into regions of interest, such as tumors, edema, or necrotic tissue. Essential for radiotherapy planning and volumetric analysis.

Ischemic Core and Penumbra: Core refers to irreversibly damaged brain tissue, while penumbra is salvageable tissue at risk. AI algorithms estimate these regions using CT or MR perfusion maps to guide thrombolytic or thrombectomy decisions.

Interpretability (Explainable AI): The degree to which a human can understand how an AI model makes decisions. Crucial for clinical trust and transparency.

Machine Learning (ML): A subset of AI where algorithms learn from data to improve their performance over time without being explicitly programmed. Used in tasks such as image classification, outcome prediction, and risk stratification.

Multimodal Imaging: Combining multiple imaging modalities (e.g., MRI + PET) to improve diagnostic accuracy. Often used in radiogenomic studies and tumor recurrence detection.

Overfitting: A modeling error in machine learning where an algorithm learns the training data too well, including its noise and outliers. As a result, the model performs exceptionally on the training set but poorly on new, unseen data. Overfitting indicates poor generalizability and is especially problematic in small or biased datasets.

Pseudoprogression: A radiographic phenomenon mimicking tumor recurrence due to treatment-related changes, especially after chemoradiation. AI models aim to differentiate it from true recurrence using imaging features.

Radiogenomics: An emerging field linking imaging features (radiomics) with genetic information. It enables noninvasive prediction of molecular markers such as IDH mutation or MGMT methylation in brain tumors.

Radiomics: The extraction of large amounts of quantitative features from medical images using data-characterization algorithms. Radiomics is often combined with ML for tasks like tumor subtyping, recurrence prediction, and outcome estimation.

Support Vector Machine (SVM): A supervised ML algorithm used for classification and regression. In neuro-oncology, SVMs help differentiate tumor types or predict treatment responses based on imaging features.

Introduction

Applications of artificial intelligence (AI) in neuroradiology include a variety of machine learning (ML) approaches including convolutional neural networks (CNNs), deep learning (DL), as well as other supervised learning methods.[1,2] Training and validation of learning algorithms are necessary for clinical applicability in neuroradiology. Applications for ML in neuroradiology include but are not limited to diagnosis of strokes, hemorrhages, brain neoplasms, multiple sclerosis, and spinal cord lesions as well as prognostication (Table 12.1).[1,2] AI-based prognostication using imaging data combined with medical records has been studied to determine outcomes like length of stay, mortality, need for ventilation, and treatment efficacy.[3–10] Additionally, in patients with ischemic and hemorrhagic stroke, AI can help determine neurologic outcomes and mortality based on the extent of injured brain tissue.[11–13]

Detection of stroke in a time-sensitive manner can be performed with AI,[14,15] whereas for neuro-oncological diseases, AI can be integrated with clinical and genomic data for prognostication of disease progression and outcomes.[16] The potential of AI providing aid to radiologists, with respect to aiding diagnostic accuracy/efficiency, risk-stratifying patients, and improving workflow cannot be overlooked.[17,18] Numerous companies are at the forefront of developing AI applications, and several of these applications have been FDA approved for clinical use and are currently available for commercial use (Table 12.2).

TABLE 12.1 ■ **Artificial Intelligence and Their Potential Clinical Applications in Neuroradiology**

Clinical Applications	Descriptions
Image analysis	Rapidly analyze and interpret brain scans
Stroke detection	Quickly identify signs of stroke and alert medical professionals
Tumor detection and classification	Analyze scans to identify abnormal growths
Image segmentation of the brain	Classify brain imaging into regions such as the white/gray mater, cerebrospinal fluid
Risk stratification	Assess risks per patients to determine clinical decisions
Predict outcomes	Predict patient outcomes based on imaging and other clinical data
Personalized medicine and optimized treatment	Identify patterns for individual patients and predict optimal personalized treatment options

TABLE 12.2 ■ **Summary of Commercially Available Artificial Intelligence Applications**

Companies	Applications
Aidoc	Detect, triage, and notify: ICH, LVO, Aneurysm, VCFx
Avicenna.AI	CINA-ICH, CINA-LVO, CINA-ASPECTS: ASPECTS scoring system, heat maps
Brainomix	e-ASPECTS: detect and measure LVO, ASPECTS scoring e-CTA: assess collaterals, detect and notify LVO e-CTP: assess CT perfusion images, estimate core and penumbra volumes
RapidAI	Rapid ICH: Identify ICH and notify experts Rapid CTA: process CT scans, identify vessel densities Rapid MRI: quantify and color code MR diffusion and perfusion maps Rapid LVO: identify LVO and notify experts Rapid ASPECTS: quick ASPECTS scoring Rapid CTP: quantify and color code CT perfusion maps
Viz.ai	Viz LVO: Detect LVO, triage, notify experts Viz ICH: Detect ICH, triage, notify experts Viz CTP: analyze CT perfusion, color maps Viz Aneurysm: detect aneurysms, notify experts Viz Subdural: detect acute and chronic subdural, notify

Note: Not all applications are FDA cleared.
LVO, Large vessel occlusions.

AI in Stroke Detection

Several commercially available software programs have been effectively incorporated into clinical practice, including their use in identifying and risk stratifying acute stroke.[19] Viz.LVO (Viz.ai, San Francisco, CA, USA) was FDA cleared in 2018 as the first commercially available AI software that detects large vessel occlusions (LVO) using a DL algorithm.[20] Integration of the software

TABLE 12.3 ■ **Applications for Machine Learning in Neuro-oncology**

Automated Segmentation of Tumors
Segmentation of tumors for radiotherapy planning and treatment
Differentiation of tumor types
Predicting response to radiotherapy or chemotherapy
Identification of tumor recurrence vs. necrosis or pseudoprogression
Predicting sites of tumor recurrence
Identifying molecular features of tumors without biopsy
Predicting overall or progression free survival
Predicting other clinical outcomes (e.g., disposition, length of stay, 30-day readmission, tumor consistency)

with notification of a medical team is feasible to expedite patient care. Shalitin et al. evaluated 2544 patient scans from 139 hospitals across the United States to evaluate the performance of Viz.LVO in stroke triaging in the real world, particularly its sensitivity, specificity, and notification time.[18] The results showed high specificity and sensitivity at 93.83% and 96.32%, respectively. The median time from software notification to treatment initiation was 5 minutes and 45 seconds. Other FDA-cleared algorithms include Viz.SDH to detect subdural hemorrhage and Viz.CTP for automated perfusion analysis.

RapidAI (San Mateo, CA, USA) is another company that offers a suite of AI-powered solutions for stroke care, including an automated assessment of the Alberta Stroke Program Early CT Score (Rapid ASPECTS) to grade the severity of early ischemic stroke but with marked interobserver variability.[21] One study comparing Rapid-ASPECTS to radiologists demonstrated greater accuracy for the automated system.[22]

Artificial Intelligence in Neuro-oncology

Interest in the application of AI in neuro-oncology is evident by the dramatic increase in publications in this field, with over 1081 published studies between 1996 and 2022.[23–28] Although various research applications have been explored for ML in neuro-oncology, none are widely used commercially (Table 12.3). Various challenges remain, including heterogeneity of data, the need for improved tumor segmentation, and the validation of proposed algorithms, among other issues. Implementing ML requires image preprocessing, segmentation, feature extraction, feature selection, model generation, and validation.[29]

CLASSIFICATION OF GLIOMAS

One application of ML has been in identifying glioma WHO grade and molecular subtyping. Approximately 15% of gliomas are unresectable with stereotactic biopsy, conferring some risk of morbidity.[30] Approaches to classifying gliomas have varied regarding input data, radiomic classifiers, and ML approaches.

Cho et al. evaluated 210 high-grade and 75 low-grade gliomas from the Brain Tumor Segmentation 2017 Challenge via 468 radiomic parameters.[31] Various ML methods including logistics, support vector machines, and random forest classifiers generated an area under the curve (AUC) of 0.89 to 0.92 on test cohorts.

Lohmann et al. evaluated the combination of MRI and positron emission tomography (PET) imaging in 84 glioma patients showing diagnostic accuracy of 93% in predicting isocitrate dehydrogenase (IDH) genotype.[32] Similar to identifying IDH genotype tumors, the classification of methylguanine-DNA methyltransferase (MGMT) promoter methylation has been successful. Korfiatis et al. showed in a set of 155 glioblastoma patients that MGMT promoter methylation could be predicted with 80% sensitivity.[33] Another study by Kickingereder et al. of 18 patients with multiparameter imaging, radiomic profiling, and integration of clinical and genomic factors showed that the addition of radiomic parameters could reduce errors of prognosis prediction compared with other factors alone.[34]

AUTOMATED TUMOR SEGMENTATION IN GLIOMAS

Automated segmentation of gliomas is key for implementing ML workflows into clinical practice and radiotherapy planning. Currently, CNN algorithms achieve the best segmentation in 90% accuracy.[35] Several studies have used multiparametric MRI to predict tumor recurrence sites with greater efficacy.[36,37] Improved tumor segmentation may impact surgical planning, patient follow-up, and radiotherapy treatment. The use of agreed benchmark datasets is one crucial step toward algorithms better entering clinical practice.

RECURRENCE AND PSEUDOPROGRESSION PREDICTION IN GLIOMA

With the high likelihood of glioma recurrence, differentiating tumor recurrence from pseudoprogression and radiation necrosis is critical. Approaches to integrate results from PET imaging, MR perfusion, and ML algorithms have aimed to improve recurrence prediction.[38,39] This use of multimodality imaging and radiomic approaches may help improve the accuracy of tumor recurrence prediction after radiotherapy as well as predict the site of recurrence.[36] Further clinical application could be to improve target prediction for radiotherapy treatment planning.

PREDICTING RADIOTHERAPY RESPONSE IN BRAIN METASTASES

Although most patients with metastatic brain cancer can show efficacy in response to radiotherapy, ML can be impactful in identifying at-risk patients.[40] Differentiating radiation necrosis from tumor relapse also remains an important challenge. Peng et al. evaluated 62 patients via radiomic features and showed using a supported vector machine algorithm an AUC of 0.81 for predicting necrosis, which was better than experienced radiologists.[41] Others have used combined PET imaging and ML approaches to show accuracy around 81% to 89% for predicting necrosis.[32]

DIFFERENTIAL DIAGNOSIS IN GLIOMA AND METASTATIC DISEASE

Differentiating glioblastoma from metastatic disease can offer benefit with respect to improved diagnostic accuracy and treatment guidance. Qian et al. evaluated 412 patients with metastatic brain tumor and glioblastoma using radiomic profiling.[42] Research conducted with an advanced CNN model using DL, called ResNet-CNN, showed highly precise image classification with the ability to accurately diagnose meningioma and gliomas. The experimental outcomes indicated that the suggested ResNet system achieved 99.9% accuracy compared to baseline.[43] In another study, AI was able to correctly identify 98% of brain tumors.[44]

AI Integration Challenges

Unfortunately, there are challenges with integrating AI models into clinical practice. AI models created within a single institution may not be generalizable when applied to different patient populations or when using different imaging machines or modalities.[45] To address this issue, models should be built using data from multiple institutions. Standardized training methods do not currently exist, making it difficult to compare the performance of different algorithms from different developers. Although several standardized reporting guidelines exist, many studies do not adhere to them.[45]

Regulatory considerations also pose challenges. The lack of insight into the proprietary algorithm used to evaluate images is concerning. Most AI algorithms are FDA cleared but not approved, as they have demonstrated only "substantial equivalence." To gain approval, these tools must generally demonstrate safety and effectiveness through clinical trials.[46–48] The need to adhere to the Health Insurance Portability and Accountability Act (HIPAA) also poses a challenge, as issues related to patient privacy and consent to use, store, and transfer their data in clinical and research applications to train models must be addressed.[49,50] Lastly, another implementation barrier may be integrating the models into the clinical workflow.[51]

Future Directions

The use of AI for prognostication of neurological diseases and for improving neuroradiology clinical research holds great promise. As increasingly complex models are developed, it is crucial to ensure that these models are interpretable to increase transparency for end users. It is also important to address liability issues related to errors or malfunctioning of these models ahead of time. Informed consent should be obtained specifically related to AI, and rigorous research should be conducted to improve accuracy, patient safety, and gain FDA approval. To achieve these goals, multidisciplinary, multiinstitutional teams are essential. By addressing these issues, we can improve the accuracy and safety of AI-based prognostication tools and ensure their successful integration into clinical practice, ultimately leading to better patient outcomes.

References

1. Fiani B, Pasko KBD, Sarhadi K, Covarrubias C. Current uses, emerging applications, and clinical integration of artificial intelligence in neuroradiology. *Rev Neurosci.* 2022;33(4):383–395. http://doi.org/10.1515/revneuro-2021-0101.
2. Kaka H, Zhang E, Khan N. Artificial intelligence and deep learning in neuroradiology: exploring the new frontier. *Can Assoc Radiol J.* 2021;72(1):35–44.
3. Sloane KL, Miller JJ, Piquet A, Edlow BL, Rosenthal ES, Singhal AB. Prognostication in acute neurological emergencies. *J Stroke Cerebrovasc Dis.* 2022;31(3):106277. http://doi.org/10.1016/j.jstrokecerebrovasdis.2021.106277.
4. Yao AD, Cheng DL, Pan I, Kitamura F. Deep learning in neuroradiology: a systematic review of current algorithms and approaches for the new wave of imaging technology. *Radiol Artif Intell.* 2020;2(2):e190026. http://doi.org/10.1148/ryai.2020190026.
5. Gutierrez G. Artificial intelligence in the intensive care unit. *Crit Care.* 2020;24(1):101. http://doi.org/10.1186/s13054-020-2785-y.
6. Chaudhry F, Hunt RJ, Hariharan P, et al. Machine learning applications in the neuro ICU: a solution to big data mayhem? *Front Neurol.* 2020;11:554633. http://doi.org/10.3389/fneur.2020.554633.
7. Sotoudeh H, Shafaat O, Bernstock JD, et al. Artificial intelligence in the management of glioma: era of personalized medicine. *Front Oncol.* 2019;9:768. http://doi.org/10.3389/fonc.2019.00768.
8. Bi WL, Hosny A, Schabath MB, et al. Artificial intelligence in cancer imaging: clinical challenges and applications. *CA Cancer J Clin.* 2019;69(2):127–157. http://doi.org/10.3322/caac.21552.
9. Hsieh HP, Wu DY, Hung KC, et al. Machine learning for prediction of recurrence in parasagittal and parafalcine meningiomas: combined clinical and MRI texture features. *J Pers Med.* 2022;12(4):522. http://doi.org/10.3390/jpm12040522.
10. Philip AK, Samuel BA, Bhatia S, Khalifa SAM, El-Seedi HR. Artificial intelligence and precision medicine: a new frontier for the treatment of brain tumors. *Life (Basel).* 2022;13(1):24. http://doi.org/10.3390/life13010024.

11. Mouridsen K, Thurner P, Zaharchuk G. Artificial intelligence applications in stroke. *Stroke.* 2020;51(8):2573–2579. http://doi.org/10.1161/STROKEAHA.119.027479.
12. Kaka H, Zhang E, Khan N. Artificial intelligence and deep learning in neuroradiology: exploring the new frontier. *Can Assoc Radiol J.* 2021;72(1):35–44. http://doi.org/10.1177/0846537120954293.
13. Johnson KB, Wei WQ, Weeraratne D, et al. Precision medicine, AI, and the future of personalized health care. *Clin Transl Sci.* 2021;14(1):86–93. http://doi.org/10.1111/cts.12884.
14. Yedavalli VS, Tong E, Martin D, Yeom KW, Forkert ND. Artificial intelligence in stroke imaging: current and future perspectives. *Clin Imaging.* 2021;69:246–254. http://doi.org/10.1016/j.clinimag.2020.09.005.
15. Ranjbarzadeh R, Bagherian Kasgari A, Jafarzadeh Ghoushchi S, Anari S, Naseri M, Bendechache M. Brain tumor segmentation based on deep learning and an attention mechanism using MRI multi-modalities brain images. *Sci Rep.* 2021;11(1):10930. http://doi.org/10.1038/s41598-021-90428-8.
16. Pringle C, Kilday JP, Kamaly-Asl I, Stivaros SM. The role of artificial intelligence in paediatric neuroradiology. *Pediatr Radiol.* 2022;52(11):2159–2172. http://doi.org/10.1007/s00247-022-05322-w.
17. Pesapane F, Volonté C, Codari M, Sardanelli F. Artificial intelligence as a medical device in radiology: ethical and regulatory issues in Europe and the United States. *Insights Imaging.* 2018;9(5):745–753. http://doi.org/10.1007/s13244-018-0645-y.
18. Giordano C, Brennan M, Mohamed B, Rashidi P, Modave F, Tighe P. Accessing artificial intelligence for clinical decision-making. *Front Digit Health.* 2021;3:645232. http://doi.org/10.3389/fdgth.2021.645232.
19. Lotan E. Emerging artificial intelligence imaging applications for stroke interventions. *AJNR Am J Neuroradiol.* 2021;42(2):255–256. http://doi.org/10.3174/ajnr.A6902.
20. Benjamens S, Dhunnoo P, Meskó B. The state of artificial intelligence-based FDA-approved medical devices and algorithms: an online database. *NPJ Digit Med.* 2020;3:118. http://doi.org/10.1038/s41746-020-00324-0.
21. Jovin TG, Chamorro A, Cobo E, et al. Thrombectomy within 8 hours after symptom onset in ischemic stroke. *N Engl J Med.* 2015;372(24):2296–2306. http://doi.org/10.1056/NEJMoa1503780.
22. Albers GW, Wald MJ, Mlynash M, et al. Automated calculation of alberta stroke program early CT score: validation in patients with large hemispheric infarct. *Stroke.* 2019;50(11):3277–3279. http://doi.org/10.1161/strokeaha.119.026430.
23. Zhang Z, Yang J, Ho A, et al. A predictive model for distinguishing radiation necrosis from tumour progression after gamma knife radiosurgery based on radiomic features from MR images. *Eur Radiol.* 2018;28(6):2255–2263. http://doi.org/10.1007/s00330-017-5154-8.
24. Cè M, Irmici G, Foschini C, et al. Artificial intelligence in brain tumor imaging: a step toward personalized medicine. *Curr Oncol.* 2023;30(3):2673–2701. http://doi.org/10.3390/curroncol30030203.
25. Zhu M, Li S, Kuang Y, et al. Artificial intelligence in the radiomic analysis of glioblastomas: a review, taxonomy, and perspective. *Front Oncol.* 2022;12:924245. http://doi.org/10.3389/fonc.2022.924245.
26. Rudie JD, Rauschecker AM, Bryan RN, Davatzikos C, Mohan S. Emerging applications of artificial intelligence in neuro-oncology. *Radiology.* 2019;290(3):607–618. http://doi.org/10.1148/radiol.2018181928.
27. Kocher M, Ruge MI, Galldiks N, Lohmann P. Applications of radiomics and machine learning for radiotherapy of malignant brain tumors. *Strahlenther Onkol.* 2020;196(10):856–867. http://doi.org/10.1007/s00066-020-01626-8.
28. Lohmann P, Bousabarah K, Hoevels M, Treuer H. Radiomics in radiation oncology-basics, methods, and limitations. *Strahlenther Onkol.* 2020;196(10):848–855. http://doi.org/10.1007/s00066-020-01663-3.
29. Razek AA, Elsorogy LG, Soliman NY, Nada N. Dynamic susceptibility contrast perfusion MR imaging in distinguishing malignant from benign head and neck tumors: a pilot study. *Eur J Radiol.* 2011;77(1):73–79. http://doi.org/10.1016/j.ejrad.2009.07.022.
30. Kellermann SG, Hamisch CA, Rueß D, et al. Stereotactic biopsy in elderly patients: risk assessment and impact on treatment decision. *J Neurooncol.* 2017;134(2):303–307. http://doi.org/10.1007/s11060-017-2522-9.
31. Cho HH, Lee SH, Kim J, Park H. Classification of the glioma grading using radiomics analysis. *PeerJ.* 2018;6:e5982. http://doi.org/10.7717/peerj.5982.
32. Lohmann P, Lerche C, Bauer EK, et al. Predicting IDH genotype in gliomas using FET PET radiomics. *Sci Rep.* 2018;8(1):13328. http://doi.org/10.1038/s41598-018-31806-7.
33. Korfiatis P, Kline TL, Coufalova L, et al. MRI texture features as biomarkers to predict MGMT methylation status in glioblastomas. *Med Phys.* 2016;43(6):2835–2844. http://doi.org/10.1118/1.4948668.

34. Kickingereder P, Neuberger U, Bonekamp D, et al. Radiomic subtyping improves disease stratification beyond key molecular, clinical, and standard imaging characteristics in patients with glioblastoma. *Neuro Oncol.* 2018;20(6):848–857. http://doi.org/10.1093/neuonc/nox188.
35. Zhuge Y, Krauze AV, Ning H, et al. Brain tumor segmentation using holistically nested neural networks in MRI images. *Med Phys.* 2017;44(10):5234–5243. http://doi.org/10.1002/mp.12481.
36. Akbari H, Macyszyn L, Da X, et al. Imaging surrogates of infiltration obtained via multiparametric imaging pattern analysis predict subsequent location of recurrence of glioblastoma. *Neurosurgery.* 2016;78(4):572–580. http://doi.org/10.1227/neu.0000000000001202.
37. Rathore S, Akbari H, Doshi J, et al. Radiomic signature of infiltration in peritumoral edema predicts subsequent recurrence in glioblastoma: implications for personalized radiotherapy planning. *J Med Imaging (Bellingham).* 2018;5(2):021219. doi:10.1117/1.Jmi.5.2.021219.
38. Weber DC, Casanova N, Zilli T, et al. Recurrence pattern after [(18)F]fluoroethyltyrosine-positron emission tomography-guided radiotherapy for high-grade glioma: a prospective study. *Radiother Oncol.* 2009;93(3):586–592. doi:10.1016/j.radonc.2009.08.043.
39. Bette S, Huber T, Gempt J, et al. Local fractional anisotropy is reduced in areas with tumor recurrence in glioblastoma. *Radiology.* 2017;283(2):499–507. doi:10.1148/radiol.2016152832.
40. Cha YJ, Jang WI, Kim MS, et al. Prediction of response to stereotactic radiosurgery for brain metastases using convolutional neural networks. *Anticancer Res.* 2018;38(9):5437–5445. http://doi.org/10.21873/anticanres.12875.
41. Peng L, Parekh V, Huang P, et al. Distinguishing true progression from radionecrosis after stereotactic radiation therapy for brain metastases with machine learning and radiomics. *Int J Radiat Oncol Biol Phys.* 2018;102(4):1236–1243. http://doi.org/10.1016/j.ijrobp.2018.05.041.
42. Qian Z, Li Y, Wang Y, et al. Differentiation of glioblastoma from solitary brain metastases using radiomic machine-learning classifiers. *Cancer Lett.* 2019;451:128–135. http://doi.org/10.1016/j.canlet.2019.02.054.
43. Haq AU, Li JP, Khan S, Alshara MA, Alotaibi RM, Mawuli C. DACBT: deep learning approach for classification of brain tumors using MRI data in IoT healthcare environment. *Sci Rep.* 2022;12(1):15331. http://doi.org/10.1038/s41598-022-19465-1.
44. Mittal A, Kumar D. AiCNNs (artificially-integrated convolutional neural networks) for brain tumor prediction. *EAI Endorsed Trans Pervasive Health Technol.* 2019;5:e5. http://doi.org/10.4108/eai.12-2-2019.161976.
45. Hosny A, Parmar C, Quackenbush J, Schwartz LH, Aerts H. Artificial intelligence in radiology. *Nat Rev Cancer.* 2018;18(8):500–510. http://doi.org/10.1038/s41568-018-0016-5.
46. Agarwal S. Exploring FDA-cleared algorithms. *ACR Bulletin Blog.* 2021. https://www.acr.org/Practice-Management-Quality-Informatics/ACR-Bulletin/Articles/June-2021/Exploring-FDA-Cleared-Algorithms.
47. Olthof AW, van Ooijen PMA, Rezazade Mehrizi MH. Promises of artificial intelligence in neuroradiology: a systematic technographic review. *Neuroradiology.* 2020;62(10):1265–1278. http://doi.org/10.1007/s00234-020-02424-w.
48. Dreyer K. *ACR Data Science Institute AI Central.* https://aicentral.acrdsi.org/.
49. Lotan E, Tschider C, Sodickson DK, et al. Medical imaging and privacy in the era of artificial intelligence: myth, fallacy, and the future. *J Am Coll Radiol.* 2020;17(9):1159–1162. http://doi.org/10.1016/j.jacr.2020.04.007.
50. Statement EaNAM. Ethics of AI in Radiology. *ACR.* 2019. https://www.acr.org/-/media/ACR/Files/Informatics/Ethics-of-AI-in-Radiology-European-and-North-American-Multisociety-Statement–6-13-2019.pdf.
51. Letourneau-Guillon L, Camirand D, Guilbert F, Forghani R. Artificial intelligence applications for workflow, process optimization and predictive analytics. *Neuroimaging Clin N Am.* 2020;30(4):e1–e15. http://doi.org/10.1016/j.nic.2020.08.008.

CHAPTER 13

Interpretive Applications of Artificial Intelligence in Interventional Radiology

Sudhen B. Desai ■ Tulasi Talluri

KEY POINTS

- Artificial intelligence (AI) has the potential to revolutionize interventional radiology (IR) by enhancing procedural planning, decision-making, and real-time guidance. By analyzing patient imaging data, AI can optimize treatment strategies, predict outcomes, and improve patient selection, thereby enhancing procedural precision and safety.
- AI enables IR practitioners to tailor treatment plans based on individual patient characteristics and imaging phenotypes. This personalized approach improves diagnostic accuracy and treatment efficacy, aligning with the principles of precision medicine and reducing unnecessary procedures and healthcare costs.
- Despite promising advancements, integrating AI into IR faces challenges such as data standardization, regulatory compliance, and maintaining ethical standards. Overcoming these challenges requires continued research, collaboration between AI developers and healthcare professionals, and adherence to regulatory guidelines to ensure safe and effective AI implementation in clinical practice.

GLOSSARY OF TERMS AND DEFINITIONS

TACE: transarterial chemoembolization

Introduction

Interventional radiology (IR) leverages imaging techniques such as fluoroscopy (continuous x-ray), computed tomography (CT) scans, ultrasound, and magnetic resonance imaging (MRI) to guide minimally invasive surgical procedures. These procedures often involve the use of catheters, guide wires, and other devices to diagnose and treat a variety of conditions, including vascular disease, cancer, and organ abnormalities. The primary advantages of IR over traditional surgery include reduced risk, less pain, and quicker recovery times, making it a preferred option for many patients.[1]

Despite these benefits, IR faces significant challenges, particularly in predicting procedural outcomes and optimizing treatment plans; this is where artificial intelligence (AI) can play a transformative role. Much like surgical subspecialties, IR has been slow to adopt AI solutions. Unlike most surgical subspecialties, however, IR has the advantage of being data rich with the massive trove of imaging information available. IR procedures are recorded and stored in a standardized format and can be accessed retrospectively.[2]

Recent years have seen innovative approaches to AI in IR, such as procedural planning and guidance, where it can analyze patient imaging data to plan the most effective procedural approach, predict potential complications, and provide real-time guidance during procedures.[3]

Additionally, AI can predict the success rates of specific treatments for individual patients by learning from historical data, thereby reducing unnecessary procedures and associated risks. Workflow optimization is another area where AI can streamline scheduling and resource allocation, ensuring that IR teams are utilized efficiently and patient wait times are minimized. Furthermore, AI can assist in post-procedure analysis by evaluating the effectiveness of procedures, monitoring patient recovery, and identifying areas for improvement in future interventions.[4]

Although these AI applications are still developing, they hold significant potential for future integration into IR practice. As AI technologies continue to advance, their potential to revolutionize interventional radiology becomes increasingly evident. This chapter will describe interpretive AI applications in IR, divided into pre- and periprocedural uses.

Preprocedural Uses

Image analysis has the potential to improve diagnostic accuracy and efficiency in the workflow. For example, AI algorithms are being developed to automatically identify and segment specific structures in images, such as tumors or blood vessels. This can help radiologists more quickly and accurately identify areas of interest and make treatment decisions. Aidoc Medical, Inc. (Tel Aviv, Israel) is the manufacturer of many FDA-cleared algorithms for identifying abnormalities on angiography (BriefCase Pulmonary Embolism Triage, BriefCase Aortic Dissection, BriefCase Brain Aneurysm, BriefCase Intracranial Hemorrhage, BriefCase Large Vessel Occlusion).[5] These are all time-sensitive pathologies that may mandate emergent intervention by an IR, and such algorithms can aid in rapidly identifying vascular abnormalities and determining the best course of treatment.

Another area of medical AI development is in predictive modeling, which aims to use AI to predict patient outcomes and tailor treatment plans. This could be particularly useful in IR, where treatments can be invasive and have a wide range of potential outcomes. By incorporating AI into clinical predictive modeling, IR can estimate the benefits of a treatment prior to its completion, minimizing risk to the patient and reducing healthcare costs and unnecessary treatments. Additionally, AI can assist in the development of personalized staging systems and improved therapeutic algorithms, with specific development already performed in hepatocellular carcinoma.[6]

Abaijan et al. used AI to predict transarterial chemoembolization (TACE) outcomes in hepatocellular carcinoma (HCC) patients, achieving an 88.5% negative predictive value based on tumor signal intensity and cirrhosis presence.[7] Fig. 13.1 illustrates how the tool informs treatment selection.

Similarly, studies have successfully predicted procedural outcomes in stroke and brain arteriovenous malformations.[8] For example, AI applications can use CT perfusion and CT angiography to estimate physiologic parameters such as penumbral volume, optimizing the selection of patients for endovascular clot retrieval.[2] Although AI can identify correlations between disease and treatment, it does not provide insights into causality, which can be obtained from randomized controlled trials, making AI a complementary tool in designing optimal treatment strategies.

Periprocedural Uses

Intra-arterial therapies for HCC involve carefully selecting the branches of the hepatic artery that are supplying the tumor and embolizing those vessels for targeted radiation/chemotherapy and ischemia to the tumor cells. Careful selection of the correct vessels can be time consuming, as there is risk for damage to normal liver parenchyma if nontarget embolization is done. Liver

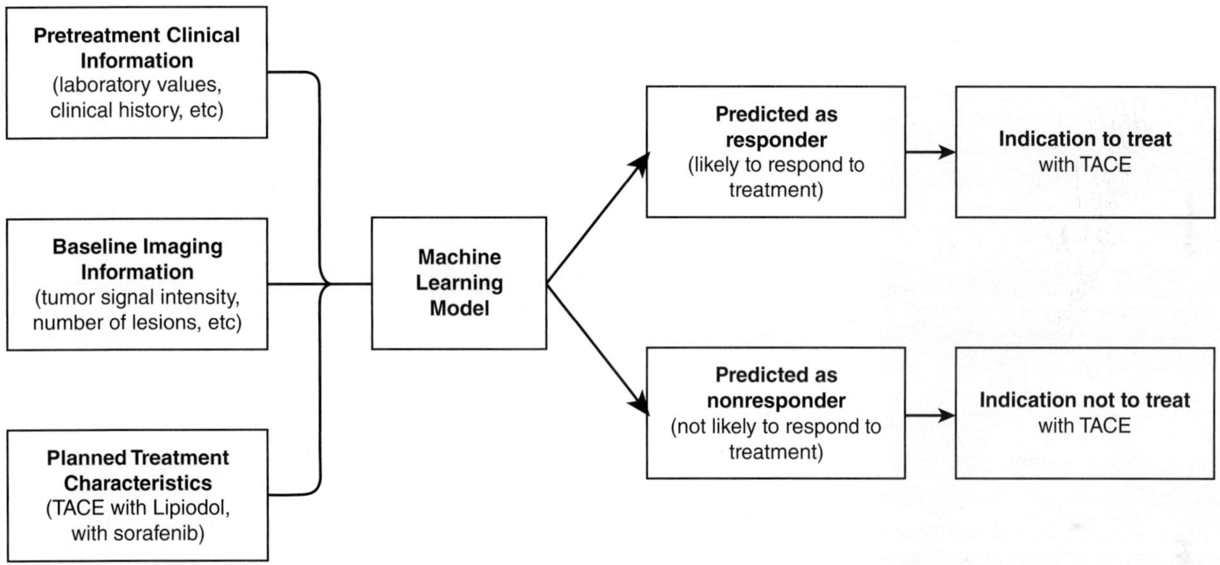

Fig. 13.1 Clinical application of machine learning models for response prediction. Illustrates the clinical application of machine learning models trained to predict response to loco-regional treatment and thereby inform treatment selection. Learning model classification of patient treatment response using pretreatment data in combination with a planned treatment protocol can be used as an indication to treat or not to treat with transarterial chemoembolization.

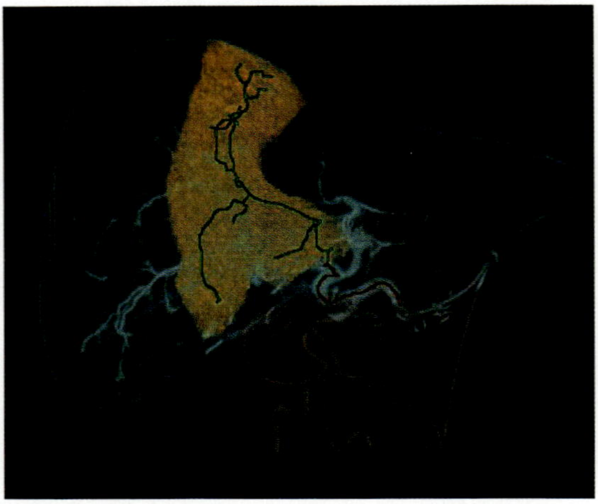

Fig. 13.2 Liver ASSIST Virtual Parenchyma (GE Healthcare) provides artificial intelligence–based virtual parenchymography, allowing the user to visualize the optimal strategy for target embolization.

ASSIST Virtual Parenchyma (GE HealthCare, Chicago, IL) is an FDA-cleared AI algorithm that allows IRs to simulate their injections dynamically, aiding them in identifying the patient's unique hepatic artery anatomy during the planning phase of their procedures (Fig. 13.2).[9] Retrospective studies have shown that this software in conjunction with a single proximal cone beam computed tomography scan (CBCT) are accurate in identifying optimal liver embolization strategy, avoiding the need for multiple selective acquisitions.[10,11] Similarly, Embo ASSIST AI (GE HealthCare) is FDA cleared to aid the interventionalist in the 3D visualization of vasculature for planning their embolization procedures in other organs.[12]

In the periprocedural phase, where real-time decision-making is crucial, AI can facilitate selection of the appropriate catheter, sheath, or implant, such as stents, for treating stenotic vascular lesions or aortic aneurysms.[13] This ensures that the most suitable devices are chosen based on precise anatomical and pathological data, reduces the time taken to select a device, and reduces waste. Furthermore, AI can estimate fractional flow reserve (FFR) in real time using fluoroscopic imaging, which is vital for identifying ischemia-related stenosis in coronary artery or venous disease.[14] This capability can be applied to IR for the treatment of peripheral vascular disease.

Although image reconstruction is technically a noninterpretive application of AI, superimposing preoperative 3D CT images onto 2D intraoperative angiography images are shown to be a valuable procedural planning tool, for example in aortic endovascular repair and embolization of an arterial bleed (Figs. 13.3 and 13.4). By integrating these AI-driven tools, IRs can achieve higher precision and efficiency during their procedures.

Challenges

There may be conflicts of interest between radiologists and AI developers, as the latter may not share the altruistic goals of healthcare and may be hesitant to share data between companies. A joint European and North American multisociety came to a consensus that AI may introduce highly consequential systemic errors and that it is not yet clear how to best integrate AI into clinical practice.[16] More research is needed to mitigate such potential systematic errors, but the use of AI must be guided by principles of freedom, dignity, privacy, transparency, dependability, responsibility, accountability, and diversity and inclusion. Examples of potential challenges and their solutions as may be encountered in interventional radiology is represented in Table 13.1.

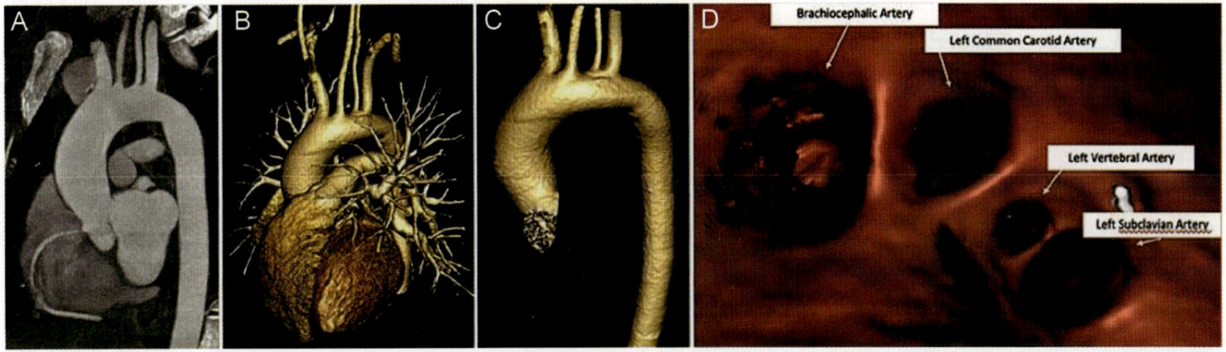

Fig. 13.3 Endovascular navigation: virtual aortoscopy. (A) Preoperative CT image; (B and C) 3D volume rendering of aorta; (D) creation of virtual angioscopy of the aorta. (From Gurgitano M, Angileri SA, Rodà GM, et al. Interventional radiology ex-machina: impact of artificial intelligence on practice. *Radiol Med*. 2021;126:998–1006.)

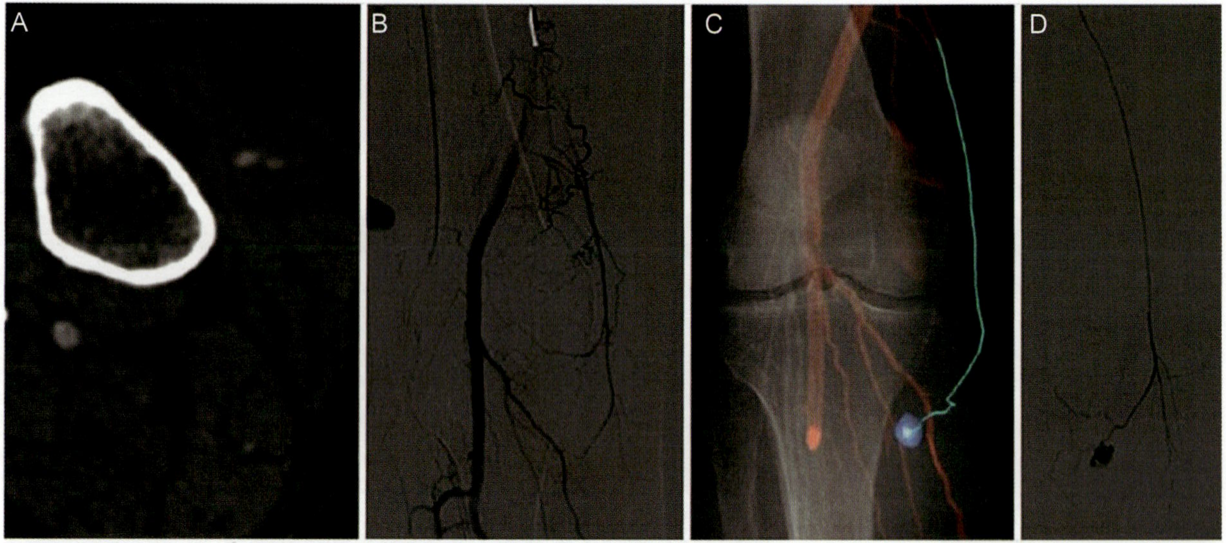

Fig. 13.4 Automatic 3D detection of arterial bleeding of the leg in a traumatic patient. (A) CT angiography (CTA) reveals arterial bleeding of the leg in a traumatic patient. (B) Initial 2D angiography does not demonstrate bleeding. (C) Target segmentation was performed on the CTA dataset after cone-beam CT (CBCT-CT) fusion; then 3D CBCT datasets were synchronized with the C-arm and overlaid on live fluoroscopy, during the intervention, to facilitate catheter navigation to the damaged vessel. (D) Once the target arterial culprit was engaged, a selective angiogram is performed to confirm correct targeting of the bleeding site. (From Gurgitano M, Angileri SA, Rodà GM, et al. Interventional radiology ex-machina: impact of artificial intelligence on practice. *Radiol Med*. 2021;126:998–1006.)

TABLE 13.1 ■ **Challenges and Solutions**

	Challenge	Example	Solution
Data Quality and Standardization	IR procedures generate vast amounts of data, but inconsistencies in data collection, storage, and formatting across institutions can hinder AI development.	Variations in imaging protocols or reporting standards between hospitals can lead to biased or ineffective AI models.	Develop and implement standardized data collection protocols and imaging standards across IR departments. Initiatives like the Society of Interventional Radiology Standardized Reports Committee can guide standardized reporting.
Data Privacy and Security	Sharing patient data for AI development raises concerns about privacy and data protection.	Multiinstitutional collaborations for AI research may be hindered by data-sharing restrictions.	Implement advanced anonymization techniques and secure data sharing platforms. Explore federated learning approaches that allow AI models to be trained across multiple institutions without directly sharing patient data.
Regulatory Compliance	Navigating the complex and evolving regulatory landscape for AI in healthcare.	The FDA's regulatory framework for AI/ML-based Software as a Medical Device (SaMD) is still evolving, creating a level of uncertainty for developers and healthcare providers.	Engage proactively with regulatory bodies. Develop AI systems with built-in mechanisms for ongoing performance monitoring and updates to align with the FDA's proposed predetermined change control plan.
Clinical Integration and Workflow Disruption	Integrating AI tools into existing clinical workflows without causing disruption or increasing workload.	An AI tool for procedure planning that requires significant additional time or steps may face resistance from time-constrained IR professionals.	Design AI systems with a focus on user experience and seamless integration. Involve end-users (interventional radiologists) in the development process to ensure tools enhance rather than complicate workflows.
Interpretability and Explainability	Many advanced AI models, particularly deep learning systems, operate as "black boxes," making their decision-making process opaque.	An AI system recommending against a particular IR procedure without clear reasoning may not be trusted by clinicians.	Develop explainable AI models that provide clear rationales for their recommendations. Implement visualization tools that highlight the features influencing AI decisions.

Continued

TABLE 13.1 ■ **Challenges and Solutions–cont'd**

	Challenge	Example	Solution
Bias and Generalizability	AI models trained on limited or biased datasets may not perform well across diverse patient populations.	An AI model for predicting outcomes of liver embolization procedures trained primarily on data from Caucasian patients may not be accurate for patients of other ethnicities.	Ensure diverse and representative datasets for AI training. Implement rigorous testing across different patient populations and regularly monitor AI performance for potential biases.
Ethical Considerations	Balancing the benefits of AI with ethical concerns such as patient autonomy and the changing role of healthcare providers.	Over-reliance on AI recommendations could potentially erode clinical judgment and doctor-patient relationships.	Develop clear guidelines for the ethical use of AI in IR. Emphasize AI as a supportive tool rather than a replacement for clinical expertise. Incorporate AI use into clinical consents. Implement ongoing ethics training for healthcare providers using AI systems.
Liability and Responsibility	Determining liability in cases where AI recommendations contribute to adverse outcomes.	If an AI system fails to flag a potential complication during an IR procedure, questions may arise about who is responsible—the AI developer, the hospital, or the interventional radiologist.	Develop clear frameworks for AI liability in healthcare. Ensure proper documentation of AI use in clinical decision-making to help determine when AI recommendations contribute to medical errors. Maintain human oversight and final decision-making authority in AI-assisted procedures.
Cost and Resource Allocation	High costs associated with AI development, implementation, and maintenance.	Smaller hospitals or rural healthcare centers may struggle to afford advanced AI systems for IR.	Explore collaborative AI development and sharing models among healthcare institutions. Develop scalable AI solutions that can be implemented at various resource levels.
Continuous Learning and Updating	Ensuring AI systems remain up to date and effective as medical knowledge and practices evolve.	An AI model for procedure planning may become outdated as new IR techniques or devices are introduced.	Implement systems for continuous monitoring and updating of AI models. Develop AI architectures that can incorporate new data and adapt to changing clinical practices. Be prepared to modify or discontinue AI tools that are found to be ineffective or harmful.

AI, Artificial intelligence; *IR*, interventional radiology; *ML*, machine learning.

A specific challenge to the implementation of AI in IR is the significant amount of data required to train the algorithms. The ever-changing nature of clinical practice can limit the pool of relevant retrospective data. Additionally, the interpretability and annotated data required for AI can pose a challenge. It has been suggested that the best approach is to combine multiple technologies with human experts and use AI as a tool to assist rather than replace radiologists. The FDA has also issued guidance on the regulation of AI instruments in medical imaging, which must be adhered to by manufacturers and healthcare providers. Despite these challenges, the potential for AI to improve patient care and assist radiologists in the diagnostic process makes it a promising area of research and development in interventional radiology.

Future Directions

As artificial intelligence continues to evolve, several emerging trends and potential developments are poised to further transform interventional radiology. Future AI models in IR are likely to employ more sophisticated deep learning architectures, such as transformer models and federated learning, potentially leading to more accurate predictions and better generalization across diverse patient populations. The integration of multiple imaging modalities (e.g., CT, MRI, ultrasound) with clinical data in AI models is an emerging trend that could provide more comprehensive insights for treatment planning and outcome prediction in complex IR procedures.

The development of AI systems capable of providing real-time guidance during IR procedures is a promising area. These systems could offer instant feedback on catheter positioning, embolization progress, or potential complications, enhancing procedural safety and efficacy. Furthermore, future AI models may incorporate genetic and molecular data alongside imaging to create highly personalized treatment plans, which could be particularly impactful in interventional oncology, allowing for tailored approaches based on tumor genetics and expected treatment response.

AI-driven systems for automated procedure reporting and intelligent follow-up scheduling are likely to emerge, streamlining workflow, ensuring consistent documentation, and optimizing patient monitoring post-procedure. The combination of AI with virtual and augmented reality technologies could revolutionize procedural planning and training in IR, generating realistic simulations for complex cases and enhancing preprocedural planning and resident education.

The development of AI-guided robotic systems for IR procedures is an exciting prospect that could potentially enhance precision in challenging anatomical locations and reduce radiation exposure to operators. AI algorithms could also be employed to predict equipment failures or maintenance needs, reducing downtime and improving resource allocation in IR suites. Advanced natural language processing models could be developed to extract relevant information from radiology reports and clinical notes, aiding in patient selection and procedure planning.

As AI becomes more integrated into clinical practice, there will likely be a push toward more transparent and explainable AI models. This could involve the development of AI systems that can provide clear rationales for their recommendations, enhancing trust and adoption among clinicians. Future AI applications may also focus on quality assurance in IR, automatically detecting deviations from best practices or identifying potential errors in procedural workflows.

Initiatives for secure, anonymized data sharing across institutions and countries could lead to more robust and generalizable AI models in IR, potentially addressing current limitations in data availability and diversity. Although these future directions hold great promise, their realization will require continued research, interdisciplinary collaboration, and careful consideration of ethical and regulatory implications. As AI technology advances, it will be crucial for the IR community to actively engage in its development and implementation to ensure that these innovations truly enhance patient care and clinical outcomes.

Conclusion

The integration of AI in interventional radiology holds great promise for revolutionizing the field. AI applications span across the planning and decision-making surrounding a procedure, enhancing the precision, efficiency, and safety of interventions. By leveraging AI algorithms for image analysis, treatment planning, and real-time guidance, IR practitioners can optimize patient selection, improve procedural outcomes, and reduce complications. Moreover, AI's ability to process and interpret vast amounts of clinical data enables personalized treatment strategies, mirroring the principles of precision medicine. Despite current challenges such as data standardization, regulatory considerations, and integration into clinical workflows, the promising results from AI-driven initiatives in IR underscore its pivotal role in shaping the future of minimally invasive procedures. Continued research, collaboration, and refinement of AI technologies will be essential to fully harness its potential and further enhance patient care in interventional radiology.

References

1. What Is Interventional Radiology? WebMD. Medically Reviewed by Poonam Sachdev. MD on February 12, 2024.
2. Seah J, Boeken T, Sapoval M, Goh GS. Prime time for artificial intelligence in interventional radiology. *Cardiovasc Intervent Radiol.* 2022;45:283–289. https://doi.org/10.1007/s00270-021-03044-4.
3. Mazaheri S, Loya MF, Newsome J, Lungren M, Gichoya JW. Challenges of implementing artificial intelligence in interventional radiology. *Semin Intervent Radiol.* 2021;38(5):554–559. http://doi.org/10.1055/s-0041-1736659.
4. von Ende E, Ryan S, Crain MA, Makary MS. Artificial intelligence, augmented reality, and virtual reality advances and applications in interventional radiology. *Diagnostics (Basel).* 2023;13(5):892. http://doi.org/10.3390/diagnostics13050892.
5. https://aicentral.acrdsi.org/Manufacturer/Aidoc-Medical–Ltd.
6. Zhong BY, Ni CF, Ji JS, et al. Nomogram and artificial neural network for prognostic performance on the albumin-bilirubin grade for hepatocellular carcinoma undergoing transarterial chemoembolization. *J Vasc Interv Radiol.* 2019;30(3):330–338. http://doi.org/10.1016/j.jvir.2018.08.026.
7. Abajian A, Murali N, Savic LJ, et al. Predicting treatment response to intra-arterial therapies for hepatocellular carcinoma with the use of supervised machine learning-an artificial intelligence concept. *J Vasc Interv Radiol.* 2018;29(6):850–857.e1. http://doi.org/10.1016/j.jvir.2018.01.769.
8. Asadi H, Kok HK, Looby S, Brennan P, O'Hare A, Thornton J. Outcomes and complications after endovascular treatment of brain arteriovenous malformations: a prognostication attempt using artificial intelligence. *World Neurosurg.* 2016;96:562–569.e1. http://doi.org/10.1016/j.wneu.2016.09.086.
9. https://aicentral.acrdsi.org/All-Ai-products/Liver-ASSIST-Virtual-Parenchyma.
10. Deschamps F, Gill A, Tselikas L, et al. Abstract no. 544 evaluation of software predicting selective liver perfusion for embolization planning. *J Vasc Interv Radiol.* 2021;32(5):S148–S149. https://www.jvir.org/article/S1051-0443(21)00739-9/fulltext.
11. Chevallier O, Yarmohammadi H, Zhao K, et al. Abstract no. 248 accuracy of a cone-beam CT-based liver-directed therapy planning software for perfused parenchyma prediction. *J Vasc Interv Radiol.* 2023;34(3):S112–S113.https://www.jvir.org/article/S1051-0443(22)01738-9/pdf.https://doi.org/10.1016/j.jvir.2022.12.311.
12. https://aicentral.acrdsi.org/All-Ai-products/Embo-ASSIST-AI.
13. Meek RD, Lungren MP, Gichoya JW. Machine learning for the interventional radiologist. *Am J Roentgenol.* 2019;213:782–784. http://doi.org/10.2214/AJR.19.21527.
14. Cho H, Lee JG, Kang SJ, et al. Angiography-based machine learning for predicting fractional flow reserve in intermediate coronary artery lesions. *J Am Heart Assoc.* 2019;8(4):e011685. http://doi.org/10.1161/JAHA.118.011685.
15. Gurgitano M, Angileri SA, Rodà GM, et al. Interventional Radiology ex-machina: impact of Artificial Intelligence on practice. *Radiol Med.* 2021;126:998–1006. https://doi.org/10.1007/s11547-021-01351-x.
16. Geis JR, Brady AP, Wu CC, et al. Ethics of artificial intelligence in radiology: summary of the joint European and North American multisociety statement. *Can Assoc Radiol J.* 2019;70:329–334.

CHAPTER 14

Artificial Intelligence in Nuclear Radiology: Unlocking the Potential for Enhanced Patient

Nadeen Aladham ■ Rajat Chand

KEY POINTS

- AI, particularly through ANNs and CNNs, is enhancing nuclear medicine by improving image quality, enabling precise dosimetry, and supporting personalized patient care with tailored radiation doses.
- Multimodal imaging combining data from CT, MRI, PET, and SPECT offers comprehensive tumor characterization, aiding in accurate diagnosis, staging, and treatment planning for oncology applications.
- Challenges for AI implementation in nuclear medicine include the need for large, high-quality datasets, model transparency, and addressing ethical concerns like data bias and algorithmic fairness.

GLOSSARY OF TERMS AND DEFINITIONS

Artificial Intelligence: The simulation of human intelligence by machines, particularly for complex problem-solving and decision-making tasks in medical imaging and diagnostics.

Convolutional Autoencoder (CAE): A type of neural network used for data compression and denoising in image processing ("which helps" versus "helping") to improve image quality.

Convolutional Neural Networks (CNNs): A type of neural network architecture particularly suited for image processing tasks, capable of detecting spatial hierarchies and features in images.

Dosimetry: The calculation and assessment of the radiation dose received by the body, essential for ensuring safe and effective nuclear medicine treatments.

Generative Adversarial Network (GAN): A machine learning model where two networks train against each other to create high-fidelity synthetic data, often used in image reconstruction.

Image Reconstruction: The process of generating high-quality images from raw imaging data, crucial for enhancing diagnostic accuracy and reducing noise in nuclear medicine.

Multimodal Imaging: The combination of multiple imaging techniques, such as CT, MRI, PET, and SPECT, to provide a comprehensive view of anatomical and functional information.

Nuclear Medicine: A medical specialty using small amounts of radioactive materials to diagnose and treat various diseases, providing insights into both anatomy and physiology.

Radiomic Analysis: The extraction and analysis of large amounts of quantitative features from medical images, aiding in diagnostic and prognostic assessments.

U-nets: A deep learning architecture designed for biomedical image segmentation, using skip connections to retain high-resolution features for enhanced image clarity.

In recent years, artificial intelligence (AI) has emerged as a disruptive force across various fields, and this includes nuclear radiology.[1] Although much attention has focused on how AI affects radiology, it is important to consider its impact on the subfield of nuclear medicine. By understanding the principles and applications of AI as well as its evolving, seemingly complex language, nuclear medicine professionals as a whole will soon be able to confidently integrate this advanced technology into their workflows. Embracing and actively educating oneself on these innovations will allow practitioners and technologists alike to adapt to future roles, optimize patient care, and ideally avoid realization of fears about AI's potentials.

AI's integration into nuclear medicine has made remarkable progress, particularly with the rise of artificial neural networks (ANNs) and convolutional neural networks (CNNs). These advanced technologies are paving the way for improved analysis of radiomic features and enhanced reporting accuracy through improved image quality, thus enabling more precise dosimetry for personalized treatment.[1]

According to a review article by Cheng et al., the integration of artificial intelligence in nuclear medicine imaging aims for a dual objective, marking a transformative shift toward precision medicine in nuclear imaging, optimizing both diagnostic efficacy and therapeutic safety. AI-based nuclear imaging and reconstruction techniques for both image creation and reconstruction aim to provide more accurate tracking of radiotracer distribution while minimizing artifacts, boosting diagnostic precision. In addition, new dosimetry models will offer personalized radiation dose mapping, considering the unique anatomical and physiological features of each patient, ensuring a safer and more effective treatment plan.[2]

Nuclear imaging has long faced technical challenges, particularly with the inherent trade-off between noise reduction and spatial resolution, which becomes even more pronounced in low-dose settings with current reconstruction methods (Fig. 14.1).[2] Nonuniform signal distribution related to attenuation and scatter also complicates current gamma photon imaging methods. These limitations underscore the need for more sophisticated approaches, yet which remain practical in real time.

One notable application of AI in nuclear medicine is the integration of multimodal imaging using structural and functional data from various modalities such as CT, MRI, positron emission tomography (PET), and single-photon emission computed tomography (SPECT) to create a more comprehensive view of oncological pathology. This integration allows for precise tumor localization and characterization, essential for effective diagnostic and therapeutic interventions. By combining anatomical details from CT and MRI with metabolic insights from PET or SPECT, multimodal imaging offers a robust approach to identifying and treating malignancies. This methodology has gained traction in oncology and nuclear medicine, as it aids in tumor detection, staging, and therapy planning, offering detailed insights that surpass the capabilities of any single imaging technique.[3]

In a multicenter radiation oncology study researchers investigated a novel deep learning framework designed to generate three-dimensional (3D) volumetric images from patient surface images, with the goal of reducing radiation exposure associated with computed tomography imaging (Fig. 14.2).[4] The dataset consisted of 500 CT image sets from 50 patients. The framework employed a generative adversarial network (GAN) model, consisting of reconstruction, verification, and refinement networks, to predict internal anatomical structures from external surface images. The

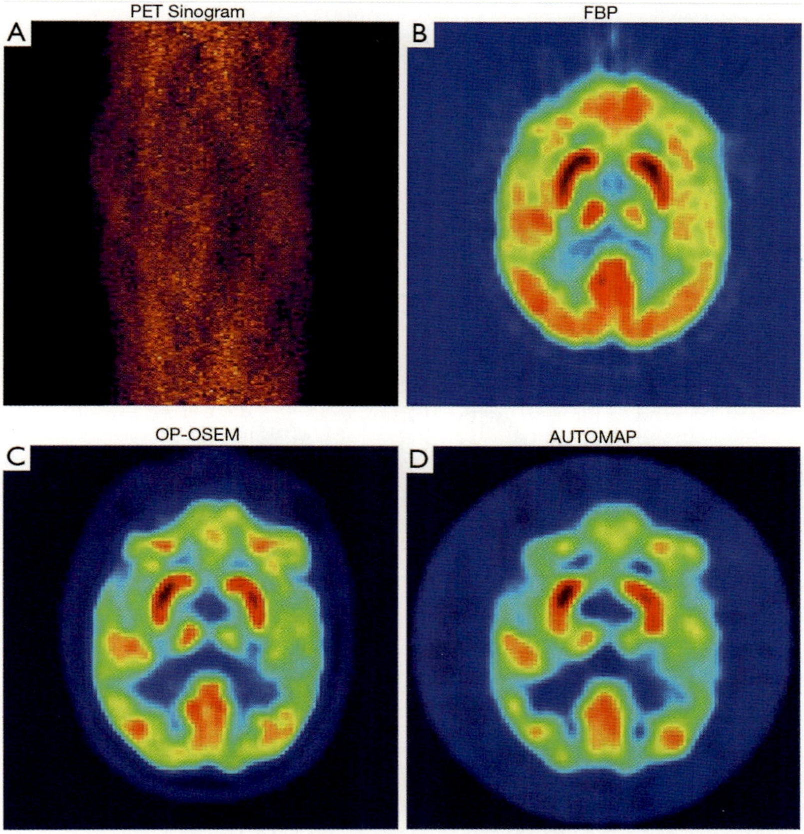

Fig. 14.1 Reconstruction results using the traditional algorithm and Zhu et al.'s method. Human FDG PET sinogram data (A) was reconstructed using (B) filter back projection (FBP), (C) ordinary Poisson ordered subsets expectation maximization (OP-OSEM), and (D) automated transform by manifold approximation (AUTOMAP). Compared with FBP, artificial intelligence results are significantly improved and can generate results that are visually similar to OP-OSEM algorithms. (From Cheng Z, Wen J, Huang G, Yan J. Applications of artificial intelligence in nuclear medicine image generation. *Quant Imaging Med Surg.* 2021;11(6):2792–2822.)

results illustrated the model's high fidelity in synthesizing CT-like images, suggesting that this approach could offer real-time, radiation-free imaging for radiotherapy guidance, enhancing patient safety by eliminating ionizing radiation risk.[5]

Machine learning application in nuclear medicine extends into thyroid disease diagnostics, addressing challenges like interobserver variability and diagnostic subjectivity in ultrasound interpretation. With the high prevalence of thyroid nodules, accurately differentiating benign from malignant ones is essential. Traditional diagnostics often rely solely on ultrasound images; however, their efficacy in distinguishing between benign follicular adenomas and malignant follicular carcinomas remains limited due to the subtlety of morphological differences.

A recent study by Lin et al. evaluating thyroid follicular adenoma or carcinoma patients at a single institution explored a novel, multimodal machine learning (ML) model that integrates both clinical and imaging data to enhance the diagnostic accuracy of thyroid pathologies. The study built an AI multimodal that incorporated both clinical variables (e.g., Bethesda classification) and

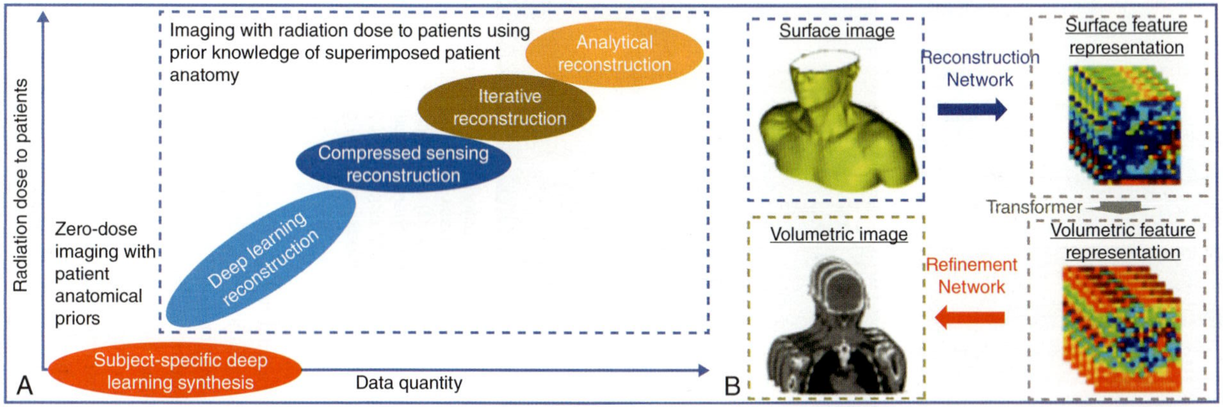

Fig. 14.2 Volumetric image reconstruction using X-ray projections and nonionizing radiation surface images. (A) Mechanical- and deep learning–based image reconstruction schemes. (B) Volumetric image reconstruction using a surface image. (From Pan S, Chang CW, Axente M, et al. Data-driven volumetric image generation from surface structures using a patient-specific deep learning model. *ArXiv*. 2023.)

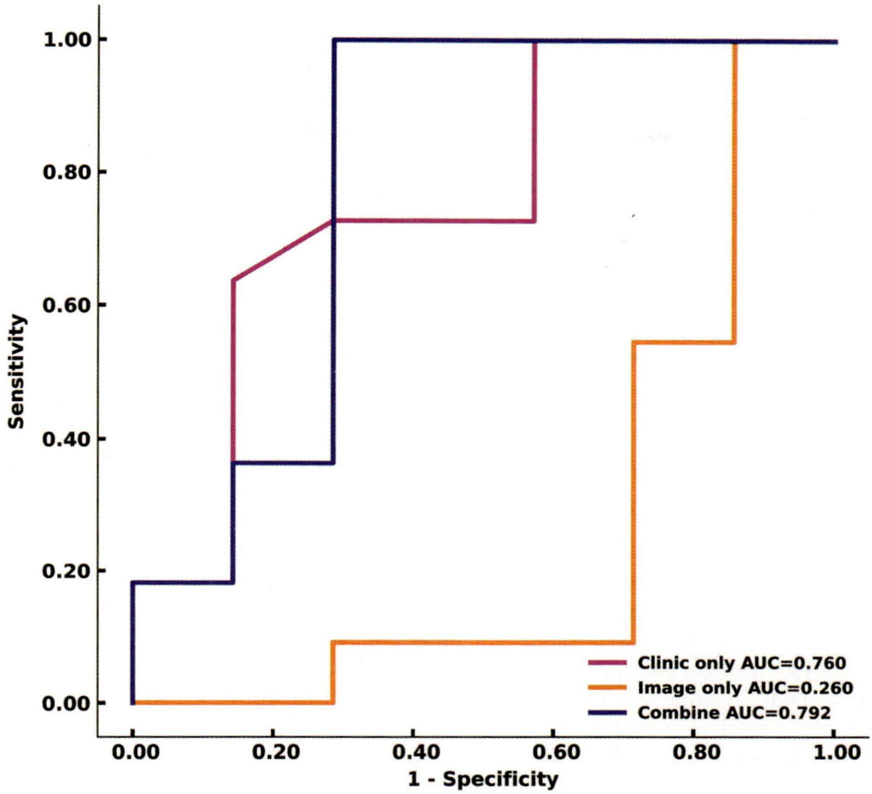

Fig. 14.3 Receiver operating characteristic curves of clinical only, image only, and multimodal model performance are shown. The area under the curve values demonstrates the improved performance of the multimodal model (0.792) in comparison with the clinical-only model (0.759) and image-only model (0.260). AUC is the area under the curve. (From Lin AC, Liu Z, Lee J, et al. Generating a multimodal artificial intelligence model to differentiate benign and malignant follicular neoplasms of the thyroid: a proof-of-concept study. *Surgery*. 2024;175(1):121–127.)

imaging features (e.g., nodule size on ultrasound) to predict malignancy. The results indicated that the multimodal combining imaging and clinical data achieved a prediction success rate of 79%, demonstrating improved predictive accuracy over models using clinical or imaging data alone. The multimodal model also showed enhanced sensitivity and specificity (Fig. 14.3). The study concluded that the combined data model using the multimodal performed better in distinguishing benign from malignant follicular neoplasms, showing promise for future applications in preoperative diagnostic support.[5]

The rapid advancement of AI in nuclear radiology has given rise to several companies developing cutting-edge solutions for the field.[6] These companies have been instrumental in shaping nuclear radiology by introducing AI applications approved by the U.S. Food and Drug Administration (FDA) that promise to transform patient care and improve workflow efficiency in nuclear radiology departments.

One organization making strides in AI-based nuclear radiology is RECOMIA, a not-for-profit dedicated to advancing AI and medical imaging research. RECOMIA has developed a cloud-based platform that fosters collaboration between medical and mathematical researchers, enabling automated analysis of 3D CT, PET/CT, and MRI scans.[7] Their platform includes deep learning tools for organ segmentation, lesion detection, and quantitative analysis, showing high accuracy and reproducibility comparable to manual work by radiologists while significantly reducing analysis time. RECOMIA's commitment to open access has made its AI applications freely available, furthering advancements in nuclear radiology.

Another key player is Aidoc, which specializes in AI-based radiology solutions. Aidoc's FDA-approved AI platform provides comprehensive support for nuclear radiology by detecting and prioritizing critical findings in CT and PET/CT scans. Their deep learning algorithms flag abnormalities, offering radiologists an AI-powered second opinion. Studies have shown this technology improves detection rates and reduces turnaround times. Aidoc's platform integrates seamlessly into existing workflows, boosting efficiency and enabling radiologists to focus on urgent cases.[8]

Lindgren Belal et al. used RECOMIA's bone segmentation tool to quantify bone metastases in PET/CT scans of prostate cancer patients (Fig. 14.4).[9] The automated tumor burden measurements were associated with overall survival. Another study used AI-based segmentation of the prostate in [18F]-choline PET/CT scans, yielding automated standardized uptake values that correlated well with manually derived measurements (Fig. 14.5).[10] These studies collectively underscore early evidence of the accuracy and efficiency of AI applications in nuclear radiology.

AI has also shown promise in the realm of myocardial perfusion imaging. ANNs trained on large datasets have outperformed traditional methods. For instance, a multicenter study involving 1638 patients from 9 different centers that evaluated the use of deep learning for predicting obstructive coronary artery disease from myocardial perfusion SPECT imaging found that deep learning outperformed the conventional total perfusion deficit (TPD) score in predicting obstructive disease (Fig. 14.6).[11] Similarly, another study used a 3D deep learning algorithm to evaluate 1861 patients who underwent myocardial perfusion imaging and found that the deep learning model significantly outperformed TPD in predicting obstructive CAD, without requiring manual correction or normal database (Fig. 14.7).[12]

One of the main challenges in nuclear medicine is to minimize patient exposure to radiation while maintaining high image quality, especially with repeated or high-dose imaging modalities. AI models, including CNNs, U-nets, and GANs, play a pivotal role in this context by supporting dose reduction while sustaining diagnostic accuracy and image quality (Fig. 14.8). These models, particularly in low-dose imaging, can effectively and more expeditiously enhance image resolution and denoise data, compensating for the reduced signal typically associated with lower radiation doses.[12]

Anatomical image-guided reconstruction is another way in which advanced AI models, such as U-nets and CNN-based architectures, can be used in the field of nuclear medicine, extracting and aligning anatomical features, allowing for more precise image reconstruction and clearer visualization of physiological processes. It integrates MRI or CT data with PET/SPECT imaging to improve diagnostic clarity by enhancing structural detail and compensating for limitations in nuclear medicine imaging alone. In this approach, MRI or CT images provide high-resolution anatomical context, which is incorporated into the reconstruction algorithms of PET and SPECT, effectively refining image quality and accuracy. This integration helps in better defining tissue boundaries, improving attenuation correction, and enhancing lesion detection, especially in low-dose scenarios.

Lastly, accurate dosimetry is crucial in nuclear therapy to ensure therapeutic effectiveness while minimizing toxicity to surrounding healthy tissues. By precisely calculating the radiation dose delivered to tumors and nearby organs, dosimetry allows for optimized treatment planning and monitoring, which is essential in achieving desired outcomes with minimal adverse effects. Traditional dosimetry methods, such as Monte Carlo simulations and Medical Internal Radiation Dose (MIRD) calculations, are highly reliable for dose estimation but can be computationally intensive and time consuming.[2] These methods model radiation transport and

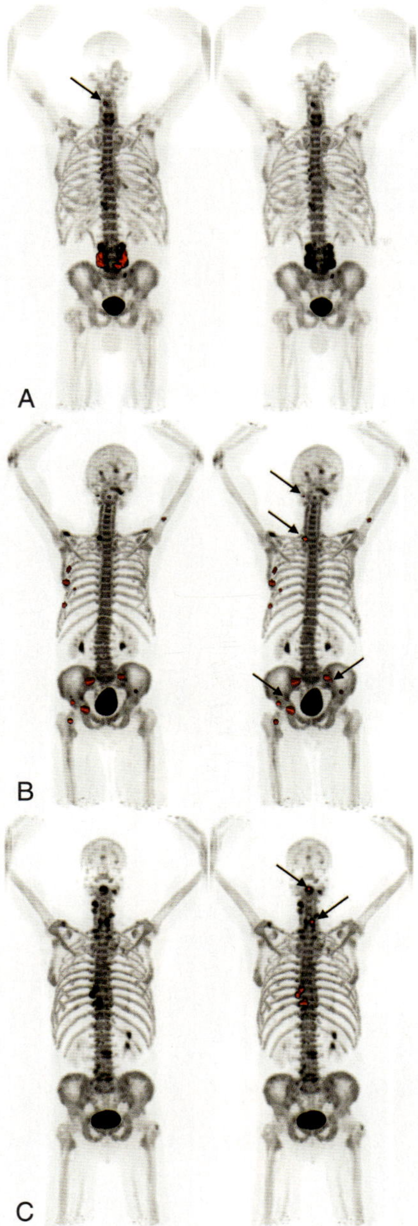

Fig. 14.4 (a) *Left:* The artificial intelligence (AI) model detects suspected metastatic uptake in the lumbar spine and a small lesion in the cervical spine (indicated by the *arrow*), highlighted in *red*. *Right*: None of the physicians identify any lesions in the same patient. (b) *Left*: The AI model identifies several foci in the right ribcage, pelvis, and right hip. *Right*: Reader D notes additional lesions in the skull, spine, and pelvis (indicated by *arrows*). (c) *Left*: Neither the AI model nor the readers detect any lesions. *Right*: Several lesions in the cervical (*arrows*) and thoracic spine. (From Lindgren Belal S, Larsson M, Holm J, et al. Automated quantification of PET/CT skeletal tumor burden in prostate cancer using artificial intelligence: the PET index. *Eur J Nucl Med Mol Imaging*. 2023;50(5):1510–1520.)

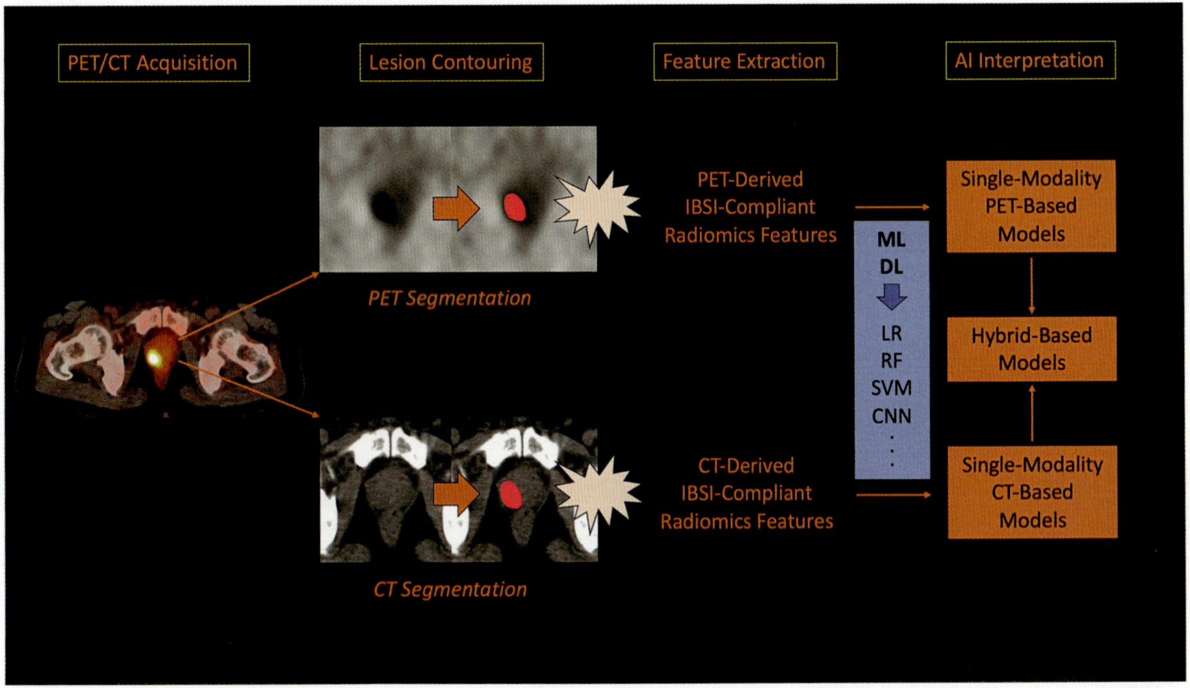

Fig. 14.5 Workflow of radiomics model using different machine/deep learning algorithms. (From Mirshahvalad SA, Eisazadeh R, Shahbazi-Akbari M, Pirich C, Beheshti M. Application of artificial intelligence in oncologic molecular PET-imaging: a narrative review on beyond [18F] F-FDG tracers-part I. PSMA, Choline, and DOTA radiotracers. *Semin Nucl Med*. 2024;54(1):171–180.)

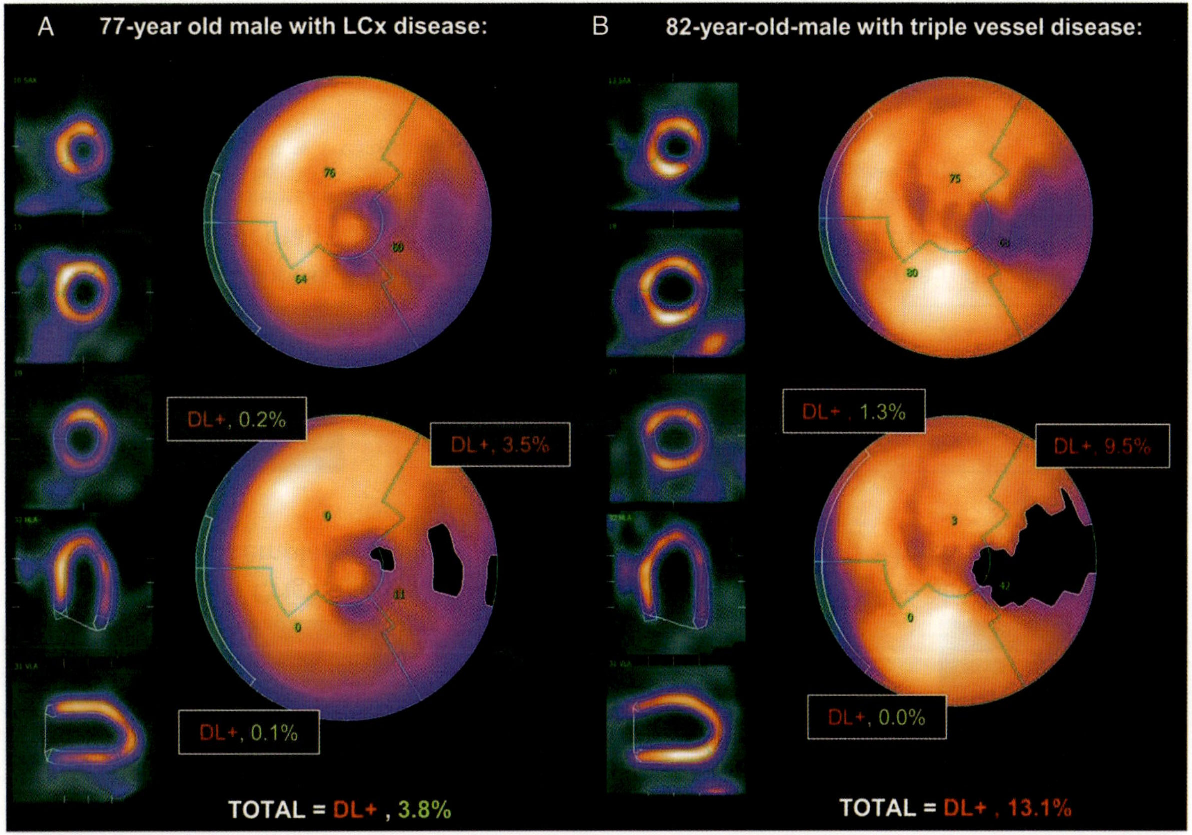

Fig. 14.6 Discrepancies in prediction of obstructive disease from stress myocardial perfusion imaging by deep learning and total perfusion deficit in (A) a patient with left circumflex coronary artery (LCx) and (B) a patient with triple vessel disease. (From Betancur J, Commandeur F, Motlagh M, et al. Deep learning for prediction of obstructive disease from fast myocardial perfusion SPECT: a multicenter study. *JACC Cardiovasc Imaging*. 2018;11(11):1654–1663.)

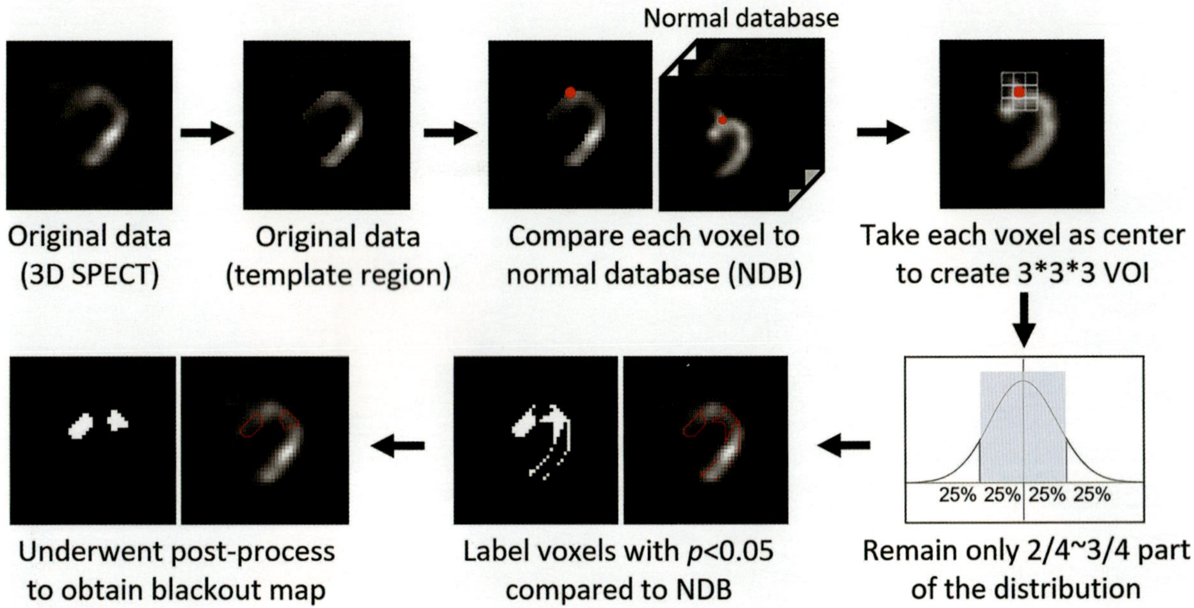

Fig. 14.7 Generation of a spatially matched blackout image to enhance the regions of hypoperfusion in cardiac SPECT. (From Ko CL, Lin SS, Huang CW, et al. Polar map-free 3D deep learning algorithm to predict obstructive coronary artery disease with myocardial perfusion CZT-SPECT. *Eur J Nucl Med Mol Imaging*. 2023;50(2):376–386.)

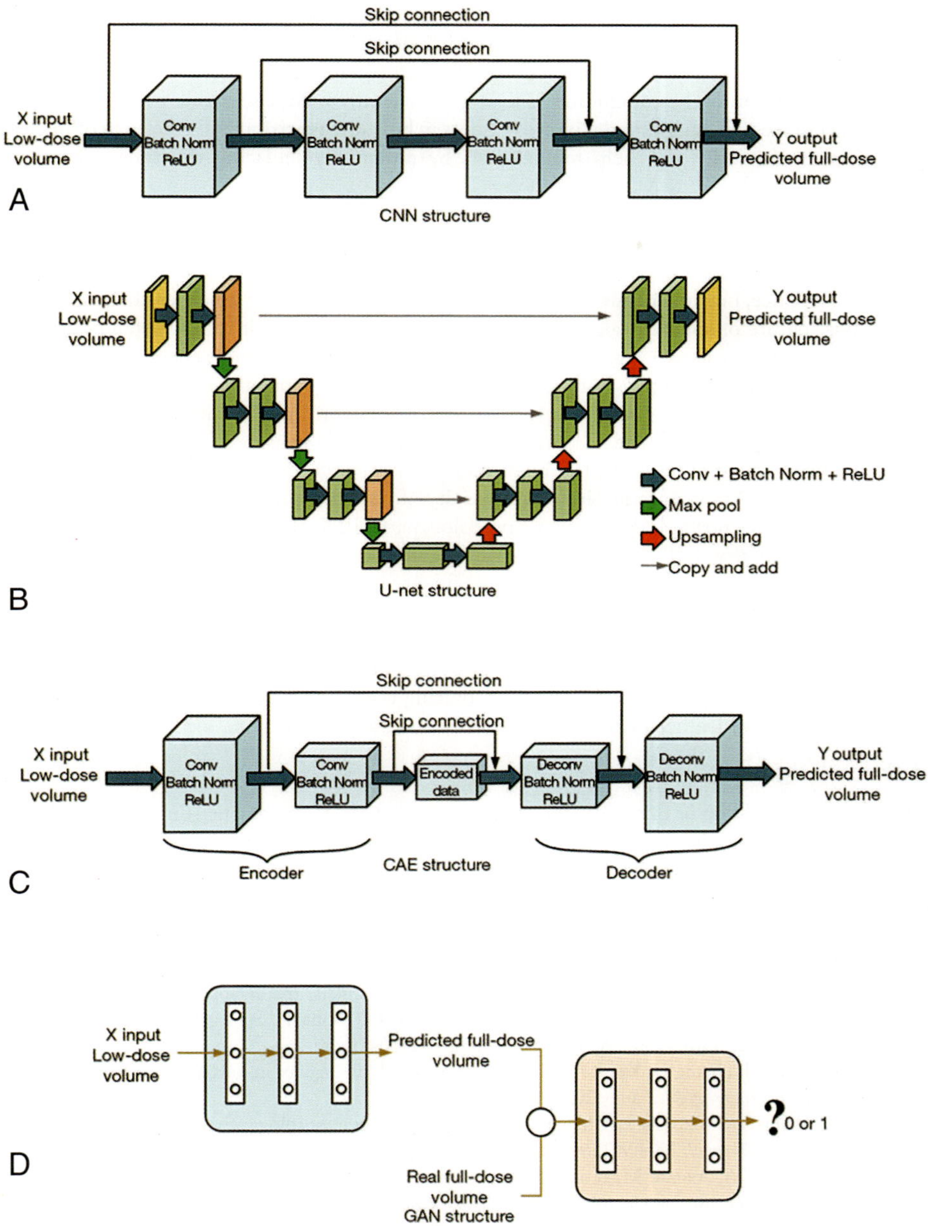

Fig. 14.8 Low-dose imaging network structure. (A) The convolutional neural networks act as a low-pass filter, using convolution to extract features. (B) In U-net, overlapping convolutional layers at each stage deepen the network. (C) Convolutional autoencoder requires specific padding and stride to maintain output size. (D) Generative adversarial network's (GAN) generator creates full-dose images, whereas the discriminator distinguishes between predicted and actual full-dose images. (From Cheng Z, Wen J, Huang G, Yan J. Applications of artificial intelligence in nuclear medicine image generation. *Quant Imaging Med Surg*. 2021;11(6):2792–2822.)

tissue interactions in detail, providing accurate but often retrospective dose assessments. In contrast, AI-based dosimetry models have recently emerged as powerful tools for real-time dose estimation, leveraging machine learning algorithms to predict dose distributions rapidly and adaptively.[13] AI approaches, including CNNs and generative models, enable personalized and timely dosimetry, offering potential improvements in both the precision and efficiency of nuclear therapy planning. They also help reduce costs by potentially replacing the time-consuming traditional methods.

Although machine learning holds immense promise for revolutionizing nuclear medicine, its implementation is not without challenges. One major hurdle is the need for large, high-quality datasets to train AI algorithms effectively. This is particularly difficult in nuclear medicine, where data can be scarce, heterogeneous, and subject to privacy regulations.[14] Another challenge is the "black box" nature of some AI algorithms, which can make it difficult to understand how they arrive at their conclusions.[15] Furthermore, ensuring the robustness and generalizability of AI models across different imaging systems, protocols, and patient populations remains a significant concern. Finally, ethical considerations such as data bias, algorithmic fairness, and the potential displacement of human expertise need to be carefully addressed to ensure the responsible development and deployment of AI in nuclear medicine.[16]

In conclusion, AI's integration into the specialty of nuclear medicine marks a transformative advancement in diagnostic and therapeutic precision, particularly through improvements in imaging quality, dosimetry, and multimodal imaging. By leveraging models like CNNs, U-nets, and GANs, nuclear medicine can now achieve high-fidelity images with reduced radiation exposure, enhancing patient safety without compromising diagnostic accuracy. Although challenges remain in terms of data requirements, model interpretability, and ethical considerations, the ongoing development and refinement of AI technologies hold the potential to revolutionize workflows and patient outcomes in nuclear radiology. Embracing these innovations will be essential for the future of personalized, efficient, and safer nuclear medicine practices.

Acknowledgment

During the preparation of this work, the author(s) used chatGPT, a writing source that uses generative AI technology, in order to generate chapter layouts and content specific to the referenced articles. After using this tool/service, the author(s) reviewed and edited the content as needed and take(s) full responsibility for the content of the publication.

References

1. Decuyper M, Maebe J, Van Holen R, Vandenberghe S. Artificial intelligence with deep learning in nuclear medicine and radiology. In: *EJNMMI Physics* (Vol. 8, Issue 1). Springer Science and Business Media LLC; 2021. https://doi.org/10.1186/s40658-021-00426-y.
2. Cheng Z, Wen J, Huang G, Yan J. Applications of artificial intelligence in nuclear medicine image generation. *Quant Imaging Med Surg*. 2021;11(6):2792–2822.
3. Zong Y, Wang S, Cui Z, Lin L, Chen Y. Multimodal imaging in oncology: challenges and future directions. *Acad J Sci Technol*. 2024;9(2):66–71.
4. Pan S, Chang CW, Axente M, et al. Data-driven volumetric image generation from surface structures using a patient-specific deep learning model. *ArXiv*. 2023.
5. Lin AC, Liu Z, Lee J, et al. Generating a multimodal artificial intelligence model to differentiate benign and malignant follicular neoplasms of the thyroid: a proof-of-concept study. *Surgery*. 2024;175(1):121–127.
6. Nensa F, Demircioglu A, Rischpler C. Artificial intelligence in nuclear medicine. *J Nucl Med*. 2019;60(Supplement 2):29S–37S. Society of Nuclear Medicine. https://doi.org/10.2967/jnumed.118.220590.
7. Trägårdh E, Borrelli P, Kaboteh R, et al. RECOMIA—a cloud-based platform for artificial intelligence research in nuclear medicine and radiologyEJNMMI Physics7. Springer Science and Business Media LLC; 2020. https://doi.org/10.1186/s40658-020-00316-9.
8. Aidoc. *Aidoc: AI for Radiology*; n.d. https://www.aidoc.com/.

9. Lindgren Belal S, Larsson M, Holm J, et al. Automated quantification of PET/CT skeletal tumor burden in prostate cancer using artificial intelligence: the PET index. *Eur J Nucl Med Mol Imaging*. 2023;50(5):1510–1520. https://pubmed.ncbi.nlm.nih.gov/36650356/.
10. Mirshahvalad SA, Eisazadeh R, Shahbazi-Akbari M, Pirich C, Beheshti M. Application of artificial intelligence in oncologic molecular PET-imaging: a narrative review on beyond [18F] F-FDG tracers-part I. PSMA, Choline, and DOTA radiotracers. *Semin Nucl Med*. 2024;54(1):171–180. https://doi.org/10.1053/j.semnuclmed.2023.08.004.
11. Betancur J, Commandeur F, Motlagh M, et al. Deep learning for prediction of obstructive disease from fast myocardial perfusion SPECT: a multicenter study. *JACC Cardiovasc Imaging*. 2018;11(11):1654–1663. https://doi.org/10.1016/j.jcmg.2018.01.020.
12. Ko CL, Lin SS, Huang CW, et al. Polar map-free 3D deep learning algorithm to predict obstructive coronary artery disease with myocardial perfusion CZT-SPECT. *Eur J Nucl Med Mol Imaging*. 2023;50(2):376–386. https://doi.org/10.1007/s00259-022-05953-z.
13. Brosch-Lenz JF, Delker A, Schmidt F, Tran-Gia J. On the use of artificial intelligence for dosimetry of radiopharmaceutical therapies. *Nuklearmedizin*. 2023;62(6):379–388.
14. Sahiner B, Pezeshk A, Hadjiiski LM, et al. Deep learning in medical imaging and radiation therapy. *Med Phys*. 2019;46(1):e1–e36.
15. Poon AI, Sung JJ. Opening the black box of AI-medicine. *J Gastroenterol Hepatol*. 2021;36(3):581–584.
16. Reddy S, Allan S, Coghlan S, Cooper P. A governance model for the application of AI in health care. *J Am Med Inform Assoc*. 2020;27(3):491–497.

PART III

Noninterpretive Applications

PART OUTLINE

CHAPTER 15

Patient Facing Noninterpretive Artificial Intelligence Applications

Sudhen B. Desai ■ Shahrukh Naseer

KEY POINTS

- The vast majority of current AI applications that are FDA approved to date are not geared toward the patient. Although there exists a plethora of AI assistants in development or pending approval for use, there is a much smaller field for patient-facing noninterpretive uses
- Patient-facing use cases of AI in radiology can fall into the categories of online portal management, peri-appointment communications, virtual consultations and patient education, and symptom checking software.
- Radiologic AI assistants must be able to provide accurate information with empathetic communication to a diverse population of patients while maintaining safety, confidentiality, and ethical delivery of this information.

GLOSSARY OF TERMS AND DEFINITIONS

Optimization: The process of finding the most efficient solution among a set of choices and alternatives, with the goals of maximizing benefits, minimizing costs, or achieving specific goals.

Predictive Analysis: The practice of using algorithms, data, and machine learning to make predictions about future events or outcomes. This utilizes historical data to identify patterns that can be analyzed in the future.

Healthcare literacy: The ability for individuals to obtain, understand, and apply health-related information to make informed decisions about their own healthcare.

Evidence-based medical practices: Healthcare decisions and treatments that are based on scientific evidence and clinical data. This is done to ensure that patient care is informed by proven methods and outcomes.

Introduction

Noninterpretive applications of artificial intelligence (AI) in medical radiology refer to the ways in which artificial intelligence technology is utilized to improve various aspects of the radiology workflow and processes beyond the direct interpretation of medical images. Noninterpretive applications of AI in medical radiology cover a wide range of areas, including workflow optimization for technologists, image enhancement algorithms, enterprise operational efficiencies, and radiologists/clinicians.

Current focus areas of AI in radiology include[1]:

- Diagnostic aids that can automatically identify critical findings

- Automation of time-consuming functions such as quantification, contouring, and auto completion of text in reports
- Workflow improvements and automation
- Data mining applications
- Clinical decision support for next steps in a patient's care or to ensure imaging exam meets the guidelines
- Modality specific AI to iso-center patients, choosing imaging protocols, or speeding MRI exam time
- AI to enhance image reconstruction, to improve image quality and resolution, and to identify and fix imaging artifacts.
- Guidance AI to help imagers get the best possible images, even if they are novice users of the system or are unfamiliar with the anatomy.
- Automatic anatomical identification, labeling and contouring of organs or specific types of tissue.

Patient-facing applications of AI in radiology aim to directly benefit patients by enhancing their experience, engagement, and understanding of medical imaging. Although there is a plethora of undiscovered utilizations of AI in radiology for the patient-facing sector, the key topics we will briefly explore are online portal management/electronic medical records/picture archiving and communication system (EMR/PACS), peri-appointment communications, virtual consultations, patient education, and symptom checking software.

Online Portal Management/EMR/PACS

In the modern landscape of healthcare, AI-powered online portals can transform the way patients interact with their medical information and take an active role in their treatment journey. Online portals provide patients with secure access to their imaging data, reports, and potential AI-powered educational resources, which can help foster a sense of involvement in their healthcare decisions.[2]

Intelligent search functionalities powered by AI can enable patients to quickly locate specific information within the portal. Furthermore, integrating AI-powered voice assistants into these portals enhances accessibility, allowing patients to interact with the platform through natural language commands, making the experience more intuitive and user-friendly. Usability and accessibility are critical factors to ensure that patients of varying technological backgrounds can navigate their portal with ease. This also includes addressing the needs of individuals with disabilities, ensuring that the portal remains accessible to all users. Furthermore, seamless integration with electronic health record (EHR) systems is vital to offer comprehensive patient data access experience, allowing patients and healthcare providers to have a unified view of the patient's medical journey inclusive of their imaging records/reports. A list of the best-performing PACS systems (>300k imaging studies/year) is available in Table 15.1.[3] These vendors are all involved in various AI initiatives, with various levels of EMR integration. There is further recognition that radiology reports can benefit from AI review toward a more patient-centric output. The potential benefits of using generative AI assistants to generate imaging reports include improved report quality, greater efficiency in radiology workflow for producing summaries, patient-centered reports and recommendations, and a move toward patient-centered radiology.[4] Patient access to these reports via their portal is another opportunity to encourage patient involvement with their healthcare.

As this integration and patient-facing work product continues to develop, AI-driven portal management systems must excel in security and privacy, which are paramount in healthcare. By enhancing data security protocols and ensuring compliance with patient privacy regulations, these portals can provide patients with the confidence that their sensitive medical information is safeguarded.[5]

TABLE 15.1 ■ **Best-Performing Large Health System PACS (>300K Imaging Studies Per Year)**

Rank	Vendor
1.	Sectra PACS
2.	Merative (formerly IBM Watson Health) Merge PACS
3.	Change Healthcare Radiology Solutions
4.	Fujifilm Synapse
5.	Agfa Healthcare, Enterprise Imaging for Radiology
6.	GE Healthcare Centricity PACS

From Nashwan AJ, AbuJaber AA. Harnessing the power of large language models (LLMs) for electronic health records (EHRs) optimization. *Cureus*. 2023;15(7):e42634.

Peri-Appointment Communications

Predictive analytics powered by AI represent another avenue for innovation in radiology with peri-appointment communications. AI tools can be designed to anticipate instances that patients are likely to overlook or delay appointments. By proactively sending targeted messaging during these moments, healthcare providers can minimize missed appointments and enhance patient compliance with prescribed care regimens.[6] Furthermore, AI can facilitate multichannel communication to be delivered through a variety of channels such as text messages, emails, and app notifications, aligning with patients' preferred modes of communication.

AI can play a pivotal role in improving appointment compliance by not only managing communications and confirmations but also predicting patient follow-through. By analyzing historical patterns of patient behavior, AI can identify factors influencing attendance such as travel distance, appointment timing, or other individual barriers that are related to patients' show/no-show rates. Furthermore, postappointment AI tools can include summaries of appointments, what follow-up appointments may entail, and explanations of the importance of follow-up in appointment specific cases. This predictive capability allows providers to proactively address potential no-shows, such as by offering more convenient appointment scheduling.

The utilization of these tools is beneficial at the enterprise level but takes on particular import at the imaging level, where efficient utilization of expensive technologies is important from throughput, expedient diagnostics delivery and resource utilization standpoints.

Virtual Consultations

The diagnostic radiologist/patient interaction remains limited but is increasing in demand and popularity, in particular within high-end or multidisciplinary imaging domains (e.g., fetal radiology, interventional radiology). Telemedicine has become an essential component of modern post-COVID healthcare. With the ability to facilitate remote interactions between patients and clinicians, virtual consultations offer the convenience of discussing medical imaging and patient concerns from the comfort of their homes, as is standard in other disciplines.[7] As the use of AI increases, there is an opportunity for radiologists to develop and maintain close relationships with their patients and to become further involved in their care.[8] Utilization of image-enhancing AI tools to enable annotation and highlighting of specific areas of interest on medical images can foster more comprehensive and insightful virtual interactions.

Patient Education

As virtual interactions in radiology become more commonplace, the subcomponents of patient education and healthcare literacy with respect to medical imaging can similarly undergo a transformative shift with the integration of AI-powered tools. These tools can generate easily understandable explanations of intricate medical images and procedures, enabling patients to comprehend their diagnoses and treatment plans following physician analysis. The global nature of healthcare necessitates the inclusion of multilingual support within AI applications, allowing programs to cater to a diverse patient population by providing educational materials in various languages.[9] Customized content delivery is another avenue ripe for innovation, with AI capable of tailoring explanations to each patient's unique level of medical understanding. Companies have developed a framework around these technological concepts, one example being Vision SR, in addition to literature conversation around this concept.[10]

There are challenges and areas for improvement in the realm of AI utilization for virtual consultations and patient education to support widespread adoption. There needs to be an importance placed on designing user-friendly interfaces that seamlessly connect healthcare providers with AI tools during virtual consultations and in educational materials. The augmentation of AI algorithms to deliver highly accurate and clinically relevant information during virtual consultations also remains integral for understanding in virtual settings. Ensuring the accuracy and comprehensiveness of AI-generated explanations is crucial to building patient trust and understanding. Moreover, the emotional aspect of patient education should not be overlooked, necessitating the development of AI tools that deliver information with empathy and sensitivity to patient emotions.

Symptom Checking Software

In the modern healthcare landscape, AI-powered symptom checkers can be valuable tools that empower patients to gain insights into their health conditions and make informed decisions about seeking medical attention.[11] These AI-driven platforms can assist individuals in understanding potential causes of their symptoms, offering guidance on whether medical intervention is necessary. One avenue involves the development of intelligent questionnaires powered by AI, which can efficiently gather detailed information from patients about their symptoms and medical history, thereafter assisting in the determination if patients would benefit from radiologic services.

Additionally, AI algorithms can significantly enhance symptom checking by correlating reported symptoms within the EHR from other patients reporting similar symptoms. This could then be cross-referenced to the PACS. AI-driven systems can generate lists of potential diagnoses based on reported symptoms and clinical data, assisting both patients and physicians in the decision-making process using local data support that accounts for local health trends.

Conclusion

In conclusion, patient-facing AI applications in radiology are currently less common than those that deal with operational or clinical use cases but can be leveraged to improve patient engagement, enhance education, and deepen involvement in care. AI-driven tools can generate tailored, easy-to-understand radiology reports, helping patients better comprehend complex imaging findings through in-home consultative reviews. Predictive scheduling algorithms can optimize appointment management, minimizing delays and no-shows while improving resource allocation. AI-powered EHR data mining can assist radiologists by integrating relevant clinical information directly into reports, streamlining workflows and enabling more accurate and comprehensive care.

As this field evolves, a commitment to accuracy, empathy, accessibility, seamless workflow integration and data security will be pivotal to successfully embedding patient-centric AI into radiology. By combining these innovations with virtual consultations and patient education, AI is positioned to reshape radiology's role in healthcare, fostering greater accessibility, efficiency, and patient-centered care.

References

1. Fornell D. FDA has now cleared 700 AI healthcare algorithms, more than 76% in radiology. *Health Imaging*. Artificial Intelligence; 2023. https://healthimaging.com/topics/artificial-intelligence/fda-has-now-cleared-700-ai-healthcare-algorithms-more-76-radiology.
2. Nashwan AJ, AbuJaber AA. Harnessing the power of large language models (LLMs) for electronic health records (EHRs) optimization. *Cureus*. 2023;15(7):e42634. http://doi.org/10.7759/cureus.42634.
3. Fornell D. *Rankings of Radiology IT Solutions by End-Users in the 2023 Best in KLAS Program*. Radiology Business, Imaging Informatics; 2023. https://radiologybusiness.com/topics/health-it/enterprise-imaging/imaging-informatics/rankings-radiology-it-solutions-end-users-2023-best-klas-program.
4. Park J, Oh K, Han K, Lee YH. Patient-centered radiology reports with generative artificial intelligence: adding value to radiology reporting. *Sci Rep*. 2024;14(1):13218. http://doi.org/10.1038/s41598-024-63824-z.
5. Fournier-Tombs E, McHardy J. A medical ethics framework for conversational artificial intelligence. *J Med Internet Res*. 2023;25:e43068. http://doi.org/10.2196/43068.
6. Retson TA, Eghtedari M. Expanding horizons: the realities of CAD, the promise of artificial intelligence, and machine learning's role in breast imaging beyond screening mammography. *Diagnostics (Basel)*. 2023;13(13):2133. http://doi.org/10.3390/diagnostics13132133.
7. Randazzo G, Reitano G, Carletti F, et al. Urology: a trip into metaverse [published online ahead of print, 2023 Aug 8]. *World J Urol*. 2023;41(10):2647–2657. http://doi.org/10.1007/s00345-023-04560-3.
8. Borondy Kitts A. Patient perspectives on artificial intelligence in radiology. *JACR*. 2023;20(9):863–867.
9. Badawy MK, Kharmwan K, Carrion D. A pilot study of generative AI video for patient communication in radiology and nuclear medicine. *Health Technol*. 2025;15:395–404. https://doi.org/10.1007/s12553-025-00945-z.
10. Folio LR, Machado LB, Dwyer AJ. Multimedia-enhanced radiology reports: concept, components, and challenges. *Radiographics*. 2018;38(2):462–482. https://doi.org/10.1148/rg.2017170047.
11. Wiedermann CJ, Mahlknecht A, Piccoliori G, Engl A. Redesigning primary care: the emergence of artificial-intelligence-driven symptom diagnostic tools. *J Pers Med*. 2023;13(9):1379. http://doi.org/10.3390/jpm13091379.

CHAPTER 16

Navigating the Radiologic Technologist's Landscape: Current Innovations and Future Directions of Artificial Intelligence in Radiology

Maria Bach Nielsen ■ Robert Lauritzen ■ Janus Uhd Nybing ■ Michel Christian Nemery ■ Martin Lillholm

KEY POINTS

- This chapter explores the impact of AI on radiologic technologists' roles, highlighting the implications for workflow efficiency and diagnostic precision.
- While acknowledging the challenges of technology adaptation and the need for ongoing research, this chapter advocates for a gradual deployment strategy to optimize impact and outcomes. It also emphasizes that the synergy between AI and human expertise is crucial, with AI serving as a tool to support, not replace, radiologic technologists.
- This chapter describes the importance of continuous professional development and adaptability in radiography. It encourages radiologic technologists to embrace educational opportunities, develop AI literacy, and adapt to new technological advancements.

GLOSSARY OF TERMS AND DEFINITIONS

Artificial Intelligence (AI): the simulation of human intelligence processes by machines, especially computer systems, used in radiology for image analysis, diagnosis, and workflow enhancement.

Digital Imaging and Communications in Medicine (DICOM): a standard for handling, storing, printing, and transmitting information in medical imaging.

Emergency Room (ER) Applications: the use of radiology in emergency settings, often requiring rapid and accurate diagnostic imaging to inform patient care decisions.

Quality Assurance (QA): processes and procedures used to ensure the quality and safety of diagnostic imaging.

Radiologic Technologists (RTs): a radiologic technologist, also known as a radiographer, is a healthcare professional specialized in operating radiologic imaging equipment. They possess extensive knowledge of radiological tools. They are skilled in preparing patients for imaging procedures, positioning them accurately to obtain optimal imaging results, and adhering to safety protocols to protect patients and staff from unnecessary radiation exposure.

Workflow Efficiency: the effectiveness and efficiency of the workflow in radiology departments, including patient throughput, image processing, and diagnostic reporting.

Introduction

In the rapidly evolving radiology landscape, the emergence of artificial intelligence (AI) offers many opportunities to revolutionize the field. This chapter focuses on how AI is developed and integrated to change radiologic technologist (RT) procedures, tasks, requirements, and workflows. Although the recent trajectory in radiology has been toward deeper specialization of modalities and imaging, the rapid surge of AI applications could counter that by enabling RTs to take on broader, cross-sectional roles. In parallel, some RTs may shift toward further specialization, becoming ultra-specialist RTs as operators of advanced AI multimodal systems. This chapter aims to provide an overview of the RT landscape, showcase examples of areas where AI applications contribute to the current work practice, and discuss potential future AI applications through a case study.

The Current Radiologic Technologist Landscape

This section considers the role of RTs in the modern clinical environment. It aims to establish a framework for further discussion of the incorporation of AI into their processes and the associated challenges.

HISTORICAL PERSPECTIVE

The current role of RTs has been driven in large part by the advancement of imaging modalities. Since the initial discovery of x-rays and the birth of radiology, the field has witnessed the development of imaging modalities including ultrasound, computed tomography (CT), magnetic resonance imaging (MRI), positron emission tomography (PET), and nuclear medicine.[1] Each modality demands knowledge of various anatomic structures and clinical states in order to produce high-quality images. The complexity of modalities additionally continues to evolve, including with functional MRI, spectral CT, and photon counting. The education and training of RTs has transformed to meet such demands, with modern RT training programs providing comprehensive education in anatomy, physiology, radiation physics, and imaging techniques.[2] Many programs also offer specialized training in certain modalities, such as CT or MRI, to enable RTs to operate complex imaging equipment proficiently.[3] Beyond modality-specific knowledge, RTs must ensure patient comfort and confidentiality during imaging procedures. They also play a crucial role in minimization of radiation exposure, administration of contrast media, and adherence to established safety protocols.[4,5] Additionally, they closely collaborate with radiologists, physicists, multiple vendors, and other physicians and healthcare professionals.[6,7]

A critical element of the historical context for RTs relates to the documented rise in radiological workloads over the last few decades. One reason for this heightened demand is the increase in multimodal cross-sectional examinations due to revised standards of care[8]; these standards of care often reflect innovations made within medical imaging, whereby technology enables optimized analysis for clinical outcomes but frequently necessitates a trade-off with extended examination durations. Other reasons include aging populations, increasing rates of comorbidity, and comprehensive screening programs.[9] Consequently, radiology departments must acquire and analyze significantly larger volumes of imaging data to meet this demand.[10,11] Alongside the increased demand, there have often been declining reimbursements for imaging services yet increased costs associated with acquiring and processing images. Radiology departments are therefore compelled to enhance productivity to sustain income levels while reducing budgetary resources for personnel.[12] This situation has contributed to a complex and time-sensitive working environment for RTs; in some parts of the world, they are even assessed on targets of the volume of patients that have imaging performed.

TABLE 16.1 ■ **Critical Areas of Focus for RTs**

Area of Focus	Description	Impact
Patient Care and Imaging Procedures	Effective performance impacts patient outcomes, satisfaction, and departmental efficiency. Challenges include complex imaging acquisition, emergency cases, and fluctuating volumes.	Improves patient outcomes, increases satisfaction, enhances departmental efficiency.
Technical Proficiency and Adaptability	Handling and maintaining both traditional and advanced radiologic equipment. This expertise allows precise execution of complex imaging procedures.	Ensures precise imaging, reduces errors, facilitates adaptation to new technologies.
Quality Assurance and Control	Maintaining high imaging quality and safety standards, ensuring accurate and reliable radiological practices.	Provides high-quality images and patient safety, promotes reliable radiological practices.
Contextual Awareness	Differentiating approaches and priorities in routine and emergency radiological scenarios.	Enhances decision-making in diverse clinical situations, improves response in emergencies.
Preliminary Reporting	Initial documentation, interpretation, and reporting of imaging results (e.g., in the United Kingdom and Scandinavia).[17]	Streamlines workflow, provides timely information for further clinical decisions.

This evolving role of RTs reflects the dynamic nature of the medical field. It also underscores the importance of continuous learning and adaptation to technological advancements, to ensure the broadening of their skillset.[13–15] To this end, as AI in radiology ushers in a new era of technological sophistication and efficiency, there will be further redefining of RT roles, capabilities, and responsibilities.[16]

CURRENT SCOPE OF PRACTICE AND THE AI REVOLUTION

The current critical areas of focus for RTs, which provide the foundation for many future applications of AI, are displayed in Table 16.1.

The contribution of AI to RTs' workflows has the potential to extend across multiple areas, as shown in Table 16.2.

Areas of AI Impact on Radiologic Technologists' Workflows

Integrating AI in radiology presents both opportunities and challenges that need careful implementation to meet end users' needs. The effectiveness of AI is influenced by differences in patient populations, radiological settings, equipment, and imaging protocols. Continuous research and development are crucial to overcoming implementation challenges and realizing AI's potential.

TABLE 16.2 ■ **Contribution of AI to RTs' Workflows**

Area of Contribution	Description	Potential Impact
Clinical Decision Support	AI algorithms can interpret images, detect subtle abnormalities, and provide diagnostic recommendations. They may augment decision-making in clinical settings and enable real-time acquisition of supplemental imaging.[18]	Enhances diagnostic accuracy, improves decision-making, increases ability to perform timely interventions.
Advanced Imaging Technologies	AI technologies can optimize image quality and parameter selection through acquisition automation.	Improves image quality, optimizes imaging parameters, reduces need for manual adjustments.
Triaging and Prioritization	AI algorithms can triage and prioritize cases in emergency settings, particularly for critical conditions such as stroke or internal injuries.[19–23] These technologies enable faster decision-making and treatment initiation.	Improves patient outcomes, decreases response times in emergencies, ensures efficient resource allocation.

Applying human-centric approaches ensures that AI delivers tangible value to RTs and healthcare professionals.[24–26] The following sections expand on the RT's components of practice and showcase examples of how AI is transforming these areas.

PATIENT CARE AND IMAGING PROCEDURES

AI-powered technology may fundamentally alter RTs' methodologies for patient care and imaging techniques. AI could optimize operational efficiency and raise the standard of patient care by automating and enhancing several facets of the imaging workflow.

Automating Manual Processes

Significant developments in AI-driven technologies, such as Vista AI's One Click MRI™ (FDA 510(k) cleared), are redefining traditional practices of imaging adjustment planning. A pivotal study at Brigham and Women's Hospital by Dr. Raymond Kwong demonstrated the efficiency of the One Click MRI, with AI-assisted scans being 31% shorter than non-AI scans.[27] This technology allows a one-click acquisition and is integrated with GE Healthcare, using AI both to compute acquisition parameters tailored to individual patient needs and adjust scan plane location through auto localizer sequence programming. These AI automations address bottlenecks like lengthy examination times and the need for specialized RT skills to adjust the equipment for each patient. They thereby significantly streamline these MRI processes, enhancing the operational efficiency of RTs and improving patient throughput.[28] They may also improve diagnostic accuracy for radiologists by minimizing human error during acquisition.

Enhancing Imaging Quality

AI applications like SyntheticMR's SyMRI (FDA 510(k) cleared) and Subtle Medical's SubtleSYNTH (FDA 510(k) cleared) have introduced innovations including artificial sequence enhancement and synthesized sequences, which will be discussed in more detail later in this chapter. They can enhance the quality of MRI imaging sequences without requiring additional hardware or highly specialized RT resources, resulting in more precise and more detailed images needed for diagnosis.[29–34] The impact of such AI technologies on RTs' ability to produce high-quality scans in less time mainly revolves around increased throughput. However, potential challenges could emerge if the preexisting workflow is not considered part of the implementation process. An unmonitored implementation could require RTs to manage a larger number of patients within the same time frames; without proper procedural considerations, this situation could increase operational pressure and stress levels as RTs do their best to ensure each patient receives adequate care and attention.

New Optimized Workflows

Another avenue for AI application in radiology is automating time-demanding tasks in high-volume but low-risk settings. Radiobotics' RBknee™ (FDA 510(k) cleared), an AI-powered tool designed for knee radiography analysis, provides an example. It leverages advanced machine learning algorithms to automatically detect and analyze radiographic features of knee osteoarthritis, providing RTs and clinicians with detailed, accurate, and automated standardized reports. These reports could also create new patient flows, as the auto-generated reports allow reporting RTs to immediately determine whether the patient qualifies for further imaging with an MRI or can be sent home.[35] To this end, the patient experience can be optimized as patients either are flagged for same-day MRI imaging without a need to wait a period of time to be recalled. This approach also optimizes resource utilization by ensuring that only those patients who need an MRI receive one.

QUALITY ASSURANCE, QUALITY CONTROL, AND ERROR REPORTING

Radiology can utilize AI for quality assurance, imaging process standardization, and decision support. A current obstacle for optimizing image acquisition processes is the development and consistent use of standardized guidelines for patient preparation and acquisition protocols. AI applications can play a pivotal role by assisting in the creation and implementation of these guidelines and protocols.

Reducing Technical Recalls: Automating and Refining Acquisition Processes

A component of quality assurance improvements that AI can enable is the reduction of technical recalls. Technical recalls occur when images are insufficient for diagnosis, requiring additional imaging. These scenarios may inconvenience patients, incur costs for healthcare providers, and increase patient radiation exposure. AI algorithms have been developed to aid RTs by offering immediate feedback throughout the image acquisition. The RT is notified if the positioning or settings are suboptimal or if issues could affect image quality. For instance, AI can identify whether a patient has shifted position or if there is a potential for motion artifacts and recommend modifications to address these concerns.

Preacquisition Phase Application

During the preacquisition phase of radiologic imaging, AI can be essential to customize scan settings for better image quality and patient safety. GE Healthcare's AIR™ Recon DL and Siemens Healthineers' myExam Autopilot are good examples of this category. AIR™ Recon DL (FDA 510(k) cleared) is marketed as a deep learning algorithm that improves signal-to-noise ratio, sharpens images by up to 60%, and optimizes scan time by up to 50%.[36] myExam Autopilot

(FDA 510(k) cleared) customizes the scanning process for each patient by modifying contrast quantity, angle of image acquisition, and scan time based on patient-specific data like size, shape, and clinical indication.[37]

Postacquisition Phase Application

Postacquisition artifact mitigation is another area where AI can have powerful applications for quality enhancement. Artifacts may result from multiple factors, such as metal implants, patient movement, or technical malfunctions in the imaging equipment. These distortions in the images may conceal clinical data and diminish the quality of the image. AI-powered artifact mitigation techniques function by detecting and separating the artifacts present in the images; once identified, the AI may reduce or remove the effects of these artifacts by reconstructing the affected portion of the image.[38] Utilizing these AI technologies can reduce the necessity for further scans, saving time.[39] Siemens Healthineers' FlowMotion AI (FDA-510(k) cleared) solution for motion control and artifact reconstruction demonstrates AI's postacquisition potential: it integrates continuous bed motion technology, which moves a patient smoothly through the scanner, providing a more comfortable experience and reducing scan times without compromising image quality.[40] This technology also minimizes unnecessary CT exposure by precisely defining scan regions, adhering to the ALARA (As Low As Reasonably Achievable) principle.

Quality Assurance Protocols and Error Reporting

AI has become increasingly significant in fleet management and business intelligence in radiology quality control. AI can analyze massive datasets to improve service delivery and equipment efficiency, with this use often not constituting a medical device as defined by the FDA. Solutions like Volpara Analytics™ monitor how hospital staff utilize imaging equipment.[41] Fleet management AI technologies can monitor imaging equipment at several sites, identify usage trends, predict maintenance requirements, and suggest process improvements. AI may identify underutilized equipment and advise schedule changes to maximize utilization of resources. Business intelligence AI can evaluate operational data to assist healthcare providers in making informed decisions regarding their services. AI can identify opportunities to improve radiological services or suggest when to purchase new equipment by predicting service demand and patient throughput. These systems help identify patterns and implement corrective measures by auto-generating reports that structure the information and highlight key areas of improvement. Merative AI is another example of this type of AI with its advanced data processing and analytical features including Merge and Health Insights, which can consistently monitor and evaluate images.[42,43] Such systems also allow for systematic error reporting and analysis by scanning imaging data for discrepancies and deviations from a clinic's protocols.

ROUTINE VERSUS EMERGENCY SCENARIOS

In both routine and emergency radiology settings, workflow efficiency and prioritization are paramount. With the many components of the imaging workflow including patient preparation, image acquisition, and interpretation, there are many opportunities for bottlenecks. AI has the potential to increase efficiency in these settings through the streamlining of processes while enabling triage for more urgent clinical scenarios.

Remote Scanning

GE Healthcare's Digital Expert Access (FDA 510(k) cleared) and Ionic Health's nCommand platform (FDA 510(k) cleared) are innovative technologies that enable specialist RTs to perform image acquisition without being physically present at the imaging device site. This approach can be particularly beneficial in rural areas where specialist RTs are in short supply, enabling centralized expertise to cater to many locations and guaranteeing broader access to high-quality, highly specialized imaging services. Other healthcare personnel are physically present at the imaging site in order to prepare the patient and assist them into the scanner. In parallel, these remote services can double as a practical training opportunity for the local RTs as they observe the complex operational maneuvering by their specialized remote colleagues. Remote scanning technologies reduce the need to move patients and may enable earlier clinical decision-making, which can be vital for critically ill or immobile patients. In routine clinical settings, these technologies may decrease waiting times for nonurgent scans, improve patient satisfaction, and enhance resource allocation by enabling radiology departments to handle a larger breadth of elective imaging requests.

Triaging of Patients

In emergency departments, AI can be a useful tool for rapidly assessing and prioritizing patient treatment in time-sensitive settings.[19–23] Aidoc and Viz.ai's solutions provide examples of triaging algorithms designed to detect irregularities and allow for faster detection of significant pathology. Both platforms have been developed to seamlessly interact with current radiology workflow applications and promptly evaluate images after acquisition. When the system identifies a potential severe abnormality like intracranial hemorrhage (Aidoc's intracranial hemorrhage algorithm; FDA 510(k) cleared) or large vessel occlusions (Viz.ai's large vessel occlusion algorithm; FDA *de novo* request granted), it promptly notifies the radiologists or emergency room specialists.[22,40] In addition to their use in emergent situations, similar algorithms may aid routine clinical workflows by flagging cases with abnormal findings for earlier interpretation by radiologists such that clinical management can commence sooner.

TECHNOLOGICAL PROFICIENCY AND ADAPTABILITY

Implementing AI in radiology presents significant challenges that require continuous learning and adaptability by RTs beyond the other advances in imaging technology that they must stay updated on.[23] This training may come through continuous professional development and certification, and is supported by the recent creation of AI curricula for RTs and radiologists.[44]

A known challenge in existing workflows is the volume and variety of technologies utilized in radiology departments. These differences span scanner manufacturers, IT infrastructures, and user interfaces, which can each have their own configuration, design, and setup. The integration of software into these technical ecosystems becomes progressively more challenging as a result. This effect is currently exacerbated for AI applications, as they are often cutting edge with novel technology that lacks broader industry-recognized standards for integration and deployment. Consequently, the path to implementing such technologies is often tedious and time-consuming, frequently necessitating significant workflow practice modifications on the end user's part and potentially decreasing the value of AI applications. In the future, a transition toward greater technological convergence and standardization will be required to achieve streamlined clinical practices that incorporate AI.

RTs may have differing confidence and interest in incorporating new technology into their workflow. As such, it is essential to adjust the complexity of the technology to smoothly integrate with current workflow procedures and infrastructure, in order to minimize interruption and maximize the possibility of user approval. Breaking down the workflow into smaller modules or steps is typically perceived as more suitable for end users, as making extensive, overarching modifications to the workflow at once can lead to resistance. A pilot-like approach, using iterative adoption and including end users, can establish trust and acceptance of the technology.[45–47] A gradual approach to implementation also allows a more controlled assessment of AI's influence on effectiveness and patient care.

A Case Study in AI-Enhanced Brain MRI Analysis

AI has transformed radiology by enhancing accuracy, reducing time, and supporting decision-making across various imaging modalities. However, brain MRI analysis presents unique challenges due to the complexity of neurological structures and the critical nature of neurological disorders. Technological advances have enabled complex multisequence protocols, improving diagnostic imaging but also leading to longer scanning durations and the need for highly specialized RTs and radiologists. Examining the integration of AI in brain MRI analysis through real-world applications illustrates the tangible benefits of these technologies. AI can refine this intricate imaging process, offering insights that significantly influence treatment pathways. The benefits include enhancing on-table protocol adaptation, contributing to personalized medicine, and improving patient experiences. In this section, we investigate how CEREBRIU's Apollo Brain can address some of the complexities and challenges through both its current incarnation and future potential.

Apollo provides automated AI-based brain MRI analysis while patients are still in the scanner and offers real-time decision support (Fig. 16.1).[48] It is (at the time of writing this chapter) CE-marked for clinical use in Europe, whereas FDA 510(k) clearance is in progress. Its core AI algorithm supports the detection of candidate findings of infarcts, hemorrhages, and tumors based on the acquisition of three initial Digital Imaging and Communications in Medicine (DICOM) sequences: FLAIR, DWI, and SWI (or T2*GRE). Its analysis runs as sequences are acquired and typically finishes before a potential fourth placeholder sequence is completed.

Apollo's core functionality, Smart Protocol, leverages the real-time detection of candidate findings to suggest relevant protocol adaptations that tailor the subsequent sequences, including the potential use of contrast, to a patient's underlying condition. This approach could reduce the need for patient recall by acquiring additional sequences at that point in time. It could allow short exam times and avoidance of unnecessary contrast use when candidate findings are not identified without compromising the standard of care. These factors could address some of the inherent resource challenges associated with the increased need and use of comprehensive brain MRI exams.

Apollo's second core functionality, Smart Alert, notifies radiologists, clinicians and RTs about detected candidate findings via a triaging mechanism while the patient is in the scanner and after the acquisition of the initial three sequences (FLAIR, DWI, SWI). For potentially acute findings, RTs are empowered to page attending radiologists to assess the need for immediate intervention or specialized protocol adaptations, whereas the MRI examination is ongoing. Furthermore, such alerts could be propagated downstream in the radiological workflow, facilitating general triaging and worklist prioritization for study interpretation including to enable stroke-related treatment workflows.[49] A study on 995 patients, which involved comparing the detection of acute ischemia by Apollo with a ground truth interpretation from an experienced neuroradiologist, showed its potential clinical utility: it exhibited both high sensitivity (89%) and specificity (90%).[50]

Looking ahead, the combination of Cerebriu Apollo with preacquisition automation functionality like myExam Autopilot (Siemens Healthineers) or One Click MRI (Vista AI) could lead to substantial automation of brain MRI acquisition. It could enable automated initialization and adaption, including personalized acquisition protocols. It could be integrated directly into existing scanner systems (both hardware and software) to truly enable real-time analysis while circumventing deployment and interoperability challenges. There is also the opportunity for downstream integration including alert-based triaging and worklist prioritization. A vision of automated brain MRI and associated radiological workflows is therefore no longer science fiction. At the same time, it is crucial to recognize that systems like Apollo are designed to complement, not replace, the expertise of RTs and radiologists, whose judgment and experience will still be critical for the radiology workflow.

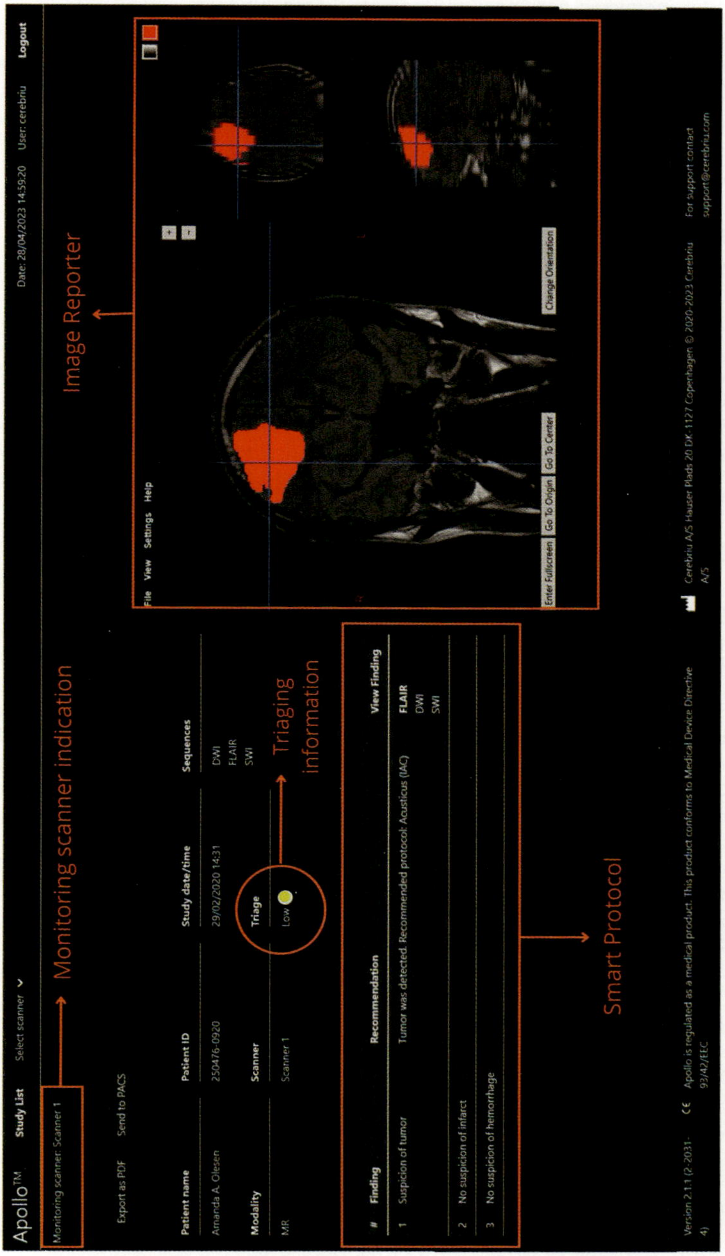

Fig. 16.1 Apollo study interface with explanations for a deidentified patient.

Conclusion

The incorporation of artificial intelligence in radiology provides opportunities to greatly enhance the efficiency of radiologic personnel and potentially revolutionize patient care. We have presented examples of how current and future AI-driven technologies can contribute by optimizing the quality of imaging, automating manual tasks, aiding clinical decision-making, and expediting triage and case prioritization. There will inevitably be challenges, but an open dialogue in the adoption process and a step-by-step deployment strategy can lead to favorable outcomes that will improve clinical care. The continuous implementation of AI into radiology techniques shows significant potential for advancing medical imaging into the future.

References

1. Sakano Y, Muroi K, Goto M, et al. A contribution to the history of Japanese education systems for radiological technologists. *Juntendo Med J.* 2021;68(1):44–51. http://doi.org/10.14789/jmj.jmj21-0028-r.
2. Abuzaid MM, Elshami W, Noorajan Z, Khayal S, Sulieman A. Assessment of the professional practice knowledge of computed tomography preceptors. *Eur J Radiol Open.* 2020;7:100216. http://doi.org/10.1016/j.ejro.2020.01.005.
3. Dong GQ, wen Wang W, Deng K, Wang G. The pilot study of radiology nursing intervention in abdominal 3-T magnetic resonance examination. *Rev Esc Enferm Usp.* 2016;50(6):961–964. http://doi.org/10.1590/s0080-623420160000700012.
4. Tsapaki V. Radiation dose optimization in diagnostic and interventional radiology: current issues and future perspectives. *Phys Med.* 2020;79:16–21. http://doi.org/10.1016/j.ejmp.2020.09.015.
5. Linet MS, Kim KP, Miller DL, Kleinerman RA, Simon SL, de González AB. Historical review of occupational exposures and cancer risks in medical radiation workers. *Radiat Res.* 2010;174(6):793–808. http://doi.org/10.1667/rr2014.1.
6. Alzahrani NM, Paddock M, Jeanes A, Shuweihdi F, Offiah AC. Professional practice and awareness of child abuse among radiologists and radiologic technologists: results from Saudi Arabia. *Pediatr Radiol.* 2023;53(5):832–843. http://doi.org/10.1007/s00247-022-05561-x.
7. Neri E, Souza ND, Brady AP, et al. What the radiologist should know about artificial intelligence – an ESR white paper. *Insights Imaging.* 2019;10(1):44. http://doi.org/10.1186/s13244-019-0738-2.
8. Brink JA, Hricak H. Radiology 2040. *Radiology.* 2023;306(1):69–72. http://doi.org/10.1148/radiol.222594.
9. Abernethy A, Adams L, Barrett M, et al. The promise of digital health: then, now, and the future. *NAM Perspect.* 2022;2022. http://doi.org/10.31478/202206e.
10. McDonald RJ, Schwartz KM, Eckel LJ, et al. The effects of changes in utilization and technological advancements of cross-sectional imaging on radiologist workload. *Acad Radiol.* 2015;22(9):1191–1198. http://doi.org/10.1016/j.acra.2015.05.007.
11. Bruls RJM, Kwee RM. Workload for radiologists during on-call hours: dramatic increase in the past 15 years. *Insights Imaging.* 2020;11(1):121. http://doi.org/10.1186/s13244-020-00925-z.
12. Kwee TC, Kwee RM. Workload of diagnostic radiologists in the foreseeable future based on recent scientific advances: growth expectations and role of artificial intelligence. *Insights Imaging.* 2021;12(1):88. http://doi.org/10.1186/s13244-021-01031-4.
13. Arai T, Murata S, Watanabe Y, et al. Fact-finding survey on the competencies and literacy of radiological technologists regarding radiation disasters. *J X-Ray Sci Technol.* 2023;31(2):237–245. http://doi.org/10.3233/xst-221341.
14. Cabrera AG. Defining the role of a PACS technologist. *J Digit Imaging.* 2002;15(Suppl 1):120–123. http://doi.org/10.1007/s10278-002-5095-9.
15. Kakinuma R, Ashizawa K, Kobayashi T, et al. Comparison of sensitivity of lung nodule detection between radiologists and technologists on low-dose CT lung cancer screening images. *Br J Radiol.* 2012;85(1017):e603–e608. http://doi.org/10.1259/bjr/75768386.
16. Tajaldeen A, Al-Ghamdi S. Evaluation of radiologist's knowledge about the artificial intelligence in diagnostic radiology: a survey-based study. *Acta Radiol Open.* 2020;9(7):205846012094532. http://doi.org/10.1177/2058460120945320.

17. Pedersen MRV, Jensen J, Senior C, Gale N, Heales CJ, Woznitza N. Reporting radiographers in Europe survey: an overview of the role within the European Federation of Radiographer Society (EFRS) member countries. *Radiography*. 2023;29(6):1100–1107. http://doi.org/10.1016/j.radi.2023.09.005.
18. Pesapane F, Codari M, Sardanelli F. Artificial intelligence in medical imaging: threat or opportunity? Radiologists again at the forefront of innovation in medicine. *Eur Radiol Exp*. 2018;2(1):35. http://doi.org/10.1186/s41747-018-0061-6.
19. Reyes M, Meier R, Pereira S, et al. On the interpretability of artificial intelligence in radiology: challenges and opportunities. *Radiol Artif Intell*. 2020;2(3):e190043. http://doi.org/10.1148/ryai.2020190043.
20. Jha S. Value of triage by artificial intelligence. *Acad Radiol*. 2020;27(1):153–155. http://doi.org/10.1016/j.acra.2019.11.002.
21. Soun JE, Chow DS, Nagamine M, et al. Artificial intelligence and acute stroke imaging. *AJNR Am J Neuroradiol*. 2021;42(1):2–11. http://doi.org/10.3174/ajnr.A6883.
22. Abedi V, Khan A, Chaudhary D, et al. Using artificial intelligence for improving stroke diagnosis in emergency departments: a practical framework. *Ther Adv Neurol Disord*. 2020;13:175628642093896. http://doi.org/10.1177/1756286420938962.
23. Al-Dasuqi K, Johnson MH, Cavallo JJ. Use of artificial intelligence in emergency radiology: an overview of current applications, challenges, and opportunities. *Clin Imaging*. 2022;89:61–67. http://doi.org/10.1016/j.clinimag.2022.05.010.
24. Cavaliere C, Tramontano L, Fiorenza D, Alfano V, Aiello M, Salvatore M. Gliosis and neurodegenerative diseases: the role of pet and mr imaging. *Front Cell Neurosci*. 2020;14:75. http://doi.org/10.3389/fncel.2020.00075.
25. Sadek M, Calvo RA, Mougenot C. Designing value-sensitive AI: a critical review and recommendations for socio-technical design processes. *AI Ethics*. 2023;4(4):949–967. http://doi.org/10.1007/s43681-023-00373-7.
26. Gerdes A. A participatory data-centric approach to AI ethics by design. *Appl Artif Intell*. 2022;36(1):2009222. http://doi.org/10.1080/08839514.2021.2009222.
27. Kwong DR. Clinical study shows Vista.ai significantly reduces cardiac MRI scan time. *Vista.ai*. 2023. https://vista.ai/evidence/.
28. Hardy M, Harvey H. Artificial intelligence in diagnostic imaging: impact on the radiography profession. *Br J Radiol*. 2020;93(1108):20190840. http://doi.org/10.1259/bjr.20190840.
29. Synthetic MR. Accessed February 2, 2024. https://syntheticmr.com/resources/clinical-studies/
30. Kim E, Cho HH, Cho SH, et al. Accelerated synthetic MRI with deep learning-based reconstruction for pediatric neuroimaging. *AJNR Am J Neuroradiol*. 2022;43(11):1653–1659. http://doi.org/10.3174/ajnr.A7664.
31. Warntjes JBM, Lundberg P, Tisell A. Brain parcellation repeatability and reproducibility using conventional and quantitative 3D MR imaging. *Am J Neuroradiol*. 2023;44(8):910–915. http://doi.org/10.3174/ajnr.A7937.
32. Radiology AI research and publications. *Subtle Med*. Accessed February 2, 2024. https://subtlemedical.com/publications/.
33. Bash S, Wang L, Airriess C, et al. Deep learning enables 60% accelerated volumetric brain MRI while preserving quantitative performance: a prospective, multicenter, multireader trial. *Am J Neuroradiol*. 2021;42(12):2130–2137. http://doi.org/10.3174/ajnr.A7358.
34. Tanenbaum LN, Bash SC, Zaharchuk G, et al. Deep learning–generated synthetic MR imaging STIR spine images are superior in image quality and diagnostically equivalent to conventional STIR: a multicenter, multireader trial. *Am J Neuroradiol*. 2023;44(8):987–993. http://doi.org/10.3174/ajnr.A7920.
35. Brejnebøl MW, Hansen P, Nybing JU, et al. External validation of an artificial intelligence tool for radiographic knee osteoarthritis severity classification. *Eur J Radiol*. 2022;150:110249. http://doi.org/10.1016/j.ejrad.2022.110249.
36. GE Healthcare. *MR Image Reconstruction with AIRTMRecon DL*. MR Image Reconstruction with AIR AIRTM Recon DL. Accessed February 8, 2024. https://www.gehealthcare.com/products/magnetic-resonance-imaging/air-recon-dl.
37. myExam Companion – Intelligence That Works with You. Accessed February 19, 2024. https://www.siemens-healthineers.com/magnetic-resonance-imaging/technologies-and-innovations/my-exam-companion.

38. Huang JY, Kerns JR, Nute JL, et al. An evaluation of three commercially available metal artifact reduction methods for CT imaging. *Phys Med Biol.* 2015;60(3):1047–1067. http://doi.org/10.1088/0031-9155/60/3/1047.
39. Ma JJ, Nakarmi U, Kin CYS, et al. Diagnostic image quality assessment and classification in medical imaging: opportunities and challenges. In: *2020 IEEE 17th International Symposium on Biomedical Imaging (ISBI).* IEEE; 2020:337–340. http://doi.org/10.1109/ISBI45749.2020.9098735.
40. FlowMotion AI – Moving the Standard to Personalized Care. Accessed February 19, 2024. https://www.siemens-healthineers.com/molecular-imaging/options-and-upgrades/software-applications/flowmotion-technology.
41. Mammography Analytics | Analytics. *Volpara Health.* Accessed February 19, 2024. https://www.volparahealth.com/breast-health-software/products/analytics/.
42. Healthcare Analytics Solutions | Merative. Accessed February 19, 2024. https://www.merative.com/healthcare-analytics.
43. Enterprise Imaging Solutions and Software | Merative. Accessed February 19, 2024. https://www.merative.com/merge-imaging.
44. Lindqwister A, Hassanpour S, Levy J, Sin J. Ai-rads: successes and challenges of a novel artificial intelligence curriculum for radiologists across different delivery formats. *Front Med Technol.* 2023;4:1007708. http://doi.org/10.3389/fmedt.2022.1007708.
45. Bajgain B, Lorenzetti D, Lee J, Sauro K. Determinants of implementing artificial intelligence-based clinical decision support tools in healthcare: a scoping review protocol. *BMJ Open.* 2023;13(2):e068373. http://doi.org/10.1136/bmjopen-2022-068373.
46. Lambert SI, Madi M, Sopka S, et al. An integrative review on the acceptance of artificial intelligence among healthcare professionals in hospitals. *NPJ Digit Med.* 2023;6(1):111. http://doi.org/10.1038/s41746-023-00852-5.
47. Magrabi F, Ammenwerth E, McNair JB, et al. Artificial intelligence in clinical decision support: challenges for evaluating AI and practical implications: a position paper from the IMIA technology assessment & quality development in health informatics working group and the EFMI working group for assessment of health information systems. *Yearb Med Inform.* 2019;28(01):128–134. http://doi.org/10.1055/s-0039-1677903.
48. Solutions – Cerebriu – Excellence in MRI Acquisition. Published online November 2023. Accessed February 27, 2024. https://cerebriu.com/.
49. Johansen J, Offersen CM, Carlsen JF, et al. An automatic DWI/FLAIR mismatch assessment of stroke patients. *Diagnostics.* 2023;14(1):69. http://doi.org/10.3390/diagnostics14010069.
50. Krag CH, Müller FC, Gandrup KL, et al. Diagnostic test accuracy study of a commercially available deep learning algorithm for ischemic lesion detection on brain MRIs in suspected stroke patients from a non-comprehensive stroke center. *Eur J Radiol.* 2023;168:111126. https://doi.org/10.1016/j.ejrad.2023.111126.

CHAPTER 17

Business-Facing Approaches

Michael M. Gilbert Bodell ■ Reid Fursmidt ■ Robert Short

KEY POINTS

- Several businesses are working on incorporating AI into radiology, which can be categorized into two complementary divisions: workflow applications and diagnostic solutions.
- The publication of the FDA's ethical and legal guidelines for regulating AI-based tools as medical devices or software as medical devices (SaMDs) has resulted in an increase number of FDA-approved AI/ML-enabled algorithms, driving more business and capital investment.
- Initiatives have emerged to ensure clinical relevance, empower AI developers, and build trust with healthcare partners.
- Businesses promote the implementation of AI in radiology via their ability to provide funding, market and promotion, a technical infrastructure, and enhance the user experience.

GLOSSARY OF TERMS AND DEFINITIONS

Business-Facing: services, or products in a company that interact with other businesses that aid in enhancing processes, budgeting, predicting outcomes, and forecasting performances that are critical to improve customer experience.

Diagnostic Approaches: processes used to identify the cause of the disease or system in question.

Food and Drug Administration (FDA): responsible for protecting the public health by ensuring the safety, efficacy, and security of human, biological products and medical devices.

FDA-approved Algorithms: refers to algorithms that have been reviewed and cleared by the FDA.

Good Machine Learning Practice: A set of principles that can be used to ensure machine learning models are accurate, ethical. and appropriate for use in the medical setting.

Software as Medical Devices (SaMDs): software intended to be used for one or more medical purposes that perform these purposes without being part of a hardware medical device.

Workflow Application: software or tools that help automate and streamline the process or task.

Introduction

Artificial intelligence (AI) and machine learning technologies have the opportunity to transform the field of radiology through a multitude of different approaches. The use of these technologies is spreading rapidly. In the coming future, AI has the potential to significantly enhance the precision and effectiveness of diagnostic procedures (or processes), as well as streamline the workflow of radiologists. However, this integration has been complex, with many challenges and limitations. Businesses are playing an increasingly important role in addressing some of these challenges, and are transforming the field, as they develop and deploy AI solutions for a range of radiology tasks and diagnostic approaches.

The term "artificial intelligence" was originally coined by John McCarthy, the creator of the LSIP programming language, during the Dartmouth Summer Research Project on Artificial Intelligence in 1956.[1] Although the earliest applications of AI in medicine were developed by a diverse group of computer scientists, engineers, and medical experts in the 1960s and 1970s, the first iterations of AI in radiology emerged after the advent of microcomputers and CT scanners in the 1970s.[2] This was soon followed by the introduction of the picture archiving and communication system (PACS), which laid the groundwork for an electronic image platform, remote access, and workflow management. The Digital Imaging and Communications in Medicine (DICOM) standardization later enabled PACS image storage and transfer across networks.

In addition to the PACS system, research was conducted on computer-aided detection and diagnosis software in the 1980s at the Kurt Rossman Laboratories for Radiologic Image Research in the Department of Radiology at the University of Chicago. These systems created large datasets that would eventually allow for the first attempts at identifying subtle changes in images. The combination of these events led to the first AI application in radiology to detect microcalcifications in mammography in 1992.[2] More recently, deep learning algorithms such as convolutional neural networks (CNNs) have become increasingly popular in radiology, expanding on the initial work product from the Rossman Labs.

Despite the many advances in AI in radiology, there were obvious challenges and limitations in its deployment in the early 2000s. The most notable of these limitations include the development of AI primarily at academic centers. These academic centers lacked the proper infrastructure to support widespread adoption and importantly, scalability to the wider public. Further, ethical and legal considerations were not clearly defined in any domain. This led to two important evolutions: the commercialization of AI in radiology by private interests that began in the 2010s, and the Food and Drug Administration (FDA) developing a framework for machine learning practices and how to obtain approval of machine learning algorithms. In subsequent sections below we will discuss the current FDA guidelines around AI and the role of business-facing applications. We will expand on this by examining the current market, including examples. We will conclude with ethical and legal considerations and a discussion of the importance of industry in the AI radiology space.

FDA Consideration

In the early 2010s, there were an increasing number of businesses that were creating AI-based technologies for the radiology workflow. However, there was a lack of FDA guidance on these AI-based tools. As a result, the FDA issued guidelines to regulate AI-based tools as medical devices or Software as a Medical Device (SaMD).[3] Before the FDA's SaMD program was established, the agency regulated medical devices based on their physical hardware components, such as implants, pacemakers, and x-ray machines. Software that was integrated with these hardware devices was also regulated as part of the device. However, standalone medical software or software that learned with the user was not well-defined under the FDA's regulatory framework, initially leading to confusion and uncertainty. These products had to go through traditional review through an appropriate premarket pathway, de novo classifications, or premarket approval. To address this gap, SaMD was created as a guidance for the development and regulation of standalone medical software, including the use of AI and machine learning.[3] The program established a clear set of guidelines for SaMD manufacturers to follow, including recommendations for validation, performance monitoring, and post-market surveillance. This new framework has allowed for the number of AI-enabled devices approved by the FDA to drastically increase. As of November 2024, the FDA had approved 949 AI/machine learning (ML)-enabled devices and 723 were radiology based.[3] A majority of these have been in neuroradiology and breast platforms (Fig. 17.1).[4] This has helped lead to an explosion of intellectual and capital investment. The diagnostic radiology market is projected to grow at a compound annual growth rate of 5.5% reaching a predicted value of 34.6 billion dollars by 2028.[5]

Current Landscape

The ever-evolving world of AI in radiology involves a number of types of businesses. Startups, well-known IT firms, and healthcare providers are all competing within the AI-radiology space. These businesses typically focus on two main aspects: workflow application and diagnostic solutions, both of which aim to improve clinical treatment in light of the increasing volume of imaging studies to read. Although they share this common goal, these two aspects are fundamentally different. Workflow applications, which can be easily integrated into existing platforms, provide a more immediate disruption to radiologists by reducing the number of clicks needed, organizing scans in a specific way, and providing tools such as tracking scans over time. These solutions may be less sophisticated but allow for quick implementation of real-world AI solutions. In contrast, diagnostic solutions that allow one to identify cancer or other pathologies are more challenging, require more complex models and large datasets, and typically need clinical correlation. Both of these applications are crucial for creating better patient care, but businesses will be needed to create scalable platforms that can reach a wide range of radiologists. These approaches provide ways to increase both the efficiency and quality of the radiologist's reports, saving time and resources while improving accuracy. Some of these businesses are highlighted below and showcase the wide variety of ways AI can be integrated into Radiology. These companies are already having an impact in radiology with their early adoption and dissemination of AI-based workflows and diagnostic approaches. This is not a comprehensive resource and more information can be found at FDA.gov for approved SaMD's.

1. **Tempus:** Recently called Artery's, a precision medicine artificial intelligence company. Before their Tempus's acquisition, Artery's was the first company to receive FDA approval for deep learning algorithms and cloud computing in a clinical setting in 2017. Tempus then purchased Artery's in 2022. Tempus provides a variety of solutions that can aid radiologist in their workflow and diagnostic approaches including in cardiology, lung, neuroradiology, and breast. Their technology has also published a variety of scientific journals focusing on of cardiology, neurology, and their deep learning platform.[6–8]
2. **GE Healthcare**: One of the major participants in the medical imaging sector, they are addressing AI solutions from a range of sources, including tools for automated image interpretation and predictive analytics. More specifically, these include methods for reconstructing MR images using deep learning, AI x-ray algorithms for prioritizing urgent situations, and enhancing CT workflow operational effectiveness.[9]
3. **Aidoc**: With a need for solutions that increase efficiency and expediting care, Aidoc seeks to improve turnaround time using deep learning technology. The constant running of the system in the background allows for immediate flagging of acute pathologies including rib fractures, aortic dissections, and brain aneurysms.[10] Furthermore, their platform has shown potential benefits in aiding diagnostic capabilities in topics related to acute intracranial hemorrhage and pulmonary embolisms.[11–13]
4. **Philips**: Another major player in healthcare, Philips invests in a wide range of AI tools. They recently developed an Intellispace AI Workflow Suite that allows for AI-based workflow for optimization data transferring between devices and AI applications. It is a

Specialty	Number of FDA AI-Machine Learning Devices
Radiology	723
Physical Medicine	1
Pathology	8
Orthopedic	5
Ophthalmic	10
Obstetrics and Gynecology	1
Neurology	34
Microbiology	5
Immunology	1
Hematology	18
General Hospital	4
General and Plastic Surgery	6
Gastroenterology-Urology	14
Ear Nose & Throat	2
Clinical Chemistry	8
Dental	3
Cardiovascular	98
Anesthesiology	8
Grand Total	**949**

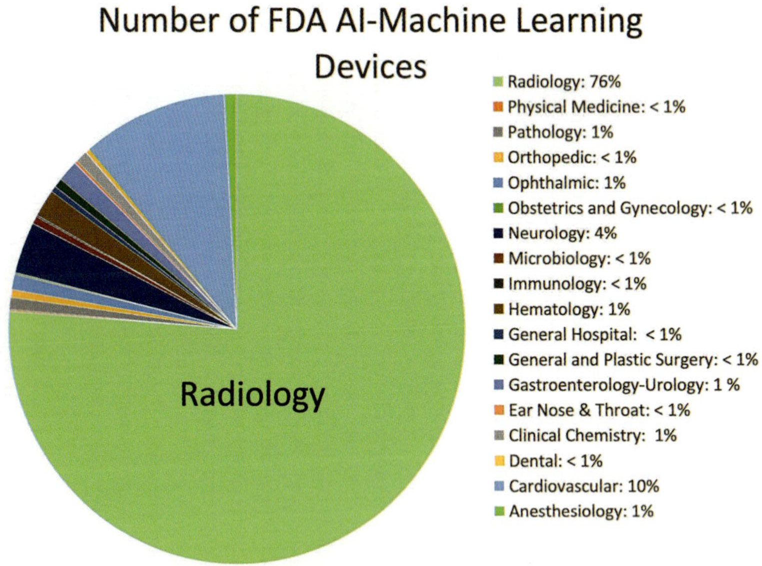

Fig. 17.1 Approval of medical specialties for AI-machine learning devices. The pie chart shows the breakdown of medical specialties approved for FDA AI-machine learning devices by the US Food and Drug Administration as of November 9, 2024.

platform that integrates scheduling, image acquisition, data interpretation, and reporting into one system.[14]

5. **Nuance**: Recently acquired by Microsoft, this company utilizes its Powerscribe One platform to improve reporting quality and workflow through a variety of features. These include ambient mode and clinical guidance which will auto-populate guidelines and populate markers that can be incorporated into the radiologist report. For example, advance language processes understand how a thyroid nodule might be described on a report and will alert the radiologist to the clinical guidelines and appropriate recommendations can subsequently populate the report.[15]
6. **RapidAI**: Rapid AI utilizes AI diagnostic approaches to examine perfusion images to determine the likehihood of success of intra-arterial interventions such as stroke therapy. Doing so aids both in appropriate selection of candidates for therapy but also expedites diagnosis for more rapid mobilization of resources. They have validated their tool through a multitied of published literature focusing on strokes and anuerysms.[16,17]

Legal and Ethical Considerations

The integration of AI technology in radiology raises various ethical and legal issues that require careful consideration. In terms of ethics, it is crucial that businesses train their AI algorithms on diverse and representative patient populations to avoid biases and ensure equity. It is the responsibility of both businesses and the healthcare system to create machine learning algorithms that do not perpetuate existing health disparities. From a legal standpoint, liability and accountability are of great concern. Who bears responsibility in the event of an AI algorithm error—is it the radiologist or the company, especially if AI in the future becomes semi or fully autonomous? Finally, what framework should be used by companies that encompasses these considerations? Within the FDA's framework of SaMD's, 10 guiding principles were introduced to set the foundation for Good Machine Learning Practice (GMLP). These are shown below, and more information can be found at FDA.gov.[3] The guiding themes of the list should be used by all businesses and partners alike.

1. Multidisciplinary Expertise Is Leveraged Throughout the Total Product Life Cycle
2. Good Software Engineering and Security Practices Are Implemented
3. Clinical Study Participants and Datasets Are Representative of the Intended Patient Population
4. Training Datasets Are Independent of Test Sets
5. Selected Reference Datasets Are Based on Best Available Methods
6. Model Design Is Tailored to the Available Data and Reflects the Intended Use of the Device
7. Focus Is Placed on the Performance of the Human-AI Team
8. Testing Demonstrates Device Performance during Clinically Relevant Conditions
9. Users Are Provided Clear, Essential Information
10. Deployed Models Are Monitored for Performance and Re-training Risks are Managed

A Case for Businesses

The development and implementation of AI in radiology requires significant investment if these tools are going to be used on a wide scale to improve patient outcomes. Although academic centers can be a source of research and development, the infrastructure necessary for implementation likely requires the involvement of commerce. Businesses can provide the necessary funding and marketing efforts and are motivated to accelerate the adoption of these technologies. Furthermore, industry can work with a wide range of healthcare providers to implement AI systems that are

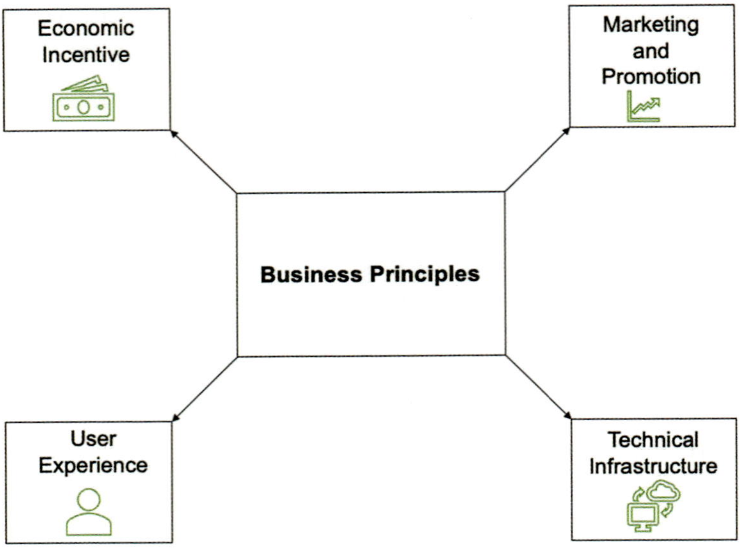

Fig. 17.2 Four business principles that enhance AI in radiology.

tailored to the specific needs of a hospital system. By driving innovation and developing cost-effective and user-friendly products, businesses can lower the barriers to adoption. In summary, the need for businesses in the implementation of AI in radiology may be driven by four proposed themes discussed below: economic incentives, marketing and promotion, user experience, and technical infrastructure (Fig. 17.2).

Economic incentive: Businesses are motivated to invest in the development and implementation of AI in radiology due to the potential economic incentives. By developing AI technologies for radiology, businesses can create new revenue streams, differentiate themselves in a crowded market, and gain a competitive advantage.

Marketing and promotion: By raising awareness of the benefits of AI-based products and services, businesses can help educate healthcare providers and patients about the potential of these technologies. Additionally, businesses can develop educational materials that highlight the unique features and benefits of their products. Although a radiologist must be cautious of advertisements, demonstrable, digestible information can inform in efficient ways that can lead to technology adoption.

User experience: Developing AI-based products for radiology requires a deep understanding of user needs and workflows. Companies can trial run products with different groups and academic centers and implement these changes relatively quickly. Competitive advantages can be gleaned by improving the user experience, drive innovation, and strive for an improved user experience in hopes of commercial success.

Technical infrastructure: Businesses that have experience in developing and managing technical infrastructure such as GE Healthcare and Philips can help ensure that AI-based systems for radiology are scalable, reliable, and secure. This requires expertise in cloud computing, data management, and cybersecurity, as well as an understanding of regulatory requirements and industry standards. By providing technical infrastructure and support, businesses (particularly those with the prior experience in these arenas) can help healthcare providers implement AI-based systems that are tailored to their specific needs and ensure that these systems meet the highest standards of quality and safety.

Empowering AI Developers

Identifying clinically relevant, ethical, and effective solutions can be challenging for groups developing AI-based tools. To support these efforts, the American College of Radiology Data Science Institute has created use case scenarios that guide AI developers in producing algorithms that are thoughtful, applicable, and can be integrated into daily workflows, ultimately enhancing patient care.[18] These specific clinical examples highlight important features to gain trust and support for AI from the medical community. Each case spells out how the AI should be able to reach its specific goal through five carefully designed sections: overview, clinical implementation, dataset considerations, technical specifications, and future developments. Examples are included from all fields ranging from abdominal, prostate, breast, cardiac, and musculoskeletal. Due to these types of initiatives, businesses, radiologists, and developers can have a framework for describing relevant algorithmic functions and have a greater understand for what is clinically relevant.

In summary, the future of AI in radiology will be interwoven between academic centers and AI-engaged healthcare companies. The early developments of AI in academic centers have led to major companies investing in these technologies. However, caution must be used as more and more businesses enter the market. The FDA's SaMD framework is crucial moving forward into the AI age. Within this framework, initiatives that empower AI developers to make more clinically useful and ethical products and support systems will continue to advance. As such, it is vital for businesses to utilize the key ethical framework laid out by the FDA. At the core of all companies should be patient outcome, which will pave the way for a better future. Industry involvement in advancing AI is a necessary driver of innovation; however, safeguards should be in place that ensure the human experience remains paramount.

References

1. Mintz Y, Brodie R. Introduction to artificial intelligence in medicine. *Minim Invasive Ther Allied Technol.* 2019;28(2):73–81. http://doi.org/10.1080/13645706.2019.1575882.
2. El Naqa I, Haider MA, Giger ML. Ten Haken RK. Artificial intelligence: reshaping the practice of radiological sciences in the 21st century. *Br J Radiol.* 2020;93(1106):20190855. http://doi.org/10.1259/bjr.20190855.
3. Software as a Medical Device (SaMD). FDA. Updated December 4, 2018. Accessed March 28, 2023. https://www.fda.gov/medical-devices/digital-health-center-excellence/software-medical-device-samd.
4. American College of Radiology. Accessed March 28, 2023. https://aicentral.acrdsi.org.
5. Bok GL. Investing in artificial intelligence and digital health—What radiology innovators need to know. *J Am Coll Radiol.* 2024;21(10):1595–1600. http://doi.org/10.1016/j.jacr.2024.06.019.
6. Hahn LD, Hall K, Alebdi T, Kligerman SJ, Hsiao A. Automated deep learning analysis for quality improvement of CT pulmonary angiography. *Radiol Artif Intell.* 2022;4(2):e210162. http://doi.org/10.1148/ryai.210162.
7. Raimondi F, Martins D, Coenen R, et al. Prevalence of venovenous shunting and high-output state quantified with 4D flow MRI in patients with Fontan circulation. *Radiol Cardiothorac Imaging.* 2021;3(6):e210161. http://doi.org/10.1148/ryct.210161.
8. Zhao MY, Fan AP, Chen DY-T, et al. Cerebrovascular reactivity measurements using simultaneous 15O-water PET and ASL MRI: impacts of arterial transit time, labeling efficiency, and hematocrit. *NeuroImage.* 2021;233:117955. https://doi.org/10.1016/j.neuroimage.2021.117955.
9. GE HealthCare; 2024. https://www.gehealthcare.com/.
10. Aidoc; 2024. https://www.aidoc.com/solutions/radiology/.
11. Davis MA, Rao B, Cedeno PA, Saha A, Zohrabian VM. Machine learning and improved quality metrics in acute intracranial hemorrhage by noncontrast computed tomography. *Curr Probl Diagn Radiol.* 2022;51(4):556–561. http://doi.org/10.1067/j.cpradiol.2020.10.007.
12. Wismüller A, Dsouza AM, Abidin AZ, et al. Early-stage COVID-19 pandemic observations on pulmonary embolism using nationwide multi-institutional data harvesting. *NPJ Digit Med.* 2022;5(1):120. http://doi.org/10.1038/s41746-022-00653-2.

13. Wiklund P, Medson K, Elf J. Incidental pulmonary embolism in patients with cancer: prevalence, underdiagnosis and evaluation of an AI algorithm for automatic detection of pulmonary embolism. *Eur Radiol.* 2023;33(2):1185–1193. http://doi.org/10.1007/s00330-022-09071-0.
14. Philips; 2024. https://www.usa.philips.com/healthcare/specialty/radiology.
15. The New Era of AI-Infused Reporting Is Here; 2024. https://www.nuance.com/healthcare/campaign/ppc/powerscribe-one/on-demand-demo.html?cid=7016T0000030pegQAA&utm_campaign=NHD-AO-2025-PSO_OnDemand_Demo_PPC&utm_medium=CPC&utm_source=google&gad_source=1-&gclid=Cj0KCQiArby5BhCDARIsAIJvjIQstZHaNfViQ7yFCV5T2plzCRmQdGE1VV3Nz0HOMV92–bVzKY8XasaAlJkEALw_wcB.
16. Sahlein DH, Gibson D, Scott JA, et al. Artificial intelligence aneurysm measurement tool finds growth in all aneurysms that ruptured during conservative management. *J Neurointerv Surg.* 2023;15(8):766–770.
17. Heit JJ, Honce JM, Yedavalli VS, et al. RAPID aneurysm: artificial intelligence for unruptured cerebral aneurysm detection on CT angiography. *J Stroke Cerebrovasc Dis.* 2022;31(10):106690. http://doi.org/10.1016/j.jstrokecerebrovasdis.2022.106690.
18. American College of Radiology; 2024. https://www.acrdsi.org/DSI-Services/Define-AI.

CHAPTER 18

Non-interpretive Application of Artificial Intelligence in Radiology: Population Health

Vishaal Kondoor ■ Jonathan Antony Stone ■ Tulasi Talluri ■ Heather Mattie

KEY POINTS

- Artificial intelligence (AI) facilitates opportunistic screening by analyzing incidental findings in routine imaging studies, thereby enhancing population health through earlier detection of conditions such as osteoporosis, cardiovascular disease, and metabolic disorders. This approach can optimize healthcare resources and improve preventive care strategies.
- AI technologies democratize access to radiology expertise by automating complex image analysis and providing decision support tools. Particularly in underserved regions and low-resource settings, AI can enable timely diagnostics, support remote consultations, and enhance healthcare delivery efficiency.
- Although AI offers promise in mitigating racial disparities by improving diagnostic accuracy across diverse populations, it also poses challenges related to bias perpetuation. Addressing these concerns requires transparent model development, diverse training datasets, and stringent regulatory oversight to ensure fairness and equity in healthcare outcomes.

GLOSSARY OF TERMS AND DEFINITIONS

Population Health: The study of health outcomes of a group of individuals through understanding and addressing diverse factors that influence health outcomes in different populations, such as social determinants of health, access to healthcare, and disease prevention.

Opportunistic Screening: The use of imaging studies performed for unrelated clinical reasons to detect incidental findings that may indicate undiagnosed conditions.

Global Burden of Disease (GBD): A comprehensive research initiative that quantifies the impact of diseases, injuries, and risk factors on populations worldwide using metrics like Disability-Adjusted Life Years (DALYs) and Years of Life Lost (YLL).

Introduction

Although major advancements in medicine and technology have led to an increase in life expectancy worldwide, healthcare systems face new challenges that come with an aging population: the growing burden of chronic diseases and increasing healthcare costs. The World Health Organization (WHO) predicts that by 2050, 80% of older people will live in low- and middle-income countries (LMICs), and by 2030, one in six people worldwide will be aged 60 or over.[1] With this demographic shift comes an increase in noncommunicable diseases, as evidenced by the results of the Global Burden of Disease Study in 2017.[2] Radiology's integral role in the continuum of care—from population-level screening initiatives to image-guided therapies—provides a large opportunity to enhance population health, especially as imaging has become an indispensable part of the management of both communicable and noncommunicable diseases.

Health expenditure has consistently grown faster than economic growth in Organization for Economic Co-operation and Development (OECD) countries over the past half-century. Although this increased spending has improved health outcomes and driven economic growth and job creation, financial sustainability is a growing concern, especially because most funding comes from public sources.[3] From 2000 to 2015, annual health spending growth in the OECD averaged 3.0%, compared to gross domestic product (GDP) growth of 2.3%. In 2015 to 2030, health expenditure is expected to continue outpacing GDP growth across all OECD countries. Radiology is a major driver of these healthcare costs. The number of computed tomography (CT) and magnetic resonance imaging (MRI) scans ordered between 2000 and 2016 in OECD countries increased by 60% and 80%, respectively. This increase underscores the importance of optimizing the cost effectiveness and diagnostic yield of these studies. In preventive health, artificial intelligence (AI) can support population-level screening for major diseases through opportunistic screening, democratize radiology expertise to increase access to radiological services in low-resource settings, and reduce healthcare costs. AI algorithms can analyze large amounts of imaging data quickly and accurately, enabling real-time monitoring of disease patterns across populations. Earlier detection and proactive management of morbidities can reduce healthcare costs by preventing progression and managing conditions more effectively. These opportunities all make AI a vital tool in the future of radiological and population health care.

To date, the U.S. Food and Drug Administration (FDA) has cleared (or otherwise authorized for marketing) 882 AI and machine learning (ML) medical devices, of which 671 are for radiology.[4] Many of these AI/ML algorithms can enhance population health by aiding with disease detection, risk stratification, and providing recommendations based on existing public health guidelines. Table 18.1 highlights the key features, current regulatory status, and potential use for population health of some of these devices.[5,6]

In addition to FDA-cleared devices, several companies are at the forefront of developing AI/ML solutions for radiology in the context of population health.[7] The potential applications include earlier detection, risk assessment, and intervention strategies for various conditions. Table 18.2 provides an overview of some of these companies including their key innovations, current impact, and potential future directions.

Preventive Health Screening

AI/ML algorithms, particularly those based on deep learning, have demonstrated remarkable proficiency in identifying malignancies across imaging modalities, including CT, MRI, and mammography. For instance, convolutional neural networks (CNNs) have shown superior performance in detecting breast cancer in mammograms. Similarly, Google's AI/ML system can reduce both false positives and false negatives in mammographic screening, achieving an area under the curve (AUC) of 0.889, compared to 0.810 by human radiologists.[8] AI/ML algorithms have additionally been developed for lung cancer screening using low-dose CT scans, where they have proven effective in identifying early-stage nodules that might be missed by radiologists.[9]

AI/ML also plays a crucial role in optimizing population-level cancer screening programs. By analyzing vast amounts of imaging and clinical data, AI/ML systems can stratify patients based on their risk profiles, enabling personalized screening protocols. For example, the application of AI/ML in colorectal cancer screening has led to the development of algorithms that predict the likelihood of advanced neoplasia based on patients' demographic, clinical, and

TABLE 18.1 ■ **Examples of FDA-Cleared AI/ML Devices in Radiology That Could Be Utilized for Population Health**

Application Name	Key Features	Current Regulatory Status With the FDA	Potential Use for Population Health
ABMD Software (HeartLung Corporation)	This bone densitometer application uses AI/ML to estimate bone mineral density within the spine based on CT scans that are ordered for reasons other than bone mineral density measurement.	Received 510(k) clearance on July 29, 2022.	It could opportunistically screen for low bone density and allow clinicians to intervene earlier to optimize patients' bone health.
Deep Learning Image Reconstruction (GE Healthcare Japan Corporation)	This AI/ML-powered system generates CT images with enhanced quality including for image noise and streak artifact suppression.	Received most recent 510(k) clearance on April 20, 2023.	It could improve the image quality of CT images obtained especially in settings with older technology or less radiology expertise (albeit noting the FDA clearance of this device is specific to certain CT scanner models).

From US Food & Drug Administration. *510(k) premarket notification (ABMD software)*. Updated July 29, 2022. https://www.accessdata.fda.gov/scripts/cdrh/cfdocs/cfpmn/pmn.cfm?ID=K213760; and
US Food & Drug Administration. *510(k) premarket notification (Deep learning image reconstruction)*. Updated April 20, 2023. https://www.accessdata.fda.gov/scripts/cdrh/cfdocs/cfpmn/pmn.cfm?ID=K230807.

TABLE 18.2 ■ **Examples of Companies Developing AI/ML Solutions for Radiology in Population Health**

Company	Key Features or Innovations	Current Impact	Potential Future Directions
IBM Watson Health	IBM Watson Health utilizes AI/ML for rapid processing and analysis of radiology images, enabling population-level insights for health management and intervention strategies.	As a pioneer in healthcare AI/ML applications, IBM Watson Health has contributed to population health initiatives by providing data-driven decision support and risk assessment capabilities.	Future directions may involve refining AI/ML algorithms to provide personalized health recommendations and interventions based on radiology findings.
Butterfly Network	This company provides a handheld whole-body ultrasound device capable of real-time disease detection while scanning, with a focus on population health applications such as prenatal care and remote screenings.	Butterfly Network's innovative approach to portable ultrasound imaging has the potential to expand access to population-level screenings and interventions, particularly in underserved areas.	Future developments may involve expanding the range of population health applications and integrating AI/ML algorithms to enhance diagnostic accuracy and risk stratification for specific health conditions.

previous screening data. Such predictive models help in identifying individuals who might benefit from more frequent colonoscopies while reducing the screening burden on low-risk individuals.[10]

The implementation of AI/ML in radiology has shown promise in reducing the rates of false positives and negatives, which are critical concerns in oncologic screening. False positives can lead to unnecessary biopsies, patient anxiety, and increased healthcare costs, whereas false negatives can delay diagnosis and treatment, adversely affecting patient outcomes. A notable example is the use of AI/ML in prostate cancer screening. Prostate MRI scans analyzed by AI algorithms have shown a significant reduction in false-positive rates by accurately distinguishing between benign and malignant lesions.[11] This capability can lead to more precise biopsy recommendations and better patient management.

The vast datasets generated through oncologic screening programs provide a rich resource for AI/ML-driven research and insights. By leveraging AI/ML techniques, researchers can uncover novel associations and patterns that may not be apparent through conventional statistical methods. For example, AI/ML models have been utilized to analyze large-scale genomic and imaging datasets in the context of breast cancer, leading to the identification of new imaging biomarkers that correlate with genetic mutations such as BRCA1 and BRCA2.[12] These biomarkers can potentially guide personalized treatment strategies and improve prognostic assessments.

Although the use of AI/ML algorithms in routine oncologic screening is increasingly common, an emerging use of them is in opportunistic screening, where incidental findings that might otherwise be overlooked can be identified. For instance, over 80 million CT scans are completed every year in the United States, and they could be used to screen for several conditions without additional radiation exposure or costs.[13,14] Radiology departments can set up automated protocols where imaging studies performed for specific indications are concurrently analyzed for common incidental findings. This concurrent analysis maximizes the utility of each imaging study and enhances the overall value of radiologic examinations. The integration of the algorithms with electronic health records and other healthcare data sources could also enable multimodal algorithms with the potential to enhance predictive accuracy.

The following examples depict how CT could be used to opportunistically stratify disease risk[15]:

- Osteoporosis: bone mineral density assessments could be made based on bones (especially vertebrae) captured within a CT scan to help in diagnosing osteoporosis and assessing fracture risk.
- Cardiovascular risk: aortic calcification can be measured on noncontrast chest CT studies to serve as a marker for atherosclerosis and predict cardiovascular events.
- Metabolic syndrome: visceral fat, which correlates closely with metabolic syndrome and cardiovascular risk, can be measured on abdominal CT scans.
- Sarcopenia: sarcopenia can be assessed through measuring muscle mass, density, and composition on muscles captured within a CT study.
- Hepatic steatosis: liver fat content can be based on attenuation measurements from abdominal CT scans to assist with diagnosing and managing hepatic steatosis.

These imaging-based assessments could play a pivotal role in clinical practice through earlier detection, risk stratification, and management of medical conditions. AI/ML use in opportunistic screening also supports personalized patient care by identifying risk factors and guiding preventive measures tailored to individual patient profiles. A notable example is the use of AI/ML in detecting coronary artery calcifications, where stratification of patients based on their cardiovascular risk can be used to recommend further diagnostic evaluations or lifestyle modifications.[16] This personalized approach to patient care may also foster patient engagement and adherence to preventive strategies.

Despite the promising potential of AI/ML in opportunistic screening, several challenges must be addressed to fully realize the benefits. One major challenge is the integration of AI/ML algorithms into diverse technical settings with varying imaging protocols. It will be critical to ensure the generalizability and robustness of AI/ML models in these different settings. Another challenge is the potential for perpetuating biases as described further below.

Democratizing Radiology Expertise

The global shortage of radiologists, particularly in LMICs, can exacerbate health disparities through delays in diagnosis and treatment. AI/ML technologies facilitate the democratization of radiology expertise by automating complex image analysis, enhancing diagnostic accuracy, and providing decision support. AI/ML algorithms can be deployed on portable imaging devices and smartphones, enabling widespread access to high-quality diagnostic imaging and interpretation. Projects like the Global Initiative on AI for Health by the WHO aim to leverage AI/ML to enhance diagnostic capabilities in LMICs.[17] By facilitating the earlier detection and intervention of conditions that have an increased burden in LMICs, such as tuberculosis, pneumonia, and malignancies, these tools could contribute to improved health outcomes and reduced mortality rates.

AI/ML-driven radiology platforms can be integrated into telemedicine frameworks, facilitating remote consultations and second opinions. This integration is particularly beneficial in low-resource settings where access to radiologists is limited. AI/ML algorithms can preanalyze imaging studies and generate preliminary reports, which can then be reviewed by radiologists in centralized locations. This approach may not only expedite the diagnostic process but also optimize the utilization of radiology expertise.

For instance, teleradiology services augmented with AI/ML capabilities have been successfully implemented in rural and underserved regions, providing timely and accurate diagnostic support.[18] These services leverage AI/ML to triage imaging studies, prioritize urgent cases, and ensure that critical findings are promptly addressed. This model enhances the efficiency of radiological services and reduces the burden on overworked radiologists in urban centers. These tools can also be deployed in primary care settings and remote clinics, potentially enabling healthcare providers without specialized training in radiology make informed decisions based on reliable diagnostic insights.

AI/ML technologies also play a pivotal role in the ongoing education and training of healthcare professionals. AI/ML-driven educational platforms can provide radiologists and other healthcare providers with access to curated databases of annotated images, interactive learning modules, and real-time feedback on diagnostic performance. These resources facilitate continuing professional development and help bridge the knowledge gap between urban and rural healthcare providers. For example, platforms like Radiology Assistant and AI/ML-based training simulators offer comprehensive learning experiences that enhance diagnostic skills and keep practitioners updated with the latest advancements in radiology.[19] By democratizing access to high-quality educational resources, AI/ML could contribute to the equitable distribution of radiological expertise and improve the overall standard of care.

Algorithmic Bias and Ethical Considerations

AI/ML algorithms in radiology are trained on extensive datasets, and using racially diverse datasets during training can help reduce biases that exist in healthcare. However, if the training data contain biases, these biases can be perpetuated by the AI/ML system. Therefore AI in radiology has the dual potential to both mitigate existing racial disparities in healthcare by improving diagnostic accuracy across diverse populations and exacerbate disparities if algorithms are not properly developed and validated. One study exemplified AI/ML's potential to reduce disparities by deploying a deep learning model on knee x-rays to predict pain levels.[20] The model significantly reduced unexplained racial disparities in pain levels; in contrast, underserved populations have historically reported higher pain levels even when accounting for objective assessment of disease severity using medical images. Although radiologists' severity assessments explained only 9% of racial pain disparities, the AI/ML model's predictions accounted for 43%, indicating a 4.7-fold improvement. This result was attributed to the model's ability to capture nuanced factors within the knee not visible in standard radiographic evaluations. Moreover, the use of racially and socioeconomically diverse training data enhanced the model's effectiveness across diverse patient groups, potentially equalizing access to treatments such as arthroplasty.

Conversely, AI/ML in radiology can perpetuate racial bias, as evidenced by a study called "AI recognition of patient race in medical imaging."[21] This study revealed that AI/ML models unintentionally learned to identify and predict patient race from medical images. Such capabilities raise ethical concerns about fairness and justice in healthcare, as biased algorithms may lead to differential treatment based on race. The unintended recognition of race in medical imaging underscores the need for rigorous algorithmic development and validation protocols. Addressing biases requires diverse and representative training datasets, transparent model development processes, and ongoing evaluation to mitigate unintended consequences.

Issues such as patient consent, data privacy, and equitable access to AI/ML technologies must be carefully managed to protect individual rights and prevent disparities in healthcare outcomes. The growing breadth of clinical AI/ML applications, compounded by the need for adaptations to accommodate diverse local health systems and the inevitable evolution of data over time, poses a significant regulatory challenge. Regulation is essential for ensuring patient safety and data security. Commercial availability of AI/ML systems typically requires approval or clearance by centralized regulatory bodies such as the FDA in the United States. These bodies often have guidelines for AI/ML algorithm development, validation, and postmarket surveillance. However, some argue that the current centralized regulatory model, when scaled, may not be able to account for the demographic and technical diversity across all implementations of an AI/ML algorithm. Therefore a hybrid regulatory approach that combines centralized oversight with decentralized mechanisms has been proposed. This approach could allow for flexibility in regulatory requirements that better align with local healthcare contexts, promoting innovation by facilitating iterative improvements in AI/ML systems and supporting equitable access to advanced healthcare technologies tailored to diverse populations. However, implementing such a model requires robust coordination between centralized regulatory bodies and local stakeholders, clear guidelines for data governance and algorithm transparency, and continuous monitoring to ensure ongoing compliance with safety and efficacy standards.

Conclusion

As healthcare systems worldwide confront the challenges posed by aging populations, increasing chronic diseases, and escalating healthcare costs, AI/ML in radiology can mitigate these challenges by enabling earlier detection and intervention through sophisticated screening algorithms that analyze vast amounts of imaging data. These capabilities can empower healthcare providers to identify diseases at their earliest stages, potentially reducing the need for invasive procedures and improving prognosis for patients. Moreover, AI/ML-driven technologies facilitate personalized medicine by tailoring diagnostic and treatment plans to individual patient profiles, thereby optimizing healthcare delivery and resource allocation.

However, the widespread adoption of AI/ML in radiology requires careful consideration of ethical implications and regulatory frameworks. Concerns regarding algorithmic bias, data privacy, and equitable access must be addressed to ensure that AI/ML technologies benefit all patient populations equally. Transparency in AI/ML algorithm development, rigorous validation processes, and collaboration among stakeholders are essential to mitigate risks and maximize the benefits of AI/ML in healthcare. Continued research and innovation in AI/ML-driven radiology hold the potential to revolutionize population health strategies, making healthcare more efficient, accessible, and patient centered. Future research should focus on enhancing the interpretability and transparency of AI/ML algorithms, fostering interdisciplinary collaboration between radiologists, data scientists, and clinicians, and exploring the potential of AI/ML in detecting a broader range of incidental findings across various imaging modalities. By fostering interdisciplinary collaboration and ethical stewardship, healthcare systems can leverage AI/ML to navigate complex challenges and improve health outcomes worldwide.

References

1. World Health Organization. Ageing and health. Updated October 1, 2022. Accessed June 14, 2024. https://www.who.int/news-room/fact-sheets/detail/ageing-and-health.
2. Collaborators GBDRF. Global, regional, and national comparative risk assessment of 84 behavioural, environmental and occupational, and metabolic risks or clusters of risks for 195 countries and territories, 1990–2017: a systematic analysis for the Global Burden of Disease Study 2017. *Lancet*. 2018;392(10159):1923–1994. http://doi.org/10.1016/S0140-6736(18)32225-6.
3. OECD. Finance for sustainable development. Accessed June 14, 2024. https://www.oecd.org/en/topics/policy-issues/finance-for-sustainable-development.html.
4. U.S. Food & Drug Administration. Artificial intelligence and machine learning (AI/ML)-enabled medical devices. Updated May 13, 2024. Accessed June 14, 2024. https://www.fda.gov/medical-devices/software-medical-device-samd/artificial-intelligence-and-machine-learning-aiml-enabled-medical-devices.
5. U.S. Food & Drug Administration. 510(k) premarket notification (ABMD software). Updated July 29, 2022. Accessed June 14, 2024. https://www.accessdata.fda.gov/scripts/cdrh/cfdocs/cfpmn/pmn.cfm?ID=K213760.
6. U.S. Food & Drug Administration. 510(k) premarket notification (Deep learning image reconstruction). Updated April 20, 2023. Accessed June 14, 2024. https://www.accessdata.fda.gov/scripts/cdrh/cfdocs/cfpmn/pmn.cfm?ID=K230807.
7. Dilmegani C. Top companies in AI-powered medical imaging. AIMultiple. Updated January 12, 2024. Accessed June 14, 2024. https://research.aimultiple.com/looking-for-better-medical-imaging-for-early-diagnostic-and-monitoring-contact-the-leading-vendors-here/.
8. McKinney SM, Sieniek M, Godbole V, et al. International evaluation of an AI system for breast cancer screening. *Nature*. 2020;577(7788):89–94. http://doi.org/10.1038/s41586-019-1799-6.
9. Ardila D, Kiraly AP, Bharadwaj S, et al. End-to-end lung cancer screening with three-dimensional deep learning on low-dose chest computed tomography. *Nat Med*. 2019;25(6):954–961. http://doi.org/10.1038/s41591-019-0447-x.
10. Nartowt BJ, Hart GR, Muhammad W, Liang Y, Stark GF, Deng J. Robust machine learning for colorectal cancer risk prediction and stratification. *Front Big Data*. 2020;3:6. http://doi.org/10.3389/fdata.2020.00006.
11. Litjens GJ, Barentsz JO, Karssemeijer N, Huisman HJ. Clinical evaluation of a computer-aided diagnosis system for determining cancer aggressiveness in prostate MRI. *Eur Radiol*. 2015;25(11):3187–3199. http://doi.org/10.1007/s00330-015-3743-y.
12. Beck AH, Sangoi AR, Leung S, et al. Systematic analysis of breast cancer morphology uncovers stromal features associated with survival. *Sci Transl Med*. 2011;3(108). 108ra113. http://doi.org/10.1126/scitranslmed.3002564.
13. Bredella MA. Opportunistic osteoporosis screening with cardiac CT: can we predict future fractures? *Radiology*. 2020;296(3):509–510. http://doi.org/10.1148/radiol.2020202374.
14. Aggarwal V, Maslen C, Abel RL, et al. Opportunistic diagnosis of osteoporosis, fragile bone strength and vertebral fractures from routine CT scans; a review of approved technology systems and pathways to implementation. *Ther Adv Musculoskelet Dis*. 2021;13. 1759720X211024029. http://doi.org/10.1177/1759720X211024029.

15. Pickhardt PJ, Graffy PM, Perez AA, Lubner MG, Elton DC, Summers RM. Opportunistic screening at abdominal CT: use of automated body composition biomarkers for added cardiometabolic value. *Radiographics*. 2021;41(2):524–542. http://doi.org/10.1148/rg.2021200056.
16. Isgum I, Rutten A, Prokop M, van Ginneken B. Detection of coronary calcifications from computed tomography scans for automated risk assessment of coronary artery disease. *Med Phys*. 2007;34(4):1450–1461. http://doi.org/10.1118/1.2710548.
17. World Health Organization. Artificial intelligence for health. Updated May 27, 2024. Accessed June 14, 2024. https://www.who.int/publications/m/item/artificial-intelligence-for-health.
18. Zuhair V, Babar A, Ali R, et al. Exploring the impact of artificial intelligence on global health and enhancing healthcare in developing nations. *J Prim Care Community Health*. 2024;15:21501319241245847. http://doi.org/10.1177/21501319241245847.
19. Poot CC, van der Kleij RM, Brakema EA, et al. From research to evidence-informed decision making: a systematic approach. *J Public Health (Oxf)*. 2018;40(suppl_1):i3–i12. http://doi.org/10.1093/pubmed/fdx153.
20. Pierson E, Cutler DM, Leskovec J, Mullainathan S, Obermeyer Z. An algorithmic approach to reducing unexplained pain disparities in underserved populations. *Nat Med*. 2021;27(1):136–140. http://doi.org/10.1038/s41591-020-01192-7.
21. Gichoya JW, Banerjee I, Bhimireddy AR, et al. AI recognition of patient race in medical imaging: a modelling study. *Lancet Digit Health*. 2022;4(6):e406–e414. http://doi.org/10.1016/S2589-7500(22)00063-2.

PART IV

Develop Your Application

PART OUTLINE

CHAPTER 19

Data Curation

Sijing Feng ■ Christopher McMahan ■ Anna Hu

Introduction

Data is the essential driving force for advancing artificial intelligence (AI) in radiology, often likened to the new "electricity," underscoring its transformative potential in healthcare. In 2006, Dr. Fei-Fei Li's team established the ImageNet database, which ushered in a new era for the general computer vision science community.[1] The availability of well-curated labeled datasets and growing computational capabilities catalyzed the advancement of deep learning.

Radiology embraced this data-centric revolution by adopting picture archiving and communication systems (PACS) and radiology information systems (RIS) in the 1980s, accelerating the proliferation of digital data. This surge in digital data availability allowed breakthroughs in specialized medical AI systems, positioning radiology at the forefront of AI integration within the healthcare sector. Curating radiology datasets requires collaboration between radiologists and data scientists. Radiologists and data scientists collaborate throughout all stages of the dataset life cycle (see Fig. 19.1) to prepare for diverse end users.

The sensitivity of health data necessitates strict adherence to ethical and regulatory standards during these technical processes. Governance and regulatory standards, which vary based on geographic location and institution type, maintain radiology data's integrity and ethical use.[2–6] Understanding and navigating the standards in the radiology data life cycle is essential, combining technical expertise with ethical and commercial awareness.

This chapter explores the general health data life cycle, emphasizing the objectives, methodologies, and challenges associated with data curation. It offers insights into practical tools and case studies and addresses the ethical and commercial implications of data curation. The goal is to provide radiologists with the essential knowledge for effective data management.

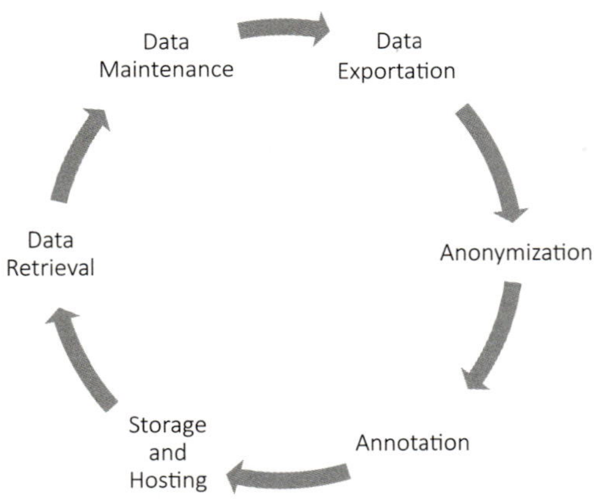

Fig. 19.1 Flowchart of the general data curation life cycle.

Purpose of Dataset Curation

Effective data curation is essential for developing AI models in healthcare, each tailored to specific clinical tasks to improve the quality of healthcare. Radiology data, comprising various content types such as images, audio, and audiovisual, showcases the field's richness and diversity (see Table 19.1). This categorization underscores the complexity and variety of data sources in radiology. The curation must align with the type of AI system to ensure data specificity and relevance, including whether the system involves supervised or unsupervised models, reinforcement learning, or generative/multimodal deep learning systems.[7]

For example, a supervised AI system can be designed to identify pneumothorax on chest X-rays. To create such a system, the dataset must include chest X-rays labeled to indicate the presence or absence of pneumothoraxes. However, if it is also important to know the location and size of any pneumothoraxes, segmentation annotations detailing size and location would become essential, furnishing the model with precise spatial learning information. In the case of large language models (LLM), thousands of radiology reports are required to train these models effectively to categorize reports based on their nuanced features.[21] The complexity of features directly influences the size of the training dataset needed to attain satisfactory inference

TABLE 19.1 ■ **Healthcare Datasets by Data Type**[8–18]

Data Type	Dataset Name	Description/Usage
Images	RSNA pneumonia, PE, intracranial hemorrhage datasets	Large multiinstitutional datasets of de-identified health data organized by RSNA.
	CheXpert	A dataset for chest radiograph interpretation, containing labeled images for training AI models.
Audio	Heart Sounds Dataset	Contains heart sound recordings for cardiac diagnosis and research.
	Respiratory Sound Database	A collection of respiratory sounds for analysis and pattern recognition in pulmonary diseases.
Audiovisual	Audio-Visual Datasets for Depression Recognition	A dataset designed for depression recognition using both audio and visual cues.
	ICU Audio-Visual Dataset	An audiovisual dataset capturing various aspects of patient care in intensive care units.
Text	Clinical Notes Dataset	A collection of anonymized clinical notes used for NLP applications in healthcare.
Multimodal	UK BioBank	Comprehensive large database containing de-identified genetic, lifestyle and health information, and biological samples from 500,000 UK participants.
	Scottish Database	Incorporates various data types, including audio, visual and textual data, for comprehensive medical research.
	MIMIC-CXR	A large dataset of de-identified health data from intensive care units. Used for various medical imaging studies.
	CANDID-PTX dataset	Large adult CXR dataset containing classification and segmentation annotations from NZ population

performance. The more complex a feature is for the model to "learn," the more training examples are generally required for the model to "learn" that feature well. Curating datasets for reinforcement learning models in radiology necessitates data that capture sequences of actions and their resulting rewards.

As such, radiology AI models are expanding to include multimodal systems, posing new challenges with combining individual data types, such as additional steps to link them. However, multimodal datasets also present new opportunities for more diverse applications in addition to their initial purpose.

Features of a High-Quality Dataset

The quality of datasets is another critical consideration early in the dataset curation process. Several important features of a high-quality dataset are worth defining (see Table 19.2). Although creating a dataset encompassing all these high-quality features is often challenging due to resource constraints, the ability to judiciously balance these elements is crucial for dataset designers.

Data Exportation

Data exportation is the initial step in the data curation process. It ensures the seamless transition of medical images from clinical systems to analytic environments, focusing on balancing accessibility, security, and compliance with healthcare regulations. Three primary methods of data exportation are utilized for curation (see Table 19.3). Each exportation method caters to specific needs and operational scenarios within radiology AI, from individual research to extensive, multiinstitutional endeavors. Selecting the most suitable method depends on the project's scope, data sensitivity, and the applicable regulatory demands.

TABLE 19.2 ■ **Features of High-Quality Datasets**

Feature	Description	Impact on AI Learning	Challenges/ Considerations
Expert Annotation	Requires domain expert input for accurate labeling of pathology, anatomical locations and segmentation.	Enhances accuracy and ground truth derivation	Requires expert domain knowledge
Dataset Size	Adequate quantity is necessary for parameter optimization and capturing clinical complexity.	Affects model generalization and performance	Limited size may hinder diversity
Multimodal Datasets	Integrates various data types (images, reports, records) for a comprehensive patient view.	Provides holistic analysis for AI	Complexity in data integration
Publicly Available Datasets	Promotes fairness, benchmarking and collaboration in AI development.	Encourages transparency and standardization	Requires open data sharing policies

TABLE 19.3 ■ **Common Data Exportation Methods**

Method	Description	Strengths	Weaknesses	Applications
PACS Integration	Direct transfer of data to research databases.	Streamlines workflow by reducing manual data handling, while maintaining data integrity and quality.	Depends on robust IT infrastructure; subject to IT constraints and security risks.	Optimal for real-time analysis and AI model training in well-resourced settings.
Encrypted External Hard Drive/ Flash Drive	Utilizes encrypted devices for secure physical data transfer.	Maximizes data security for sensitive information.	Labor-intensive with risks of data loss and storage limits.	Ideal for small-scale transfers where security is paramount.
Cloud-Based Platforms	Cloud storage integration, for example AWS, Microsoft Azure, Google Cloud	HIPAA compliance with more comprehensive data security measures, enhanced reliability, and interoperability.	Can be costly, data required to be located external to the home institution, can be subject to additional Institutional Review Board (IRB) or data governance approval.	Ideal for enterprise ready organizations or mission-critical large-scale projects.

Anonymization

PRINCIPLES OF ANONYMIZATION

Medical images are stored in the Digital Imaging and Communications in Medicine (DICOM) format as a global standard. Protected health information (PHI) may be located within various areas in the DICOM format, including structured metadata fields and pixels incorporated into the image.

Anonymization and de-identification are the processes to remove these PHIs. They are often used interchangeably in the literature, but there are distinct differences. Anonymization is defined as the process of removing PHI that cannot be linked back to the patient. In contrast, de-identification involves the removal of explicit identifiers. It is crucial to perform the anonymization process as part of data exportation to comply with regulations and protect patient privacy. The principles guiding anonymization cover various aspects of the challenge, and must align with the project's needs and the sensitivity of the information. Table 19.4 provides an overview of these core principles and their significance in preserving the confidentiality of patient data.

TOOLS FOR ANONYMIZATION

Specialized tools are required to anonymize radiological data to ensure confidentiality while retaining utility for research and AI applications. Various programs and scripts are designed for

TABLE 19.4 ■ **Core Principles of Data Anonymization**

Principle	Description
Levels of Anonymization	Adjusting the degree of identity removal to protect patient data while ensuring data utility for AI algorithm use.
Preservation of Chronological Data	Maintaining the integrity of temporal data for longitudinal studies without compromising patient identity.
Re-identification Risks	Continuously minimizing the potential for anonymized data to be traced back to individuals with evolving re-identification techniques.

TABLE 19.5 ■ **Example Tools for Anonymization**

Tool	Description	Strengths	URL
NLM's "Scrubber"	Specializes in text anonymization for medical records and reports.	Industry standard for text data, reliable and widely used.	https://lhncbc.nlm.nih.gov/scrubber/
Open-Source Tools	A variety of anonymization tools are available on GitHub.	Accessible and community-supported tools with a focus on image data anonymization.	CTP DICOM Anonymizer (https://www.rsna.org/research/imaging-research-tools) PixelMed (https://www.pixelmed.com/dicomtoolkit.html) dcm2niix (https://github.com/rordenlab/dcm2niix) RadiAnt (https://www.radiantviewer.com/) DeID (https://github.com/pydicom/deid) Orthanc (https://www.orthanc-server.com/)
Advanced AI Algorithms	AI-based methods for automating the identification and redaction of PHI from various data types.	Represents the forefront of anonymization technology with potential for high automation.	

this purpose with different functionalities and strengths (see Table 19.5). Each tool brings unique capabilities to the anonymization process, and the project's specific needs dictate the choice of tool.

ASSESSMENT OF ANONYMIZATION

Quality assessment of anonymization ensures the integrity of patient information. It involves adhering to established standards that define the method and degree to which data should be de-identified. These standards are unique and can vary depending on the regulatory body, geographic location, and institution type. For example, the Health Insurance Portability and Accountability Act (HIPAA) provides guidelines in the United States, whereas in Europe, the General

TABLE 19.6 ■ **Preprocessing Steps for Data Curation**

Preprocessing Step	Description	Importance
Standardization	Converting imaging data and metadata to a uniform format.	Ensures consistency across datasets by aligning file types, image resolution, and scale.
Cleaning	Identifying and correcting errors or inconsistencies.	Improves data accuracy by fixing mislabeled images, removing artifacts, and matching patient information.
Missing Data	Implementing imputation techniques for missing values.	Utilizes methods like interpolation or convolutional neural networks to reconstruct missing image segments, enhancing data completeness.

Data Protection Regulation (GDPR) serves as the authoritative standard.[2,3,5] Compliance with local institutional review board requirements may also be necessary to maintain data integrity.

PREPROCESSING

Preprocessing ensures that the data are clean, consistent, and properly formatted, significantly impacting the accuracy and reliability of AI applications. The preprocessing phase encompasses multiple steps, each holding distinct importance in data curation (see Table 19.6). These steps range from standardizing formats to effectively handling missing data, collectively ensuring the development of robust and reliable AI tools in radiology.

Annotation

Annotation is the process of extracting the essential features from a dataset. Annotation is typically the most labor-intensive and time-consuming curation step. The choice of annotation method depends on the specific requirements of the AI application.

LABEL DESIGN

Label design is essential in annotating images to suit specific dataset requirements. It involves selecting between two primary types of annotation: classification and segmentation. Classification broadly categorizes images or their parts, whereas segmentation provides more details by identifying specific areas within an image. Each method offers distinct advantages, catering to different analytical needs in radiology (see Table 19.7).

Selecting accurate and relevant labels influences model performance in diagnostic and patient care settings, where the labels must align with the real-world scenarios in which the model will operate. In the context of diagnostic applications, inaccurate or overly broad labels could lead to misdiagnoses, potentially causing harm to patients. However, labels that are too specific for their intended use may require more resources to create. Thus balancing the granularity of labeling is critical for model design.

MANUAL LABELING

Manual labeling varies based on the dataset's complexity and specific needs. Regarded as the gold standard in annotation quality, it ensures high accuracy when performed by subspecialty-trained

TABLE 19.7 ■ **Examples of Annotation Categories**

Annotation Type	Subcategory	Description
Classification		Labeling images or parts of images with specific categories or classes.
Segmentation	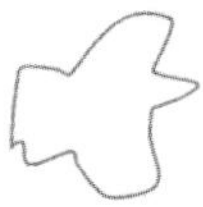 Freeform	Drawing arbitrary shapes around the area of interest. Used for flexible area marking.
	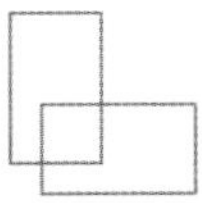 Bounding Box	Placing a rectangular box around the target feature. Suitable for clear-cut, defined areas.
	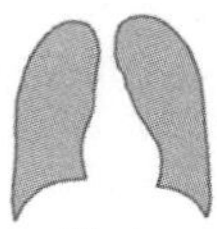 Mask	Creating pixel-level annotations to precisely cover the area of interest. Ideal for detailed tissue or lesion segmentation. It may utilize thresholding based on Hounsfield units.
	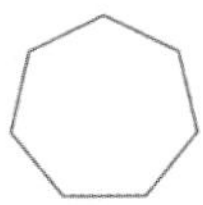 Polygon	Outlining an area/region with straight line borders connecting multiple points.
	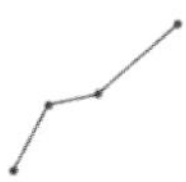 Line	A single or multiple straight lines connecting multiple points from a starting point to an end point on images.
	 Location	Single crosshair marking a single location.
	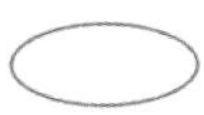 Ellipse	Oval region of interest.

Categories adapted from MD.ai.[19]

radiologists (Fig. 19.2). However, this approach is resource intensive and challenging for curating large datasets. Strategies like a tiered review system or expert crowdsourcing are often employed to enhance efficiency and maintain data quality.

AI-ASSISTED LABELING

AI-assisted labeling utilizes deep learning systems to annotate parts of the dataset automatically, leveraging features "learned" from the manually labeled data. This method can significantly expand the volume of annotated data with a reasonable level of accuracy. Care must be taken in designing the annotation models, especially for subtle or complex findings, to ensure the accuracy and reliability of AI-assisted labels. Rule-based annotation models can still outperform deep learning–based models for low-prevalence results in a dataset due to rarity of training examples.

ANNOTATION PLATFORMS

The choice of an annotation platform significantly impacts the efficiency of the overall workflow. Platforms are broadly categorized into two types: locally installed and server based. Each has distinct advantages and challenges that influence their suitability for a project.

Locally installed platforms maximize patient data security, as the data do not leave the confines of an isolated system. These platforms come with comprehensive data manipulation and analysis tools, and offer high levels of customization. They are often open-source, which can be advantageous in terms of cost. However, the requirement for technical expertise to set up and maintain a local network, along with their limited range of connectivity, can pose challenges for collaborative efforts.

On the other hand, server-based platforms (see Fig. 19.2) facilitate collaboration, particularly for geographically dispersed teams. Although these platforms have historically been limited in data manipulation capabilities, many have now evolved to include richer features. Although customization may incur additional costs, the benefits of such tools can outweigh these costs, especially for larger commercial enterprises.

For specific examples of locally installed and server-based annotation platforms, and their respective strengths and weaknesses, refer to Table 19.8.

GROUND TRUTH DETERMINATION

Ground truth determines the standard used to measure AI model predictions, with its accuracy being pivotal to a dataset's quality and an AI application's dependability. However, the subjectivity of clinical diagnoses often proves challenging to establish an objective ground truth. Ground truth considerations must be set within the clinical context, accounting for the diagnostic probabilities indicated by imaging features.

Label design is closely tied to ground truth definitions, necessitating the creation of labels directly relevant to clinical outcomes and decision-making. Labels must represent clinical judgment, factoring in the urgency of a finding or its consequential impact on patient management.

Various gold standards are adopted in clinical medicine to establish definitive ground truth. In oncology, for example, biopsy results are often considered the gold standard. However, setting a benchmark in radiology is often more subjective, usually involving a consensus among multiple fellowship-trained radiologists or validation against outcomes. This rigorous process enhances the AI model's ability to make reliable predictions that can be trusted in clinical practice.

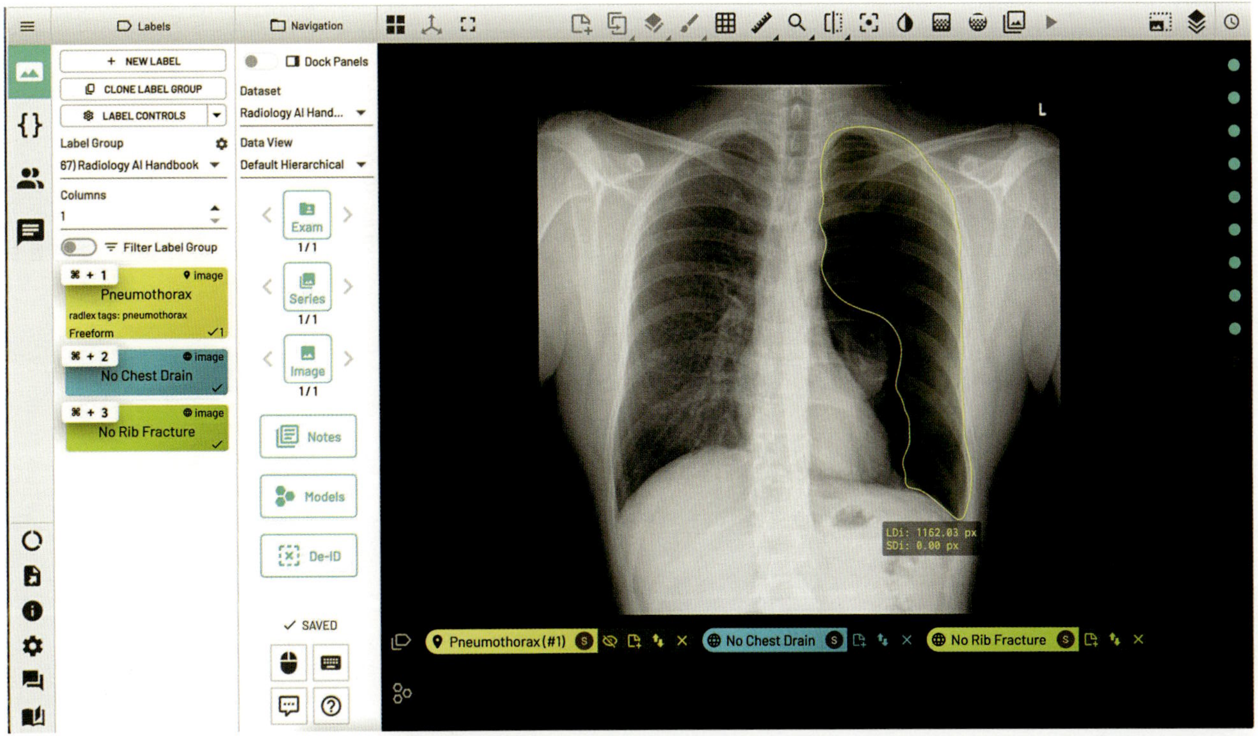

Fig. 19.2 Example of chest X-ray annotation on *MD.ai* platform, demonstrating a positive pneumothorax segmentation, and negative chest drain and negative rib fracture classification labels. (Software platform from *MD.ai*, https://www.md.ai/; chest X-ray case courtesy of Dr. Ian Bickle, rID 86926, Radiopaedia.org.)

TABLE 19.8 ■ **Examples of Common Annotation Platforms**[19–29]

Product	Type of Data	Advantages	Disadvantages	URL
Label Studio	Image/Video/Text	• High customizability	• It may require more setup time	https://labelstud.io/
Amazon SageMaker	Image/Video/Text	• Machine learning • Human annotators • Scalable, cloud based	• It could be costly • Complexity of the setup	https://aws.amazon.com/sagemaker/
Apache Annotator	Image/Video/Text	• Open-source framework • Highly customizable	• Requires technical expertise to implement	https://annotator.apache.org/
Scale AI	Image/Video/Text	• Collaborative system for labeling tasks • Emphasizes quality and consistency	• Potentially expensive for small projects	https://scale.com/
Figure Eight (Appen)	Image/Text	• Crowdsourcing • Access to a large workforce	• Quality control can be challenging	https://appen.com/
Labelbox	Image/Video	• Broad feature set for various data types • Manual and semi-automated labeling	• Complexity may be overwhelming for simple projects	https://labelbox.com/
MD.ai	Image	• Advanced features for radiology-specific tasks • RADLEX ontology integrated • Collaborative interface • HIPAA compliance	• It may be too specialized for nonradiology applications	https://www.md.ai/
VGG Image Annotator (VIA)	Image	• Good for detailed image annotation	• Limited to image data; not for video or 3D	https://www.robots.ox.ac.uk/~vgg/software/via/
3D Slicer	Image	• Free to use • Designed specifically for 3D imaging	• Relatively steep learning curve	https://www.slicer.org/
ITK-Snap	Image	• Free to use • Well designed with common useful features • Excellent community support	• Requires a level of technical knowledge	http://www.itksnap.org/pmwiki/pmwiki.php
Prodigy	Text	• Efficiency in text data labeling • Full customization of features	• Requires high level of programming skills	https://prodi.gy/
Snorkel	Text	• Large language model assisted labeling • High interoperability • HIPAA compliance	• Can be costly	https://snorkel.ai/

Model design must balance label accuracy with practical constraints like time, budget, and resources to establish a high-quality ground truth. An adjudication system is sometimes necessary to achieve consensus when conflicting views emerge within a team. Furthermore, a team can perform an inter-annotator variability analysis to guarantee the annotations' consistency and accuracy. It is crucial to ensure these aspects as an early and fundamental stage for the success of any AI-driven data curation project in radiology.

Ontology Mapping

Ontology mapping aligns medical terminologies and concepts for use in AI. This alignment is critical for ensuring that AI model labels accurately reflect medical standards and facilitate the integration of AI applications with various healthcare information systems. It also enables collaborative efforts across different institutions and countries.

The use of standard medical terminologies such as the Unified Medical Language System (UMLS), International Classification of Diseases (ICD-11), SNOMED Clinical Terms (SNOMED CT), and RadLex exemplifies this alignment in practice.[30–33] These systems are integral to ontology mapping, providing a standardized language and framework that ensures consistency and understanding across diverse medical practices. When selecting an appropriate ontology for a project, factors such as the project's specific needs, the desired level of detail, and compatibility with other data systems must be carefully considered (see Table 19.9).

Team Management

Efficient team management leads to successful data curation, particularly when utilizing crowdsourcing. Implementing a tiered annotation system (see Fig. 19.3), where junior members conduct initial annotations and senior radiologists provide oversight and review, can optimize the process. This strategy conserves time and resources, and fosters skill development among junior team members, contributing to the overall advancement of radiologic data annotation.

In large-scale projects, managing data involves balancing efficiency with available resources. An adequate system improves efficiency and reduces errors, such as annotation inaccuracies. While a clear labeling protocol is fundamental, teams should be mindful of adapting when an unexpected situation arises. For example, variable team member availability

TABLE 19.9 ■ **Commonly Used Medical Terminology Ontologies**

Ontology	Coverage Area	Strengths	Limitations
UMLS	Clinical, surgery, biomedical, life sciences	Broad coverage for translational AI systems	Complexity; requires regular updates
ICD-11	Standardized clinical diagnoses	Facilitates international data exchange	Primarily clinical focus; may lack detail in nonclinical aspects
SNOMED CT	Detailed clinical terms	Enhances electronic health records and data interoperability	Intricate hierarchy; potential for overspecification
RadLex	Imaging diagnostics in radiology	Precise terminology for radiology	Limited scope for broader clinical datasets

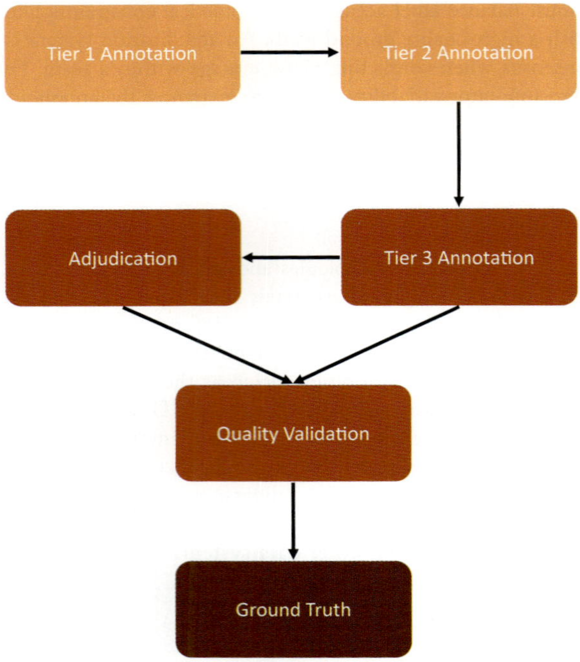

Fig. 19.3 A simplified CANDID-PTX dataset workflow diagram demonstrating the tiered annotation process. Junior annotators in tier 1 and tier 2 performed the initial read on cases. Images were then reviewed and corrected by tier 3 annotators (senior annotators) who were eligible to output ground truth labels for a case. Discordant annotations were adjudicated by a senior fellowship-trained thoracic radiologist. Annotations for all images were manually reviewed before they were finalized.

demands flexibility within the team management system. Assembling a skilled annotation team is challenging; offering incentives like monetary rewards or authorship can encourage participation. Setting clear, efficient timelines further motivates team members, ensuring steady progress.

Extended periods of annotation can lead to fatigue and compromise label quality. Establishing organizing committees is beneficial for teams with a considerable number of members. These committees oversee the progress, enhance communication through regular meetings, and conduct frequent monitoring and evaluation to address errors, thereby ensuring data quality promptly. Focusing on the ultimate goal throughout the project is vital to ensure effective data curation for AI applications in radiology.

Validation

Validation prepares datasets for AI applications, ensuring accuracy, compliance with privacy regulations, and clinical relevance. This process involves a combination of expert manual review and objective performance metrics.

Experts review the dataset as part of manual validation to verify its accuracy and reliability. This step is vital to confirm that the data meets the high standards for practical AI applications in radiology. It can include the burned-in image information and structured data fields to ensure the anonymization of all PHI in adherence to privacy standards like HIPAA. Experts can also

$$F1\ score = 2 \times \frac{Precision \times Recall}{Precision + Recall}$$

$$Recall = \frac{True\ Positive}{True\ Positive + False\ Negative}$$

$$Precision = \frac{True\ Positive}{True\ Positive + False\ Positive}$$

Fig. 19.4 Mathematical formulae for F1 score, recall, and precision.

evaluate the accuracy and consistency of annotations, ensuring they align with expected radiologic findings and clinical interpretations. This step guarantees the precision and consistency of label quality. Special attention is given to complex cases in radiologic datasets, which can often require collaborative resolution between experienced radiologists and data curators.

Objectivity in validation is further ensured by employing quantitative performance metrics, such as accuracy, precision, recall, and F1 score when a dataset is tested on common, publicly available AI models. The F1 score, also called the F-score or F-measure, is a valuable metric for evaluating machine learning models. It involves calculating precision and recall (see Fig. 19.4). Precision is akin to the positive predictive value and measures the likelihood that a positive model output will reflect a true positive output, whereas recall is similar to sensitivity and assesses the accuracy in identifying positive instances. As an example of how these statistics may be applied, in radiology-based screening programs, it is essential to prioritize high recall to avoid missed diagnoses. In cases where the positive class is rare, the F1 score becomes especially valuable as it helps balance precision and recall. These metrics are used to assess the overall quality of the dataset by providing a measurable standard to gauge the dataset's suitability for practical use in clinical settings.

Storage and Hosting

Once curated, datasets need to be hosted on an appropriate platform, especially if the goal is to make them publicly available. Options include institutional hosting (e.g., National Institutes of Health [NIH], National Health Service [NHS]) or university/institutional servers, public services (e.g., Kaggle), private cloud services (e.g., Amazon Web Services [AWS], Microsoft Azure, Google Cloud), or personal storage devices compliant with local or national regulations (see Table 19.10).[34–39]

Ethical considerations often dictate where a dataset can be hosted, and these should be respected. The ethics of data hosting involves the decision between public and private repositories. Public platforms like Kaggle democratize data access, fostering global research collaboration. However, they pose risks of potential data misuse and adherence to diverse international regulations. Private hosting options—utilizing services like AWS, Azure, and Google Cloud or institutional servers—provide tighter control over data, enhancing security and regulatory compliance. The decision between public and private hosting must reflect a project's objectives, the data's sensitivity, and a commitment to ethical standards, balancing the potential for scientific progress with the responsibility to safeguard patient information.

Data Retrieval

Data retrieval dictates how end users access and interact with the dataset. Effective retrieval mechanisms provide users with efficient and accurate data extraction for their specific applications, for research, clinical decision support, or AI model training.

TABLE 19.10 ■ **Common Currently Available Dataset Hosting Platforms**[40–42]

Server	Features	Advantages	Disadvantages	Access Method
NIH Institutional Servers	Secure research data storage, compliance with research standards	High security, specialized for research data	May be restricted to certain institutions, less flexibility for nonresearch use	Through affiliated institutions or research projects
Kaggle	Data science platform with public datasets, competitions, and community	Community support, access to diverse datasets, ideal for ML projects	Limited to data science and ML projects, data quality varies	Free, online platform registration
Microsoft Azure	Cloud computing, AI and ML integration, robust security	Wide range of services, high scalability, strong enterprise support	Can be complex to navigate for beginners, costs can escalate	Subscription-based cloud service
Google Cloud	AI and ML tools, data analytics, secure storage	Strong AI and ML capabilities, integrates with other Google services	Requires technical expertise, costs can be high	Subscription-based cloud service
AWS (Amazon Web Services)	Scalable storage, advanced security, ML and data analytics tools	Leader in cloud services, highly scalable, extensive toolset	Can be complex for beginners, pricing can be a concern	Subscription-based cloud service
TCIA (The Cancer Imaging Archive)	Public access to a large database of cancer imaging, research focused	Free access to cancer imaging data, supports research and education	Focused only on cancer imaging, limited use outside research	Free, open access through website
FigShare	Public access for medical or nonmedical datasets	Supports various datatypes (i.e., images, audio, audiovisual, text); data can be hosted institutionally or externally	May require paid subscription for some additional services	Free or subscription-based platform
PhysioNet	Collection of biomedical, clinical and physiological data.	Free access, good community resource support available	May be open or restricted access	Free, open or restricted access through website

Given downloading large datasets directly from a standard web browser can be inefficient, data retrieval software often allows users to interact with the dataset on a dedicated platform. In cases where data retrieval software is unavailable, investigators can create customized data retrieval pipelines using standard programming languages (e.g., Python).

Database query design is crucial for effective data retrieval. It involves structuring commands to return the most accurate and relevant data for user requests. Radiology queries handle complex criteria such as imaging modalities, anatomic regions, and corresponding pathologic findings. Good query design is efficient with large datasets, provides quick response times, and minimizes the risk of returning irrelevant or inaccurate data.

Data Maintenance

Dataset maintenance involves keeping the datasets accurate, up to date, and aligned with the latest medical standards and practices. Well-maintained radiological datasets ensure the continued effectiveness of AI applications in healthcare.

Keeping track of changes made to a dataset is known as versioning. This practice allows for a safe and effective method of upgrading the datasets, keeping them relevant. Versioning helps document the evolution of data and promotes reproducibility in research. Specific steps to versioning should follow the requirements of the host platform.

Proactively identifying and correcting errors is an ongoing requirement. This process may involve re-evaluating the dataset for annotation accuracy, re-verifying anonymization standards, and ensuring compliance with current data protection regulations. Error correction is vital for maintaining the dataset's integrity.

Synthetic Data Generation

There are limitations to obtaining real-world health data from patients or institutions, often due to ethical constraints. Examples include the ability to obtain retrospective consent or consent waivers. In recent years, large language models, such as ChatGPT,[43] have been used to generate health datasets. Synthetic imaging and audiovisual datasets, which derive data from computational methodologies rather than directly from patient radiologic studies, are also possible. While synthetic data are generated to represent real-world data and the associated metadata, one caveat is that they can still propagate the biases inherent in the real-world data, which requires careful design of the training dataset to minimize such negative effects. Consequently, ethical and regulatory considerations remain valid for traditional real-world data curation. Synthetic data generation has several potential benefits and drawbacks (see Tables 19.11 and 19.12).

AUGMENTED DATA

Augmented data, which reflect a subset of synthetic data, involve altering real data to produce novel datasets. Examples of data modification include, but are not limited to, rotation, geometric deformation, superimposition, and alterations of image quality (e.g., noise, contrast, sharpness). While augmented data offer the advantage of being simpler to generate than synthetic data, it is important to note that these data do not obviate the original data's ethical and privacy considerations and usage restrictions.

CURRENT EXAMPLES OF SYNTHETIC DATA GENERATION

Concerning synthetic data generation, there are several applications, both open source and proprietary, that are in active development. They have applicability to a wide range of industries, including clinical radiology. Examples include NVIDIA (with its Digital Twin and Omniverse platforms for advanced simulation), Synthea (an open-source patient population simulator), and Syntheticus and MDClone (both companies specializing in health data synthesis).[44–49]

TABLE 19.11 ■ **Benefits of Synthetically Generated Data**

Benefit	Notes
Regulatory and ethical benefits	Synthetic data can ameliorate ethical and privacy considerations linked to using real patient information in radiology datasets. Furthermore, by utilizing synthetic data, dataset owners may be able to comply more easily with regulatory frameworks like the GDPR and HIPAA.
Testing and validation	The utilization of synthetic data provides a controlled environment, enabling researchers to fine-tune and assess the performance of models in different contexts. This approach can improve model resilience and generalizability.
Resource intensity	Generating synthetic data may be more efficient than gathering real data. This situation is particularly relevant in radiology, where manual image annotation is resource intensive. Furthermore, synthetic data can reduce data storage, management, and regulatory compliance overhead.
Data scarcity	In situations where real data are scarce (for example, rare pathology) or not representative of a target population, synthetic data are a valuable supplement, enhancing dataset richness. Furthermore, synthetic data may allow clinical scenarios that are otherwise impractical to be simulated with real data.

TABLE 19.12 ■ **Drawbacks of Synthetically Generated Data**

Drawback	Notes
Accuracy	Synthetic data generation techniques may not accurately replicate the richness of real radiological data. As a result, models fine-tuned on synthetic data may be prone to overfitting and subsequently perform poorly. Furthermore, establishing a ground truth for synthetic data can be problematic.
Bias	Inherent biases in training data for synthetic datasets may be propagated or amplified to the dataset.
Regulatory and ethical drawbacks	The acceptability and trustworthiness of synthetic data are contentious issues. Consumers and regulatory bodies may have concerns regarding the utilization and transparency of algorithms trained with synthetic datasets.
Technological limitations	Synthetic generation of high-quality, multimodal radiological data is complicated and computationally intensive. This limitation may prevent synthetic data from being easily accessible to organizations and researchers.

Image synthesis

Synthetic image generation represents a cutting-edge field in machine learning, leveraging sophisticated models to generate images from textual or visual inputs. Currently, there are three main types of models being utilized for image synthesis:

1. **Denoising Diffusion Probabilistic Models (DDPMs)** gradually refine noise into detailed images via a reverse diffusion process that undergoes the progressive addition of noise ("denoising"). Examples include Google Imagen and OpenAI's DALL-E.

2. **Latent Diffusion Models (LDMs)** encode images into a latent space and then apply diffusion processes to create new images, balancing image quality and computational efficiency.[49] An example is Stability AI's Stable Diffusion.
3. **Generative Adversarial Networks (GANs)** use a dual-network architecture where one network generates images while the other evaluates them, leading to highly realistic outputs.[50] Examples include NVIDIA StyleGAN and BigGAN.

Textual synthesis

There are diverse methods for textual synthesis, represented in both closed-source (e.g., OpenAI's ChatGPT and Google's Med-PaLM2) and open-source tools (e.g., OpenLLaMA and Dolly v2). These tools vary in capabilities, offering a range of applications and abilities in interpreting and generating text. Behind these models are advanced neural networks and machine learning algorithms, enabling them to understand and generate human-like text, offering powerful tools for personal and professional use, including medical applications. For example, OpenAI's ChatGPT is designed to interact conversationally, allowing for nuanced and contextually aware text generation, and is trained using reinforcement learning from human feedback (RLHF).[51] Unlike closed-source models, open-source models are particularly significant for research and development, allowing for more extensive experimentation and customization.

Ethics, Licensing, and Commercialization

ETHICS

Beauchamp and Childress's four principles of ethics are fundamental to modern medical practice.[52] They include beneficence (doing good), nonmaleficence (avoiding harm), autonomy (an individual's own decisions regarding their care), and justice (ensuring fairness and equitable distribution of resources). Correspondingly, ethical curation of radiological data is critical, and these principles should be considered foremost in developing comprehensive and high-quality datasets.

Ethical data curation demands consideration of (1) informed consent and transparency, (2) privacy and confidentiality, (3) data security, (4) compliance with legal standards, (5) oversight by ethical review boards or committees, (6) maintaining a patient-centric approach, (7) public trust and engagement, and (8) clear protocols and equitable data access. Furthermore, it is essential that AI algorithms promote equity across demographic groups and avoid bias propagation based on gender, ethnicity, or socioeconomic status.

In utilizing data for healthcare improvement, adherence to ethical principles is essential to safeguard individual rights and promote trust in the health system. Additionally, given the rapid expansion of healthcare institutions as health data repositories, consideration must be given to the increased data exchange rate between different stakeholders. Protection of these sensitive data is crucial as they are transferred between various organizations and regions.

In summary, there are many complex factors to consider when curating radiological and AI research datasets. However, the importance of adherence to ethical curation principles cannot be overstated; these principles form the basis that allows datasets to support high-quality algorithm development and overall trust in AI applications in radiology.

DATA ETHICS IN DIFFERENT REGIONS

Ethical and regulatory frameworks for data curation are rapidly evolving and vary widely geographically. This section aims to provide a concise overview of the frameworks in different regions. However, consultation with local experts is essential to ensure compliance with ethical and regulatory standards. The information outlined is a general guide and should not substitute region-specific ethical and regulatory advice.

Although access to data is important for research and health improvement, it must be balanced with the need for data protection. Informed consent is considered the gold standard for data collection, both with prospective and retrospective analysis (often referred to as "secondary use"). However, vast data requirements for AI algorithm development can make this gold standard difficult to achieve in practice. It is particularly the case for historical data, such as data collected retrospectively from deceased patients.

Several regulatory organizations provide regional or national frameworks that allow for the secondary use of data for research purposes under specific conditions. These frameworks emphasize the principle of minimal risk and, at minimum, mandate that data be anonymized and de-identified to reduce the possibility of re-identification and privacy breaches.

Given this complexity, obtaining approval from an Institutional Review Board (IRB) is considered a standard and crucial step before accessing radiology data. This approach ensures ethical integrity and compliance with relevant standards, thus safeguarding privacy while facilitating valuable research and development.

North American Context

In the United States, the ownership of radiological examinations typically resides within the healthcare institution that conducts the procedure, which is responsible for maintaining and safeguarding these data.[53] Patients can access their medical records, including radiologic data, under the HIPAA[2] provisions. Furthermore, state-level legislation may augment these rights, mandating additional requirements concerning ownership, preservation, and access to medical records. Under Federal Law, as specified in the Code of Federal Regulations Title 45,[54] researchers can obtain a waiver for consent for using health data if specific criteria are met. The criteria include research approval by an accredited IRB[3] and that the research involves no more than minimal risk to the subjects.

In Canada, health data governance falls under provincial jurisdiction, leading to regulation variations across different regions. Health institutions conducting radiologic examinations own the associated data and are responsible for data maintenance and safeguarding. Patients are entitled to access their medical records, including radiologic data.[53] The Tri-Council Policy Statement: Ethical Conduct for Research Involving Humans (2022) provides a unified framework concerning health data across Canada. Specifically, Articles 5.5A and 5.5B outline conditions under which researchers, if specific criteria are met and subject to approval by an accredited IRB, can use de-identified secondary health data for research purposes.[54]

European context

In the European Union (EU), the GDPR[5] is a rigorous regulatory framework harmonizing European data privacy laws. This regulation ensures individuals maintain complete ownership and control of their personal and health data, introducing complexities to data curation through several key provisions.

First, the GDPR mandates explicit informed consent for data processing, emphasizing institutions' responsibility to demonstrate this consent clearly and allowing for its retraction at any time.

Second, data must be collected for "specific, explicit, and legitimate purposes," with secondary use of data typically prohibited. Exceptions for scientific or statistical research exist, subject to diverse regional laws and evolving interpretations.

Third, a data minimization provision outlines the importance of collecting only pertinent data and limiting these data to their intended purpose, avoiding broader data collection and the risk of privacy breaches.

These regulations have notably impacted the development of radiology datasets in the EU. This situation is further complicated by each member country's distinct health data regulations. Despite this complication, ongoing initiatives aim to enhance international collaboration and curate radiology datasets within the EU. These efforts reflect a recognition of the value of shared health data in advancing radiology research while adhering to the GDPR's stringent privacy requirements.

Australasian context

The Royal Australian and New Zealand College of Radiologists (RANZCR) has published a guidance document, Ethical Principles for AI in Medicine (2023).[55] This document outlines nine key ethical principles for research, implementation, and maintenance of AI in health care. Underpinning these principles is the imperative for AI applications to be both consistently safe for patients and society, and adhere to established ethical standards of health care. Furthermore, the guidelines mandate that radiology data can only be shared outside the clinical setting under specific conditions: with patient consent, approval from an ethics committee, and as allowed or required by law.

The New Zealand National Ethics Committee's National Ethics Standards[56] provide ethical guidance for data use and AI applications in health care. They include criteria for appropriate secondary use of de-identified data for research purposes. The Health Information Privacy Code (2020) outlines the legislative standards for proper health data management and disclosure in research.

In Australia, ethical research data use guidelines are outlined in the Australian Privacy Principles Guidelines, the Privacy Act of 1988, and the National Health and Medical Research Council's National Statement on Ethical Conduct in Human Research (2023).[56]

Together, these standards offer a comprehensive overview of the appropriate process for radiology data curation in Australasia, outlining the ethical and legal frameworks necessary for responsibly handling and utilizing such data.

Indigenous data sovereignty

Indigenous data sovereignty underlines the fundamental right of Indigenous people to own, control, and have governance over their data.[57] This principle aims to protect Indigenous groups' unique cultural, socioeconomic and political contexts, and ensure data are used appropriately. Researchers must consider consultation with local Indigenous communities or research councils, a frequently mandated criterion for IRB approval, to ensure that research is conducted in alignment with Indigenous interests.

LICENSING

Licensing is the process of providing permission for end users to utilize a dataset, technology, or intellectual property. It is an essential aspect of ethical data curation as it provides governance over the underlying data within a dataset. A license restricts access to a dataset to appropriate end users and specifies permissible usage of the data. A license also protects against intentional or unintentional misuse, although it does not eliminate potential liability associated with data curation. Key aspects of licensing are explored in Table 19.13.

In addition to licensing, data use agreements (DUAs) are essential in ethical data curation. DUAs are contract-based, legally binding documents that often mirror licensing terms. These documents commonly detail permissible and prohibited data usage but may expand on broader aspects such as distribution, attribution, privacy obligations, and requirements for data disposal.

When licensing datasets or developing DUAs, it is important to obtain local legal expertise as there are significant variations and evolving legal interpretations of health data frameworks. Such expertise is crucial when undertaking commercial ventures or developing proprietary datasets.

Radiology datasets often include multiple data modalities (e.g., visual, textual, and audiovisual), leading to varied licensing approaches. Licensing terms can encompass specific modalities selectively or apply to the entire dataset. For example, a common practice is to allow open-source or permissive access to radiological annotations while retaining proprietary rights over source images and underlying algorithms.

The authors emphasize the importance of publicly available, high-quality, curated radiology datasets. Open-source licensing promotes the sharing and collaboration of datasets. This collaboration benefits researchers, healthcare systems, and the broader community. Importantly,

TABLE 19.13 ■ **Key Considerations of Dataset Licensing**

Aspect	Notes
Utilization	*Guidelines and restrictions*: details usage scope and clarifies the dataset's permissible and prohibited use.
Attribution	*Acknowledgment requirements*: specifies how the original authors/owners of the dataset must be credited. It may include examples of appropriate attribution in publications or derivative works.
Adaptation	*Modification rights*: outlines the extent to which end users can alter or build upon the dataset and the scope of these modifications.
Perpetuity	*Re-licensing terms*: discusses whether modified versions of the dataset (if applicable) may be re-licensed or must be shared under the original licensing terms (also known as "share alike" or "copyleft").
Commercialization	*Commercial versus noncommercial use*: defines the terms under which the dataset can (or cannot) be used for commercial purposes, including any restrictions or conditions.

accessible datasets can help diminish inequity and mitigate bias that might otherwise complicate algorithm development through comparative analysis. Due to these advantages, various national and international bodies are working towards shared imaging datasets for research and noncommercial purposes. The Creative Commons Organization[58] provides a streamlined method for individuals and institutions to license their datasets, ensuring accessibility and collaboration. In radiology dataset curation, four main licensing categories are typically considered (see Table 19.14).

TABLE 19.14 ■ **Major Dataset Creative Commons License Types**

License Type	Creative Commons License Icons	Description
Public domain		Fully waives all copyright and related rights in a dataset. *Note*: This approach is not recommended for radiology datasets, as ethical data curation necessitates appropriate guidance on usage and permissions for the dataset.
Permissive		Permits end users to use, modify, and share the data. Typically, this approach requires attribution to the original author in derivative work. It may include restrictions on commercial use.
Copyleft (share-alike)		Permits end users to use, modify, and share the data; however, derivative works must maintain the original licensing from the principal dataset. Typically, the approach requires attribution to the original author in derivative work. It may include restrictions on commercial use.
Proprietary	N/A (custom)	Varied. Typically, this approach retains all copyright and related rights in a dataset, restricting use, modification, or sharing unless specifically allowed.

Conclusion

The role of data in advancing AI in radiology is transformative and central to healthcare innovation. The quality of data curation depends on the data accuracy, data comprehensiveness, and available resources. Although traditional methods are still widely used today, newer techniques, such as synthetic and augmented data generation methods, are emerging fields that offer innovation while adhering to ethical and privacy considerations. The data curation process will undoubtedly continue to evolve to maintain a balance between data safety and trends in AI system development.

References

1. Deng J, Dong W, Socher R, Li L-J, Li K, Fei-Fei L. ImageNet: a large-scale hierarchical image database. In: *2009 IEEE Conference on Computer Vision and Pattern Recognition*. IEEE; 2009:248–255. http://doi.org/10.1109/CVPR.2009.5206848.
2. HIPAA Home. HHS.gov. Health Information Privacy. Accessed December 31, 2023. https://www.hhs.gov/hipaa/index.html.
3. Institutional Review Board. National Institute of Health. Accessed December 30, 2023. https://orwh.od.nih.gov/toolkit/human-subjects-protections/institutional-review-board.
4. Canadian Institutes of Health Research, Natural Sciences and Engineering Research Council of Canada, Social Sciences and Humanities Research Council of Canada. *Tri-Council Policy Statement: Ethical Conduct for Research Involving Humans*. January 12, 2022. Accessed December 30, 2023. https://ethics.gc.ca/eng/policy-politique_tcps2-eptc2_2022.html.
5. Complete guide to GDPR compliance. General Data Protection Regulation (GDPR). Accessed December 31, 2023. https://gdpr.eu/.
6. National Statement on Ethical Conduct in Human Research 2023. NHMRC. National Health and Medical Research Council; 2023. Accessed December 31, 2023. https://www.nhmrc.gov.au/about-us/publications/national-statement-ethical-conduct-human-research-2023.
7. Arora A, Alderman JE, Palmer J, et al. The value of standards for health datasets in artificial intelligence-based applications. *Nat Med*. 2023;29(11):2929–2938. http://doi.org/10.1038/s41591-023-02608-w.
8. AI challenges. RSNA. Accessed December 31, 2023. https://www.rsna.org/rsnai/ai-image-challenge.
9. Irvin J, Rajpurkar P, Ko M, et al. CheXpert: a large chest radiograph dataset with uncertainty labels and expert comparison. *arXiv*. 2019. http://doi.org/10.48550/arxiv.1901.07031.
10. Shi K, Schellenberger S, Will C, et al. A dataset of radar-recorded heart sounds and vital signs including synchronised reference sensor signals. *Sci Data*. 2020;7(1):50. http://doi.org/10.1038/s41597-020-0390-1.
11. Laux H, Hallawa A, Assis JCS, Schmeink A, Martin L, Peine A. Two-stage visual speech recognition for intensive care patients. *Sci Rep*. 2023;13(1):928. http://doi.org/10.1038/s41598-022-26155-5.
12. Le an Ha M, Holdbrook R, Yaneva V. NBME – Score Clinical Patient Notes | Kaggle. Kaggle. 2022. Accessed December 31, 2023. https://www.kaggle.com/c/nbme-score-clinical-patient-notes.
13. Min K, Yoon J, Kang M, Lee D, Park E, Han J. Detecting depression on video logs using audiovisual features. *Humanit Soc Sci Commun*. 2023;10(1):788. http://doi.org/10.1057/s41599-023-02313-6.
14. UK Biobank. UK Biobank. Accessed December 31, 2023. https://www.ukbiobank.ac.uk/.
15. Johnson AEW, Pollard TJ, Berkowitz SJ, et al. MIMIC-CXR, a de-identified publicly available database of chest radiographs with free-text reports. *Sci Data*. 2019;6(1):317. http://doi.org/10.1038/s41597-019-0322-0.
16. ISD Services | Electronic Data Research and Innovation Service (eDRIS) | Data for Research | ISD Scotland. Public Health Scotland. Accessed December 31, 2023. https://www.isdscotland.org/Products-and-Services/EDRIS/Data-for-Research/.
17. Feng S, Liu Q, Ritchie S, et al. *CANDID-III Dataset*. The University of Auckland; 2023. http://doi.org/10.17608/k6.auckland.22726004.v1.
18. Feng S, Azzollini D, Kim JS, et al. Curation of the CANDID-PTX dataset with free-text reports. *Radiol Artif Intell*. 2021;3(6):e210136. http://doi.org/10.1148/ryai.2021210136.
19. MD.ai. Accessed December 31, 2023. https://www.md.ai/.
20. Machine Learning Service – Amazon SageMaker – AWS. Amazon Web Services. Accessed December 31, 2023. https://aws.amazon.com/sagemaker/.

21. Apache Annotator provides annotation-enabling code for browsers, servers, and humans. Apache Annotator. Accessed December 31, 2023. https://annotator.apache.org/.
22. Appen is the Trusted Partner for Innovative World-Class AI Applications. Accessed December 31, 2023. https://appen.com/.
23. Labelbox | Data-centric AI Platform for Building & Using AI. Accessed December 31, 2023. https://labelbox.com/.
24. Dutta A, Gupta A, Zisserman A. VGA Image Annotator. Visual Geometry Group – University of Oxford. Accessed December 31, 2023. https://www.robots.ox.ac.uk/~vgg/software/via/.
25. 3D Slicer image computing platform | 3D Slicer. Accessed December 31, 2023. https://www.slicer.org/.
26. Yushkevich PA, Hao J, Ravikumar S, Pouch AM, Kaczmarczyk L, Aggarwal A. ITK-SNAP home. ITK-SNAP. Accessed December 30, 2023. http://www.itksnap.org/pmwiki/pmwiki.php.
27. Prodigy • Prodigy • An annotation tool for AI, Machine Learning & NLP. Prodigy. Accessed December 31, 2023. https://prodi.gy/.
28. Snorkel AI | Data-centric AI for the enterprise. Accessed December 31, 2023. https://snorkel.ai/.
29. Open Source Data Labeling Platform. Label Studio. Accessed December 31, 2023. https://labelstud.io/.
30. SNOMED CT. September 18, 2019. Accessed December 30, 2023. https://www.nlm.nih.gov/healthit/snomedct/index.html.
31. RadLex Term Browser. RSNA Informatics. Accessed December 31, 2023. https://radlex.org/.
32. International Classification of Diseases (ICD). World Health Organization. Accessed December 31, 2023. https://www.who.int/standards/classifications/classification-of-diseases.
33. Bodenreider O. The Unified Medical Language System (UMLS): integrating biomedical terminology. *Nucleic Acids Res*. 2004;32:D267–D270. Database issue. http://doi.org/10.1093/nar/gkh061.
34. Hosting and Storage Services (HSS) | CIT. National Institute of Health. Accessed December 31, 2023. https://www.cit.nih.gov/about-cit/hosting-and-storage-services-hss.
35. Free Cloud Computing Services – AWS Free Tier. Amazon Web Services. Accessed December 31, 2023. https://aws.amazon.com/free/.
36. Kaggle: your machine learning and data science community. Kaggle. Accessed December 31, 2023. https://www.kaggle.com/.
37. Cloud Computing Services | Microsoft Azure. Microsoft. Accessed December 31, 2023. https://azure.microsoft.com/en-us.
38. Cloud Computing, Hosting Services, and APIs. Google Cloud. Accessed December 31, 2023. https://cloud.google.com/gcp.
39. Cloud Solutions – NHS SBS. NHS | Shared Business Services. Accessed December 31, 2023. https://www.sbs.nhs.uk/fas-cloud-solutions.
40. The Cancer Imaging Archive (TCIA). National Institute of Health | National Cancer Institute. 2011. Accessed December 31, 2023. https://imaging.cancer.gov/informatics/cancer_imaging_archive.htm.
41. figshare - credit for all your research. Accessed December 31, 2023. https://figshare.com/.
42. PhysioNet. Accessed December 31, 2023. https://physionet.org/.
43. Introducing ChatGPT. OpenAI. Accessed December 31, 2023. https://openai.com/blog/chatgpt.
44. World Leader in Artificial Intelligence Computing | NVIDIA. NVIDIA. Accessed December 31, 2023. https://www.nvidia.com/en-us/.
45. Synthea. Synthetic Mass. Accessed December 31, 2023. https://synthea.mitre.org/.
46. Syntheticus | Synthetic Data Generation Made Easy. Accessed December 31, 2023. https://syntheticus.ai/.
47. MDClone – The World's Most Powerful Healthcare Data Platform. MDClone. Accessed December 31, 2023. https://www.mdclone.com/.
48. Khader F, Müller-Franzes G, Tayebi Arasteh S, et al. Denoising diffusion probabilistic models for 3D medical image generation. *Sci Rep*. 2023;13(1):7303. http://doi.org/10.1038/s41598-023-34341-2.
49. Rombach R, Blattmann A, Lorenz D, Esser P, Ommer B. High-resolution image synthesis with latent diffusion models. *arXiv*. 2021. http://doi.org/10.48550/arxiv.2112.10752.
50. Trevisan de Souza VL, Marques BAD, Batagelo HC, Gois JP. A review on generative adversarial networks for image generation. *Comput Graph*. 2023;114:13–25. http://doi.org/10.1016/j.cag.2023.05.010.
51. Ziegler DM, Stiennon N, Wu J, et al. Fine-tuning language models from human preferences. *arXiv*. 2019. http://doi.org/10.48550/arxiv.1909.08593.
52. Shea M. Forty years of the four principles: enduring themes from beauchamp and childress. *J Med Philos*. 2020;45(4–5):387–395. http://doi.org/10.1093/jmp/jhaa020.

53. Geis JR, Brady AP, Wu CC, et al. Ethics of artificial intelligence in radiology: summary of the joint european and north american multisociety statement. *Radiology*. 2019;293(2):436–440. http://doi.org/10.1148/radiol.2019191586.
54. Code of Federal Regulations (Annual Edition). GovInfo. January 1, 2023. Accessed December 31, 2023. https://www.govinfo.gov/app/collection/cfr/2023.
55. Faculties of Clinical Radiology and Radiation Oncology Councils. Ethical Principles for AI in Medicine, Version 2.0. The Royal Australian and New Zealand College of Radiologists. January 9, 2023. Accessed December 31, 2023. https://www.ranzcr.com/college/document-library/ethical-principles-for-ai-in-medicine.
56. National Ethical Standards. National Ethics Advisory Committee. March 2, 2022. Accessed December 31, 2023. https://neac.health.govt.nz/national-ethical-standards/.
57. Rainie SC, Kukutai T, Walter M, Figueroa-Rodriguez OL, Walker J, Axelsson P. Issues in Open Data: Indigenous data sovereignty. *Zenodo*. 2019. http://doi.org/10.5281/zenodo.2677801.
58. Homepage – Creative Commons. Creative Commons. Accessed December 31, 2023. https://creativecommons.org/.

CHAPTER 20

Artificial Intelligence Network Training and Validation in Radiology: Recent Developments and Real-World Examples

Marlee Mason-Maready

KEY POINTS

- This chapter provides a concise overview of recent advancements in AI network training and research and the critical development and validation processes for AI models in radiology.
- By emphasizing the significance of rigorous and standardized procedures, the chapter underscores the importance of ensuring the accuracy and reliability of AI models in radiology.
- This chapter utilizes real-world examples to illustrate the concepts discussed, showcasing the potential of AI in radiology while underscoring the ongoing need for research and validation efforts to ensure safety and effectiveness in clinical practice.

GLOSSARY OF TERMS AND DEFINITIONS

Spatial hierarchy: how different parts of an image are structured and related to each other at various scales (e.g., in computer vision tasks like object recognition, the spatial hierarchy might involve detecting low-level features such as edges or corners in the initial layers of a neural network, then gradually combining these features to recognize higher-level patterns like shapes or textures in deeper layers).

Mapping function: the mathematical transformations or algorithms used to correlate input medical image data with corresponding output predictions or classifications. These functions essentially "map" the input data, such as radiographic images, to desired outputs, such as identifying abnormalities, segmenting structures, or making diagnostic predictions.

Generative adversarial networks (GANs): a class of deep learning frameworks consisting of two neural networks, a generator and a discriminator, trained simultaneously through a competitive process. In the context of radiology, GANs can help create more realistic images for training purposes or for augmenting existing data to improve accuracy. The generator can create fake medical images, whereas the discriminator evaluates the authenticity of the fake images compared to real ones. Through iterative training, GANs learn to produce increasingly realistic synthetic images that closely resemble real medical images. They learn from each other, and the generator gets better at creating realistic images over time.

Adversarial training: involves teaching a model to be resilient against potential challenges or adversarial attacks. It works by exposing the model to intentionally perturbed or distorted data, designed to deceive or confuse it. Through this process, the model learns to recognize and disregard such adversarial inputs, enhancing its robustness and ability to perform accurately even in the presence of unforeseen variations or manipulations in the data. This approach helps the model become more resistant to artifacts or anomalies seen in medical imaging.

Domain adaptation: adjusting a model trained on one type of data to work well with a different type of data. It helps AI models perform effectively across various datasets and imaging methods without needing extensive retraining. This adaptation ensures that AI systems can handle different situations encountered in medical practice, improving their performance and usefulness in real-world scenarios.

Area under the receiver operating characteristic curve (AUC and ROC curve): the ROC curve is a graphical plot of the true positive rate (sensitivity) against the false positive rate (1-specificity) for different threshold values, whereas the AUC is the probability that the model will rank a randomly chosen positive instance higher than a randomly chosen negative instance. The AUC score ranges from 0 to 1, where 0.5 indicates random guessing, and 1 indicates perfect discriminative ability performance of the model.

Hyperparameter: a parameter set prior to the training process that controls the behavior of the machine learning model. Unlike model parameters, which are learned during training, hyperparameters are not directly learned from the data, but instead influence the learning process, like the speed of learning or the complexity of the model. They include the learning rate, batch size, and the number of layers in a neural network architecture.

Batch prediction: the process of generating predictions or outcomes for a batch of data simultaneously instead of making predictions one by one, which allows models to process multiple inputs at once, thereby increasing efficiency. This approach is commonly used in tasks such as image classification, segmentation, and disease detection, where the model needs to analyze numerous images or data points concurrently to provide insights or diagnoses.

Introduction

What are the steps of artificial intelligence (AI) development for medical imaging purposes? How do you train an AI algorithm and how do you ensure that the outputs of these systems are generalizable and valid? These questions are all immensely important, and this chapter offers answers to them including an overview of recent advancements in AI research, network training, and the development and validation processes within the field of radiology. This chapter will also explore the utility of convolutional neural networks (CNNs) and the importance of comprehensive training and proper validation of algorithms. Recent progress in these areas has significantly bolstered the performance and capabilities of AI algorithms in medical imaging contexts, as demonstrated by real-world successful applications of AI highlighted at the end of the chapter.

AI Model Development Overview

Broadly, the development process involves identifying a clinical need; choosing and partitioning appropriate data sources; designing, training, and testing the algorithm; and validating clinical performance. The reporting of these processes has been standardized[1] and is applicable across different imaging modalities, including x-ray, ultrasound, computed tomography, magnetic resonance imaging, optical coherence tomography, fundus photography, and angiography.[2] Ideally, AI models developed for radiology must be accurate, robust, and generalizable to various populations,

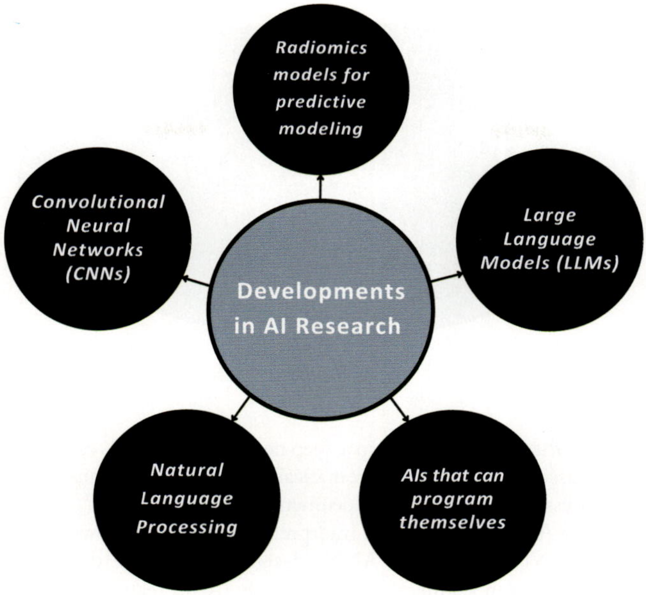

Fig. 20.1 Recent developments in artificial intelligence research as discussed in this chapter.

especially in the realm of healthcare where the consequences of decisions informed by AI can be life and death. The development of models requires a rigorous process that involves optimizing model parameters by training the model on large datasets and validating the model using independent datasets, which will be discussed later in the chapter.

Recent Developments in AI Research

Intersectional research targeting AI and radiology focuses on developing and validating algorithms for image analysis, clinical decision support, and predictive modeling. Most AI models in radiology are used to support lesion detection or quantification or to help radiologists' decision-making.[3] Some newer approaches also help with analyzing patients' history, writing reports, quantifying disease progression, and predicting patient outcomes.[4] Recent developments in AI research include the development of radiomics models for predictive modeling, the use of natural language processing (NLP) for clinical documentation, and the use of CNNs for image segmentation (see Fig. 20.1). NLP can extract relevant information from clinical notes and reports, enabling the development of decision support systems. Radiomics refers to the extraction of features from medical images using algorithms that characterize data in order to describe textures, shapes, pixel intensities, and relationships between pixels. Unfortunately, many of these features are not easily mapped to clinical situations or subjective imaging findings or are simply not very intuitive for radiologists to use.[5]

AI is an umbrella term encompassing many different subtypes, and those discussed in this chapter can be seen in Fig. 20.2. To clarify, machine learning (ML) is a subset of AI that can automatically adapt with minimal human interference by being explicitly programmed and will be referred to as AI/ML. However, complex tasks can surpass the capacities of AI/ML models and not be solved adequately. This limitation is what deep learning (DL), a domain within AI/ML, excels at. Because current DL algorithms mimic the learning processes of the human brain, one of the names that DL models go by is artificial neural networks (ANNs), which reflects the computationally encoded

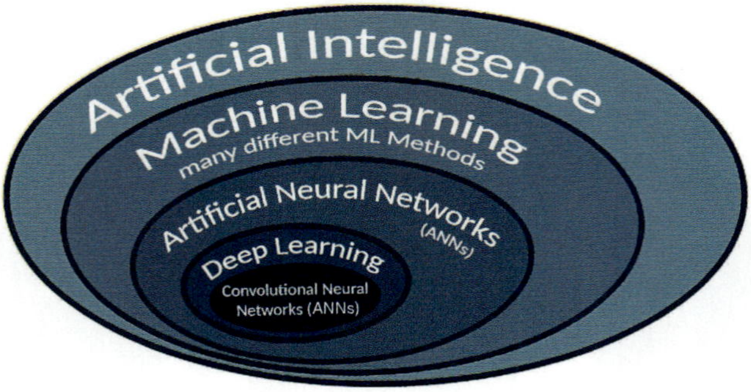

Fig. 20.2 Types of artificial intelligence.

mathematical functions that together make up a deep neural network. DL can be defined as a mathematical framework based on ANNs for automatically deriving representations from given data, which enables the processing of data such as documents, images, and text.

Understanding how AI is used in image interpretation requires knowledge of a relevant DL network architecture: CNNs, which are ANNs designed for image data that can repeatedly manipulate layers of input, can segment data to identify useful features, allowing processing of complex data sets, including images. CNNs' layered architecture is inspired by biological perception mechanisms of the human visual cortex and necessitates fewer network parameters. CNNs also require very little preprocess data compared to other DL algorithms. The results of CNNs across medicine have been impressive, with many models performing with expert or beyond-expert accuracy, sensitivity, and specificity.[6,7]

DL, and especially CNNs, are proving to be impressive tools to improve patient safety and healthcare efficiency via increased automation of routine tasks.[8–10] Accurate and reliable models have been shown to complement highly trained human assessments as a part of novel systems with equivalent or superior performance to conventional practice with the additional benefit of being less expensive.[11]

Finally, emerging AI models such as GPT-4, PaLM 2, and LLaMA 2 are increasingly able to use programming applications as tools—in other words, AI programs are getting better at learning how to program and therefore build themselves,[12] which could further speed up the process of AI system development.

AI Network Training

The current state of network training within radiology reflects a dynamic landscape characterized by rapid advancements and growing integration of AI technologies, especially DL, using large datasets for training algorithms to recognize patterns and features in images.[13]

High-quality annotated and curated datasets are paramount to training AI models effectively because they directly influence the model's performance and generalizability.[14] In radiology, these datasets consist of x-rays, CT scans, MRIs, and ultrasounds along with corresponding ground truth annotations (also known as the answer key) provided by radiologists. Once the dataset is curated, the next step is selecting an appropriate AI architecture and training strategy. CNNs are commonly used in radiology due to their ability to learn spatial hierarchies to pick up on image features. Researchers may opt for various CNN architectures, such as ResNet, DenseNet, or VGG, depending on the specific task and available computational resources.

DL models are trained with the help of advancements in capabilities such as cloud computing infrastructure, which facilitate the use of increasingly complex models on ever-enlarging datasets. However, the "black box" nature of such DL networks often impedes direct interpretation of results due to both the inherent unpredictability of mapping functions and high structural complexity of the network. Cloud-based platforms are usually more of a "black box," offering no specifics as to the model architecture, but some enable model export and batch prediction to facilitate external validation.

It is important to consider the concerns inherent in DL models' requirement of large amounts of high-quality labeled data for effective training. In radiology, obtaining such datasets can be challenging due to issues like data scarcity, data imbalance, and variations in imaging protocols. Low-quality or biased data can lead to poor model performance and generalizability.

Recent developments in AI network training that aim to enhance the generalizability and interpretability of AI models include the use of transfer learning, where an already trained model is re-used to perform a new task, which reduces the need for large annotated datasets,[15] and the use of generative adversarial networks (GANs), where two networks team up to create new data that resembles a given training dataset (e.g., using a radiological image dataset to create synthetic medical images). GANs can be used to augment small datasets, thereby improving model performance. Transfer learning has proven effective in leveraging knowledge learned from one dataset to improve performance on another.[16]

Additionally, methods like adversarial training and domain adaptation have been explored to enhance the generalizability of AI models to variations in imaging protocols, patient demographics, and scanner characteristics. Adversarial training, the AI/ML method that aims to trick models by providing deceptive input, helps the model become more resistant to said deceptive input or attacks. In radiology, this adversarial training improves models' assessment of artifacts commonly seen in medical imaging, whereas domain adaptation enables the transfer of knowledge between different imaging domains, bettering the model's performance on a greater variety of datasets, including differing imaging conditions.

Efforts to incorporate domain-specific knowledge, such as radiological expertise and clinical guidelines, into the training process are accelerating to ensure the clinical relevance and reliability of AI-based diagnostic tools. However, because AI systems rely on training data, they lack context, proceed without ethics or morals, and are more likely to exhibit bias if the training data are not representative of the system's target population. This concern is serious because AI therefore has potential to create or exacerbate healthcare disparities because training data are retrospectively procured from clinical archives, and therefore these data contain current and historical health disparities and societal inequities.[17] A recent review of 320 published studies that developed machine learning to evaluate COVID-19 on chest radiographs and CT scans concluded that "none of the models identified are of potential clinical use due to methodological flaws and/or underlying biases."[18] Identifying and addressing these biases entirely is not a straightforward task, yet it is our responsibility as physicians to actively consider, seek out, and address them.

AI Validation Process

The validation of AI algorithms is critical for ensuring their safety, reliability, and effectiveness across various patient populations, imaging protocols, and clinical scenarios. Validation is generally not a one-time occurrence but an ongoing process throughout training involving assessing the algorithm's performance on independent, ideally diverse datasets distinct from those used for training (see Fig. 20.3). Validation also subsequently evaluates the algorithm's efficacy across various imaging modalities, patient demographics, and clinical settings. Regulatory bodies, including the US Food and Drug Administration (FDA) and the European Commission have issued guidelines regarding the development and validation processes for AI algorithms in diagnostic imaging.[19,20]

The common metrics for model evaluation include sensitivity, specificity, accuracy, and the area under the receiver operating characteristic curve (AUC or ROC curve). The metrics can be applied to tasks including image classification, segmentation, and disease detection, as well as

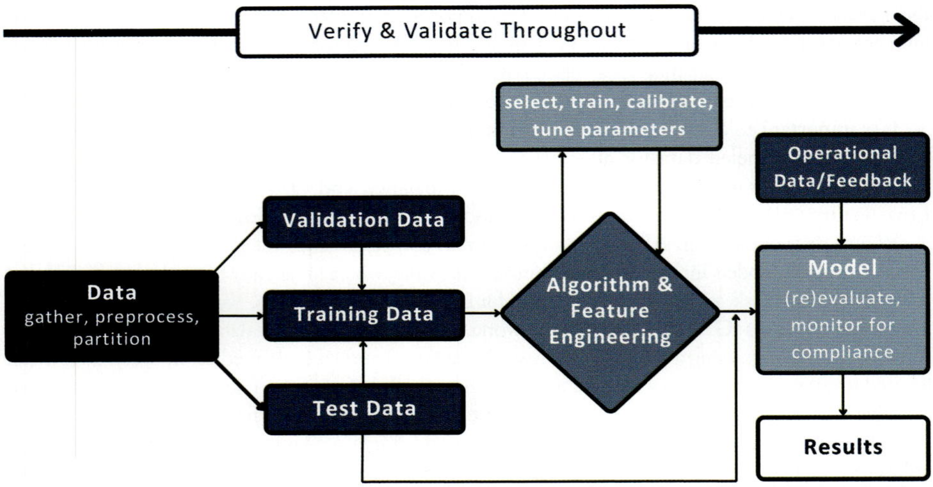

Fig. 20.3 Overview of artificial intelligence workflow. (Karunakar Budema, Dr Anna-Lena Hürter, Aritra Chakrabarti, Jocelyn Chee. (2022, August 22). Taking Shape: Artificial Intelligence Regulation and its Impact on CSV/CSA (III). KVALITO Consulting Group. https://kvalito.ch/taking-shape-artificial-intelligence-regulation-and-its-impact-on-csv-csa-iii/. Accessed May 19, 2025: Figure 1.)

improve the accuracy and generalizability of algorithms.[21] Similar metrics can be used for hyperparameter tuning and algorithm selection.[22]

Cross-validation (CV) is a resampling technique used to assess the performance of an AI/ML model by partitioning data into multiple subsets or folds. The model is trained on a portion of the data (training set) and evaluated on the remaining data (validation set). This process is repeated multiple times, with different subsets of data used for training and validation in each iteration. The performance metrics obtained from each iteration are then averaged to provide an estimate of the model's performance.

However, the larger learning capacity of newer deep networks makes them susceptible to overfitting on training data, especially if using a single or small dataset. Overfitting—when the model cannot generalize and instead fits too closely to the training dataset—can result in overoptimism regarding how a model will perform on future data.[23] This discrepancy between expectations of a model and what it can deliver in reality has become a frequent source of disappointment in clinical implementations of AI.[24,25] CV alleviates the risk of overfitting by providing more training data for models, thereby offering more dependable estimates of the model's capacity to generalize to unseen data. Choosing the correct CV approach for a given dataset (e.g., k-fold, leave-one-out, nested, bootstrapping) is important but beyond the scope of this chapter.

Conclusion

The improving data availability, coupled with advances in computing and innovative algorithms, has increased AI's potential in many respects. The training and validation of AI algorithms, consisting of meticulous data curation, selection of appropriate architectures and training strategies, and rigorous model evaluation on independent datasets are critical for ensuring their safety and effectiveness in clinical practice. However, the implementation of AI in radiology presents new challenges, such as the need for large annotated datasets for training AI algorithms, ensuring the transparency and interpretability of AI decisions, and addressing ethical and regulatory considerations. More research is required as AI continues advancing in order to maximize its potential to improve patient outcomes and transform the field of radiology.

Real-World Examples

- Ueda et al. (2023) detailed a novel deep learning-based model developed and validated across multiple institutions to classify cardiac functions and valvular heart diseases using chest radiographs.[26] By training on data from diverse sources, the model demonstrates robust performance in accurately identifying various cardiac parameters, achieving impressive AUC values ranging from 0.83 to 0.92 for different classifications, including left ventricular ejection fraction, tricuspid regurgitant velocity, and valvular pathologies. With high accuracy, sensitivity, and specificity, as well as a sizable dataset of over 22,000 radiographs, this model classified values typically obtained from echocardiography in a fraction of the time, with low system requirements and the potential to be continuously available in areas where echocardiography specialists are scarce or absent.
- Ardila et al. (2023) showcased the efficacy of an end-to-end deep learning model in lung cancer screening, achieving a notable AUC of 0.94.[27] Compared to traditional screening methods, the deep learning approach demonstrated superior performance in detecting malignant pulmonary nodules, with a sensitivity of 94.4% and a specificity of 89.8%. These compelling results highlight the significant potential of AI-driven approaches in revolutionizing lung cancer screening, by offering high accuracy and efficiency in early detection, which could ultimately translate into improved patient outcomes and reduced mortality rates.
- Arab et al. (2020) presented an expedited and entirely automated deep learning technique for precise segmentation and volume quantification of hemorrhages in noncontrast whole-head CT scans.[28] Their method achieved exceptional accuracy, with a Dice similarity coefficient of 0.874 and a mean absolute error of 4.5 mL for estimating hemorrhage volume. By automating the segmentation process, this approach eliminates the need for manual intervention and significantly reduces processing time compared to conventional methods. These findings suggest that this deep learning method holds significant potential for improving efficiency and accuracy in hemorrhage quantification, potentially enhancing clinical decision-making and patient outcomes in neurology and emergency medicine.

Resources

- Books
  - *Deep Learning in Radiology: Handbook of Radiomic Feature Selection* by Yunqiang Chen, Hongming Li, and Dinggang Shen: This book provides comprehensive coverage of deep learning techniques applied to radiology, including feature selection, image segmentation, and disease classification.
  - *Handbook of Research on AI Innovations in Healthcare and Clinical Environments* by Dilip Singh Sisodia, Ram Bilas Pachori, and Lalit Garg.
- Online Courses
  - Coursera: "AI for Medical Diagnosis": by Andrew Ng: This course covers various applications of AI in healthcare, including medical imaging analysis and diagnosis. It provides a solid foundation in machine learning techniques relevant to radiology.
  - Udacity: "AI for Healthcare Nanodegree" by Nvidia: This nanodegree program offers hands-on experience in applying AI to healthcare problems, including medical imaging tasks such as disease detection and diagnosis.
- Journals
  - *Journal of Medical Artificial Intelligence (JMAI)*: This journal publishes research articles, reviews, and case studies on the application of AI in medical imaging and radiology.

- *Radiology*: The journal regularly features articles and special issues on the use of AI and machine learning in radiology, covering topics such as image interpretation, automated diagnosis, and workflow optimization.
- Cross-Validation & Choosing an Approach by Bradshaw et al. (2023).[22]

- Conferences and Workshops
  - RSNA (Radiological Society of North America) Annual Meeting: This conference features dedicated sessions and workshops on AI in radiology, showcasing the latest research and advancements in the field.
  - MICCAI (International Conference on Medical Image Computing and Computer-Assisted Intervention): MICCAI hosts workshops and tutorials on AI techniques applied to medical imaging, including radiology-specific topics like image segmentation and disease detection.

References

1. Vasey B, Nagendran M, Campbell B, et al. Reporting guideline for the early-stage clinical evaluation of decision support systems driven by artificial intelligence: DECIDE-AI. *Nat Med*. 2022;28(5):924–933. https://doi.org/10.1038/s41591-022-01772-9.
2. Nagendran M, Chen Y, Lovejoy CA, et al. Artificial intelligence versus clinicians: systematic review of design, reporting standards, and claims of deep learning studies. *BMJ*. 2020;368:m689. https://doi.org/10.1136/bmj.m689.
3. Hosny A, Parmar C, Quackenbush J, Schwartz LH, Aerts HJWL. Artificial intelligence in radiology. *Nat Rev Cancer*. 2018;18(8):500–510. https://doi.org/10.1038/s41568-018-0016-5.
4. Shen Y, Heacock L, Elias J, et al. ChatGPT and other large language models are double-edged swords. *Radiology*. 2023;307(2):e230163. https://doi.org/10.1148/radiol.230163.
5. van Griethuysen JJM, Fedorov A, Parmar C, et al. Computational radiomics system to decode the radiographic phenotype. *Cancer Res*. 2017;77(21):e104–e107. https://doi.org/10.1158/0008-5472.CAN-17-0339.
6. Aggarwal R, Sounderajah V, Martin G, et al. Diagnostic accuracy of deep learning in medical imaging: a systematic review and meta-analysis. *NPJ Digit Med*. 2021;4(1):65. https://doi.org/10.1038/s41746-021-00438-z.
7. McKinney SM, Sieniek M, Godbole V, et al. International evaluation of an AI system for breast cancer screening. *Nature*. 2020;577(7788):89–94. https://doi.org/10.1038/s41586-019-1799-6.
8. Bash S, Johnson B, Gibbs W, Zhang T, Shankaranarayanan A, Tanenbaum LN. Deep learning image processing enables 40% faster spinal MR scans which match or exceed quality of standard of care: a prospective multicenter multireader study. *Clin Neuroradiol*. 2022;32(1):197–203. https://doi.org/10.1007/s00062-021-01121-2.
9. Kwon JM, Lee Y, Lee Y, Lee S, Park J. An algorithm based on deep learning for predicting in-hospital cardiac arrest. *J Am Heart Assoc*. 2018;7(13):e008678. https://doi.org/10.1161/JAHA.118.008678.
10. Richardson ML, Garwood ER, Lee Y, et al. Noninterpretive uses of artificial intelligence in radiology. *Acad Radiol*. 2021;28(9):1225–1235. https://doi.org/10.1016/j.acra.2020.01.012.
11. Xie Y, Nguyen QD, Hamzah H, et al. Artificial intelligence for teleophthalmology-based diabetic retinopathy screening in a national programme: an economic analysis modelling study. *Lancet Digit Health*. 2020;2(5):e240–e249. https://doi.org/10.1016/S2589-7500(20)30060-1.
12. Thirunavukarasu AJ, Ting DSJ, Elangovan K, Gutierrez L, Tan TF, Ting DSW. Large language models in medicine. *Nat Med*. 2023;29(8):1930–1940. https://doi.org/10.1038/s41591-023-02448-8.
13. Litjens G, Kooi T, Bejnordi BE, et al. A survey on deep learning in medical image analysis. *Med Image Anal*. 2017;42:60–88. https://doi.org/10.1016/j.media.2017.07.005.
14. Irvin J, Rajpurkar P, Ko M, et al. CheXpert: a large chest radiograph dataset with uncertainty labels and expert comparison. *Proc AAAI Conf Artif Intell*. 2019;33(1):590–597. https://doi.org/10.1609/aaai.v33i01.3301590.
15. Shin HC, Roth HR, Gao M, et al. Deep convolutional neural networks for computer-aided detection: CNN architectures, dataset characteristics and transfer learning. *IEEE Trans Med Imaging*. 2016;35(5):1285–1298. https://doi.org/10.1109/TMI.2016.2528162.

16. Ravishankar H, Sudhakar P, Venkataramani R, et al. Understanding the mechanisms of deep transfer learning for medical images. ArXiv, abs/1704.06040. 2016.
17. Brady AP, Allen B, Chong J, et al. Developing, purchasing, implementing and monitoring AI tools in radiology: practical considerations. A multi-society statement from the ACR, CAR, ESR, RANZCR & RSNA. *Insights Imaging*. 2024;15(1):16. https://doi.org/10.1186/s13244-023-01541-3.
18. Roberts M, Driggs D, Thorpe M, et al. Common pitfalls and recommendations for using machine learning to detect and prognosticate for COVID-19 using chest radiographs and CT scans. *Nat Mach Intell.* 2021;3:199–217. https://doi.org/10.1038/s42256-021-00307-0.
19. Larson DB, Harvey H, Rubin DL, Irani N, Tse JR, Langlotz CP. Regulatory frameworks for development and evaluation of artificial intelligence-based diagnostic imaging algorithms: summary and recommendations. *J Am Coll Radiol.* 2021;18:413–424. 3 Pt A. https://doi.org/10.1016/j.jacr.2020.09.060.
20. Recht MP, Dewey M, Dreyer K, et al. Integrating artificial intelligence into the clinical practice of radiology: challenges and recommendations. *Eur Radiol.* 2020;30(6):3576–3584. https://doi.org/10.1007/s00330-020-06672-5.
21. Wolterink JM, Leiner T, Viergever MA. Isgum I. Generative adversarial networks for noise reduction in low-dose CT. *IEEE Trans Med Imaging*. 2017;36(12):2536–2545. https://doi.org/10.1109/TMI.2017.2708987.
22. Bradshaw TJ, Huemann Z, Hu J, Rahmim A. A guide to cross-validation for artificial intelligence in medical imaging. *Radiol Artif Intell.* 2023;5(4):e220232. https://doi.org/10.1148/ryai.220232.
23. Steyerberg EW, Bleeker SE, Moll HA, Grobbee DE, Moons KG. Internal and external validation of predictive models: a simulation study of bias and precision in small samples. *J Clin Epidemiol.* 2003;56(5):441–447. https://doi.org/10.1016/s0895-4356(03)00047-7.
24. Kawaguchi K, Kaelbling LP, Bengio Y. Generalization in deep learning. ArXiv, abs/1710.05468. 2017.
25. Voter AF, Meram E, Garrett JW, Yu JJ. Diagnostic accuracy and failure mode analysis of a deep learning algorithm for the detection of intracranial hemorrhage. *J Am Coll Radiol.* 2021;18(8):1143–1152. https://doi.org/10.1016/j.jacr.2021.03.005.
26. Ueda D, Matsumoto T, Ehara S, et al. Artificial intelligence-based model to classify cardiac functions from chest radiographs: a multi-institutional, retrospective model development and validation study. *Lancet Digit Health.* 2023;5(8):e525–e533. https://doi.org/10.1016/S2589-7500(23)00107-3.
27. Ardila D, Kiraly AP, Bharadwaj S, et al. End-to-end lung cancer screening with three-dimensional deep learning on low-dose chest computed tomography. *Nat Med.* 2019;25(6):954–961. https://doi.org/10.1038/s41591-019-0447-x.
28. Arab A, Chinda B, Medvedev G, et al. A fast and fully-automated deep-learning approach for accurate hemorrhage segmentation and volume quantification in non-contrast whole-head CT. *Sci Rep.* 2020;10(1):19389. https://doi.org/10.1038/s41598-020-76459-7.

CHAPTER 21

Regulatory Considerations for Radiology Artificial Intelligence/ Machine Learning Devices

Gregory M. Ramina ■ James M. Hillis

KEY POINTS

- Radiology artificial intelligence/machine learning devices are regulated to ensure their safe and effective use.
- The United States Food and Drug Administration (FDA) provides guidance about what constitutes a device and therefore requires regulatory review.
- The two most common FDA pathways for radiology artificial intelligence/machine learning devices are the 510(k) and *de novo* pathways.

GLOSSARY OF TERMS AND DEFINITIONS

Please refer to Table 21.1 for an explanation of key regulatory language for the FDA.

TABLE 21.1 ■ **The Three Classifications of Devices Through the FDA**

	Risk Level	Review Process	Regulatory Language	Example
Class I	Low	None if exempt device; otherwise the same as Class II.	Exempt	Bandages
Class II	Moderate	*De novo* / 510(k) pathway	Granted (for *de novo*) / cleared (for 510(k))	Most radiology AI software
Class III	High	Premarket approval (PMA)	Approved	Implantable device

Medical devices are regulated worldwide in a manner to ensure their safe and effective use. These regulatory approaches are defined by regulatory frameworks, which are then administered by a presiding regulatory body. Regulatory bodies include the Food and Drug Administration (FDA) in the United States (which administers regulations encapsulated within US law), and Notified Bodies and Competent Authorities in European Union member states (which administer regulations based on the European Union Medical Device Regulation

[MDR]). Each regulatory jurisdiction has its own processes for approving the use of medical devices. Depending on the jurisdiction, the overall approach may differ. In the United States, devices are often compared to existing devices on the market and are required to conform with special rules or requirements for that type of device. In other regions, such as the European Union and Canada, medical device classification is based on a rule-based assessment; devices are expected to conform to general safety and performance requirements using applicable state-of-the-art (referred to as SOTA) practices while ensuring there is an acceptable benefit-risk ratio.

Here we focus on the FDA approach for radiology software-as-medical-devices, which includes many of the artificial intelligence/machine learning applications in medicine. The FDA typically refers to "artificial intelligence/machine learning" (AI/ML) together and uses the phrasing "AI/ML-enabled medical device."

Medical "Device" Functions

The initial distinction for a product is whether or not its functions constitute a medical "device."[1] The Food, Drug, and Cosmetic Act (FD&C Act) was amended as part of the Cures Act in 2016 to provide this distinction.[2] The criteria for being a device are included in Box 21.1A, whereas the criteria for software functions not being considered a device are described in Box 21.1B.[3,4] Commonly, device and nondevice functions can occur alongside one another as part of a device or a larger supporting system to ensure the device operates as intended.

Two important items that help determine whether a product meets the criteria of a device are "intended use" and "indications for use."[1] The intended use is the general purpose of the device or

BOX 21.1 ■ The Definition of a "Device" According to the Food, Drug, and Cosmetic Act

A. Definition of a device (adapted from the Food, Drug, and Cosmetic Act[3]):

An instrument, apparatus, implement, machine, contrivance, implant, in vitro reagent, or other similar or related article, including any component, part, or accessory, which is—

- **(A).** recognized in the official National Formulary, or the United States Pharmacopeia, or any supplement to them,
- **(B).** intended for use in the diagnosis of disease or other conditions, or in the cure, mitigation, treatment, or prevention of disease, in man or other animals, or
- **(C).** intended to affect the structure or any function of the body of man or other animals, and which does not achieve its primary intended purposes through chemical action within or on the body of man or other animals and which is not dependent upon being metabolized for the achievement of its primary intended purposes. The term "device" does not include software functions excluded pursuant to section 360j(o) of this title.

B. Criteria for software functions excluded from the definition of a device (adapted from the Food, Drug, and Cosmetic Act[4]):

The function is intended to acquire, process, or analyze a medical image or a signal from an in vitro diagnostic device or a pattern or signal from a signal acquisition system, for the purpose of:

- **(i)** displaying, analyzing, or printing medical information about a patient or other medical information (such as peer-reviewed clinical studies and clinical practice guidelines);
- **(ii)** supporting or providing recommendations to a health care professional about prevention, diagnosis, or treatment of a disease or condition; and
- **(iii)** enabling such health care professional to independently review the basis for such recommendations that such software presents so that it is not the intent that such health care professional rely primarily on any of such recommendations to make a clinical diagnosis or treatment decision regarding an individual patient.

its function, and includes the indications for use. The indications for use describe the disease or condition the device will diagnose, treat, prevent, cure, or mitigate, including a description of the patient population for which the device is intended.

The FDA has provided guidance for clinical decision support software that includes examples of device and nondevice functions.[5] The differences in these functions can often be subtle. An example of a nondevice function is "software function that analyzes a patient's age, sex, gender, and radiologist's report for findings of low bone density and micro cervical fractures in order to provide [a health care professional] with a list of follow-up options for consideration, such as performance of periodic bone-densitometry scans, nonpharmacological management (e.g., weight-bearing exercise), or referral of the patient to a specialist." An example of a device function is "software function that analyzes a radiologist's score/report of regional contrast discrepancies measured from a head CT of a suspected stroke patient to identify whether the [health care professional] should initiate a specific drug therapy based on a scoring algorithm." Although both examples describe a similar type of analytic functionality, the second example constitutes a device function because it "provides a specific treatment output or directive and supports time-critical decision making" and therefore does not fulfill the second criterion of nondevice functions (see Box 21.1B).

The FDA has also provided guidance about mobile applications as part of its Policy for Device Software Functions and Mobile Medical Applications.[6] This document similarly provides examples of device and nondevice functions. It also describes functions for which the FDA intends to exercise enforcement discretion, which means that the software function meets the statutory definition of a device, but the FDA does not intend to enforce requirements under the FD&C Act. In general, these functions automate simple tasks for healthcare professionals, or they help patients as users self-manage their disease or conditions without providing specific treatment or treatment suggestions.

Device Classification, Regulations, and Product Codes

Once it has been established that a product is a device, the next step is to determine the device classification. These classifications include Class I, Class II, and Class III (Table 21.1). Most of the current radiology AI/ML-enabled medical devices have been classified as Class II.

- Class I devices are low-risk devices.
- Class II devices are moderate-risk devices. They require premarket review by the FDA before they can be sold. This review can occur through a *de novo* or 510(k) pathway as described below. As part of the regulatory process, a *de novo* device will start as a Class III device before being reclassified to Class II as part of the granting and reclassification process.
- Class III devices are high-risk devices. Their intended use is generally life supporting and/or life sustaining. They require premarket approval by the FDA before they can be sold, which is a more intensive premarket review process where the manufacturer must demonstrate a higher standard of evidence prior to premarket authorization.

Alongside the device classification, the FDA maintains a set of regulations and product codes for different device types. These regulations and product codes refer back to the device classification and establish general regulatory controls for devices. For Class II devices, there are also special controls that are defined by the regulation for a specific product type and which apply to the different product codes within a regulation (more information is provided in the 510(k) pathway section below). These controls consider product development (e.g., minimum documentation of algorithm design) and product evaluation (e.g., required performance testing). Table 21.2 provides common terminology that is informally used to refer to regulations for radiology AI/ML-enabled medical devices. Table 21.3 includes examples of regulations and product codes based on the FDA list of AI/ML-enabled medical devices.[7]

TABLE 21.2 ■ **Informal Terminology That Is Used to Describe FDA Regulations**

Informal Term	Description	Example	Regulation Number
CADa/o	Computer-assisted acquisition/ optimization guidance device	Real-time feedback when obtaining echocardiography images	892.2100
CADe	Computer-assisted detection device[a]	Identification of lung nodules on CT chest	892.2070
CADe/x	Computer-assisted detection/ diagnosis device	Identification and diagnosis of fractures on radiographs	892.2090
CADq	Computer-assisted quantification device	Volume quantification of regions on MRI brain	892.2050[b]
CADt	Computer-assisted triage device	Prioritization of CTA head cases with suspected large vessel occlusion	892.2080
CADx	Computer-assisted diagnosis device[a]	Delineation of benign/malignant lesions on breast ultrasound	892.2060

[a]Detection can be thought of as identifying a radiographic finding within imaging, whereas diagnosis can be thought of as providing clinical characterization or diagnosis of radiographic findings and may provide insights that can only be confirmed with other testing (e.g., biopsy).

[b]The 892.2050 regulation also includes other medical image management and processing systems (MIMPS) devices and is not specific to AI/ML-enabled medical devices.

The manufacturer decides which regulation and product code a device will use at the time of submission to the FDA. This decision is heavily influenced, and in most cases determined, by devices with similar intended uses and characteristics that are already on the market and to which the manufacturer will compare itself in the premarket 510(k) application. An appropriate regulation and product code may be established through interaction with the FDA as part of a presubmission process (a type of Q-submission or "Q-sub" used to gain FDA feedback on a device's regulatory pathway, where the Q reflects the FDA letter used to track these enquiries). The FDA also considers their appropriateness during the review process of a submission and they may be changed at this stage.

Premarket Review: 510(k) Pathway

A premarket review incorporates the *de novo* and 510(k) pathways. In the context of Class II devices, the *de novo* pathway is used to establish a new regulation and associated regulation number with the special controls (requirements) that are used for a particular type of Class II device.[8] In contrast, the 510(k) pathway allows a manufacturer to demonstrate equivalence to an existing Class II device on the market, which includes demonstrating compliance to special controls that are specific to that type of Class II device.[9] Although the *de novo* pathway occurs chronologically before the 510(k) pathway, we describe the latter first, given it is more commonly used.

A 510(k) premarket notification is a notice by the manufacturer to the FDA that the manufacturer wants to market a device. The FDA in turn provides "clearance" for the manufacturer to market the device if the FDA accepts the application and finds the device substantially equivalent to a device on the market.

As part of the 510(k) application to the FDA, a manufacturer claims that its device has "substantial equivalence" to an existing device and is thus subject to the same regulations. This existing device is referred to as a "predicate device". The substantial equivalence involves demonstrating

TABLE 21.3 ■ **Common FDA Product Codes That Are Used for Radiology AI/ML-Enabled Medical Devices**

Product Code	Regulation Number	Number of Devices[a]	*De Novo* Device and Manufacturer	Date of Final Decision for Original Device	Brief Description[b]
LLZ[c]	892.2050	129	Quantra (Hologic, Inc.)	September 12, 2008	A medical image management and processing system is a device that provides one or more capabilities relating to the review and digital processing of medical images for the purposes of interpretation by a trained practitioner of disease detection, diagnosis, or patient management. The software components may provide advanced or complex image processing functions for image manipulation, enhancement, or quantification that are intended for use in the interpretation and analysis of medical images. Advanced image manipulation functions may include image segmentation, multimodality image registration, or 3D visualization. Complex quantitative functions may include semi-automated measurements or time-series measurements.
QIH[c]	892.2050	78	EchoGo Core (Ultromics Ltd.)	November 13, 2019	To provide automated radiological image processing and analysis tools. Software implementing artificial intelligence including nonadaptive machine learning algorithms trained with clinical and/or artificial data. In these devices, the algorithm training data typically impacts device performance. Adaptive AI algorithms are not within scope of this product code.

Continued

TABLE 21.3 ■ **Common FDA Product Codes That Are Used for Radiology AI/ML-Enabled Medical Devices—Cont'd**

Product Code	Regulation Number	Number of Devices[a]	*De Novo* Device and Manufacturer	Date of Final Decision for Original Device	Brief Description[b]
QVD	892.2055	1	Caption Interpretation Automated Ejection Fraction Software (Caption Health, Inc.)	February 24, 2023	A radiological machine learning quantitative imaging software with predetermined change control plan is a software-only device which employs machine learning algorithms on radiological images to provide quantitative imaging outputs. The device includes functions to support outputs such as view selection, segmentation and landmarking. The design specifications include planned modifications that may be made to the device consistent with an established predetermined change control plan.
POK	892.2060	8	QuantX (Quantitative Insights, Inc.)	July 19, 2017	A radiological computer-assisted diagnostic software for lesions suspicious of cancer is an image processing prescription device intended to aid in the characterization of lesions as suspicious for cancer identified on acquired medical images such as magnetic resonance, mammography, radiography, or computed tomography. The device characterizes lesions based on features or information extracted from the images and provides information about the lesion(s) to the user. Diagnostic and patient management decisions are made by the clinical user.
MYN	892.2070	10	QVCAD System (QView Medical, Inc.)	November 9, 2016	Medical image analyzers, including computer-assisted/aided detection (CADe) devices for mammography breast cancer, ultrasound breast lesions, radiograph lung nodules, and radiograph dental caries detection, is a prescription device that is intended to identify, mark, highlight, or in any other manner direct the clinicians' attention to portions of a radiology image that may reveal abnormalities during interpretation of patient radiology images by the clinicians. This device incorporates pattern recognition and data analysis capabilities and operates on previously acquired medical images. This device is not intended to replace the review by a qualified radiologist, and is not intended to be used for triage, or to recommend diagnosis.

TABLE 21.3 ■ **Common FDA Product Codes That Are Used for Radiology AI/ML-Enabled Medical Devices—Cont'd**

Product Code	Regulation Number	Number of Devices[a]	*De Novo* Device and Manufacturer	Date of Final Decision for Original Device	Brief Description[b]
QAS	892.2080	41	ContaCT (Viz.AI, Inc.)	February 13, 2018	Radiological computer-assisted triage and notification software is an image processing device intended to aid in prioritization and triage of time sensitive patient detection and diagnosis based on the analysis of medical images acquired from radiological signal acquisition systems. The device identifies or prioritizes time sensitive imaging for review by prespecified clinical users based on software-based image analysis but does not provide information from the image analysis other than triage and notification.
QFM	892.2080	27	Cmtriage (Curemetrix, Inc)	March 8, 2019	Radiological computer-assisted prioritization software for lesions is an image processing device intended to aid in prioritization and triage of time sensitive patient detection and diagnosis based on the analysis of medical images acquired from radiological signal acquisition systems. The device identifies or prioritizes time sensitive imaging for review by prespecified clinical users based on software-based image analysis but does not provide information from the image analysis other than triage and notification.
QBS	892.2090	6	OsteoDetect (Imagen Technologies, Inc.)	May 24, 2018	A radiological computer assisted detection and diagnostic software for suspected fracture is an image processing device intended to aid in the detection, localization, and/or characterization of fracture on acquired medical images (e.g. radiography, MR, CT). The device detects, identifies and/or characterizes fracture based on features or information extracted from images, and may provide information about the presence, location, and/or characteristics of the fracture to the user. Primary diagnostic and patient management decisions are made by the clinical user.

Continued

TABLE 21.3 ■ **Common FDA Product Codes That Are Used for Radiology AI/ML-Enabled Medical Devices—Cont'd**

Product Code	Regulation Number	Number of Devices[a]	*De Novo* Device and Manufacturer	Date of Final Decision for Original Device	Brief Description[b]
QDQ	892.2090	16	Transpara (Screenpoint Medical Bv)	November 21, 2018	A radiological computer assisted detection and diagnostic software for suspected lesions is an image processing device intended to aid in the detection, localization, and characterization of lesions suspicious for cancer on acquired medical images (e.g., mammography, MR, CT, ultrasound, radiography). The device detects, identifies and characterizes lesions suspicious for cancer based on features or information extracted from the images, and may provide information about the presence, location, and characteristics of the lesion to the user. Primary diagnostic and patient management decisions are made by the clinical user.
QJU	892.2100	4	Caption Guidance (Bay Labs, Inc.)	February 7, 2020	A radiological acquisition and/or optimization guidance system is a device that is intended to aid in the acquisition and/or optimization of images and/or diagnostic signals. The device interfaces with the acquisition system, analyzes its output, and provides guidance and/or feedback to the operator for improving image and/or signal quality.

[a]The number of devices is taken from the list on the FDA webpage "Artificial Intelligence and Machine Learning (AI/ML)-Enabled Medical Devices."[7]
[b]The brief description is taken from the "Definition" of the product code on the FDA website; for LLZ, POK and MYN, it is taken from the "Identification" of the regulation number.
[c]Although many AI/ML-enabled medical devices were initially cleared under LLZ (which is a broader code that also includes non-AI/ML-enabled medical devices), it appears that they are now being cleared more specifically under QIH.
The product codes are ordered by regulation number and then by date of final decision for original device. There are additional product codes that can be found in the FDA Product Classification Database

the similarity in the intended use and design of the applicant device. Importantly, it also includes explaining that the device does not raise new questions of safety or efficacy.

Once the FDA receives a 510(k) application, it has 90 calendar days to decide whether or not to clear the device. This timeline may be extended by the time it takes the manufacturer to respond to any formal questions from the FDA. If the FDA clears the device, the manufacturer is sent a clearance letter that cites the applicable regulation number, product code, and cleared indications for use.

As part of the submission, the manufacturer prepares a 510(k) summary that provides a device description, summary of testing, identification of the predicate, and summary of the substantial equivalence comparison to the predicate. It also commonly contains details regarding the device performance, although this item is not explicitly stated as a regulatory requirement. This 510(k) summary is made publicly available for download through a 510(k) database on the FDA website.[10]

The FDA separately has a 510(k) Third Party Review Program, which is applicable to devices with certain product codes and allows the device to instead be reviewed by a third party.[11] In this situation, the third party makes a recommendation to the FDA about the finding of substantial equivalence. The FDA then has 30 calendar days, in addition to the time it takes the manufacturer to respond to any formal questions, to make a final decision about clearance. The Product Classification Database on the FDA website, which describes the different device regulations and product codes within each regulation, identifies if devices with a particular product code are eligible for third party review.[12]

Premarket Review: *De Novo* Pathway

The *de novo* pathway is less commonly used than the 510(k) pathway, in part because there is typically a more involved regulatory process. It is used when a manufacturer cannot identify an existing predicate device with similar intended use or a device raises unique questions of safety and efficacy. The manufacturer therefore needs to propose that the FDA creates a new regulation for the new device type. The decision to proceed with a *de novo* device can be made with FDA engagement through the presubmission process prior to submission.

A *de novo* petition is submitted by a manufacturer to the FDA. It reflects that a device without a predicate will by default be classified as Class III, but that the petition requests reclassification to Class I or Class II (the latter with new special controls that are established as part of the *de novo* process).

As part of a *de novo* submission, the FDA still reviews detailed aspects of the AI/ML technology in the device including the development and testing methods. The manufacturer also needs to provide evidence of a detailed predicate search and a justification for why no acceptable predicate exists.

Once the FDA receives a *de novo* application, it has 150 calendar days to decide whether or not to "grant" the *de novo* petition. This timeline may be extended by the time it takes the manufacturer to respond to any formal questions from the FDA. If the FDA finds a favorable decision, the *de novo* petition is granted, and a new regulation, incorporating any special controls, is created. The FDA decision is incorporated into a publicly available reclassification order. The FDA also issues a public classification summary that incorporates the device description, design, development, risks, and testing.

Once the *de novo* petition for a device has been granted and the new regulation has been created, future devices can use it as a predicate via the 510(k) pathway.

Postmarket Modification

Once a device has completed regulatory approval and is on the market, a manufacturer may wish to make a change to their device. There are a number of options for doing so.

The manufacturer may not need to obtain further approvals if the changes fulfill certain criteria including not introducing a new risk or significantly affecting clinical performance. The FDA has provided guidance for software changes as part of the document "Deciding When to Submit a 510(k) for a Software Change to an Existing Device", and for nonsoftware changes, as part of the document "Deciding When to Submit a 510(k) for a Change to an Existing Device".[13,14]

If the changes do require further regulatory approval, then the manufacturer will need to submit a new 510(k) application. In this situation, it is common for manufacturers to use their prior device as the predicate for the new 510(k) application.

The manufacturer may also incorporate a predetermined change control plan (PCCP) as part of their premarket submission. This plan allows a manufacturer to predefine the changes that they wish to make and the proposed testing methods to ensure that these changes are assessed sufficiently. The components of these testing methods may include new test data collection, rotation in of new test data, rotation out of old test data, maintenance of test sets, and test endpoints. The FDA has provided draft guidance on PCCPs.[15]

Regulatory Translation to Clinical Practice

Once a device has completed the relevant regulatory review process through the FDA, it can be marketed and ultimately used clinically. A key regulatory requirement is that devices must have a user guide, which a manufacturer is required to make available to users and provide to users upon request.

The FDA maintains a number of databases of devices with marketing authorization.[10,16] There are separately non-FDA maintained lists including through the American College of Radiology.[17,18]

References

1. US Food & Drug Administration. How to determine if your product is a medical device. Updated September 29, 2022. Accessed February 28, 2024. https://www.fda.gov/medical-devices/classify-your-medical-device/how-determine-if-your-product-medical-device.
2. Woodcock J, Becerra X. Medical devices; medical device classification regulations to conform to medical software provisions in the 21st century cures act. Federal Register. Updated April 19, 2021. Accessed August 5, 2024. https://www.federalregister.gov/documents/2021/04/19/2021-07860/medical-devices-medical-device-classification-regulations-to-conform-to-medical-software-provisions.
3. United States Code. Food, drug, and cosmetic act. 21 USC 321(h)(1). Accessed August 5, 2024. https://www.govinfo.gov/content/pkg/USCODE-2023-title21/pdf/USCODE-2023-title21-chap9-subchapII-sec321.pdf.
4. United States Code. Food, drug and cosmetic act. 21 USC 360j(o)(1)(E). Accessed August 5, 2024. https://www.govinfo.gov/content/pkg/USCODE-2023-title21/pdf/USCODE-2023-title21-chap9-subchapV-partA-sec360j.pdf.
5. US Food & Drug Administration. Clinical decision support software: guidance for industry and Food and Drug Administration staff. Updated September 28, 2022. Accessed February 28, 2024. https://www.fda.gov/media/109618/download.
6. US Food & Drug Administration. Policy for device software functions and mobile medical applications: guidance for industry and Food and Drug Administration staff. Updated September 28, 2022. Accessed February 28, 2024. https://www.fda.gov/media/80958/download.
7. US Food & Drug Administration. Artificial intelligence and machine learning (AI/ML)-enabled medical devices list. Updated July 27, 2023 (final decision date of included devices). Accessed February 29, 2024. https://www.fda.gov/medical-devices/software-medical-device-samd/artificial-intelligence-and-machine-learning-aiml-enabled-medical-devices.
8. US Food & Drug Administration. De novo classification request. Updated October 4, 2022. Accessed February 28, 2024. https://www.fda.gov/medical-devices/premarket-submissions-selecting-and-preparing-correct-submission/de-novo-classification-request.

9. US Food & Drug Administration. Premarket notification 510(k). Updated December 5, 2023. Accessed February 28, 2024. https://www.fda.gov/medical-devices/premarket-submissions-selecting-and-preparing-correct-submission/premarket-notification-510k.
10. US Food & Drug Administration. 510(k) premarket notification database. Updated August 5, 2024. Accessed August 5, 2024. https://www.accessdata.fda.gov/scripts/cdrh/cfdocs/cfPMN/pmn.cfm.
11. US Food & Drug Administration. 510(k) third party review program. Updated August 19, 2022. Accessed February 28, 2024. https://www.fda.gov/medical-devices/premarket-submissions-selecting-and-preparing-correct-submission/510k-third-party-review-program.
12. US Food & Drug Administration. Product classification database. Updated August 5, 2024. Accessed August 5, 2024. https://www.accessdata.fda.gov/scripts/cdrh/cfdocs/cfPCD/classification.cfm.
13. US Food & Drug Administration. Deciding when to submit a 510(k) for a software change to an existing device: guidance for industry and Food and Drug Administration staff. Updated October 25, 2017. Accessed February 28, 2024. https://www.fda.gov/media/99785/download.
14. US Food & Drug Administration. Deciding when to submit a 510(k) for a change to an existing device: guidance for industry and Food and Drug Administration staff. Updated October 25, 2017. Accessed February 28, 2024. https://www.fda.gov/media/99812/download.
15. US Food & Drug Administration. Marketing submission recommendations for a predetermined change control plan for artificial intelligence/machine learning (AI/ML)-enabled device software functions: draft guidance for industry and Food and Drug Administration staff. Updated April 3, 2023. Accessed February 28, 2024. https://www.fda.gov/media/166704/download.
16. US Food & Drug Administration. Device classification under section 513(f)(2)(De Novo) database. Updated August 5, 2024. Accessed August 5, 2024. https://www.accessdata.fda.gov/scripts/cdrh/cfdocs/cfPMN/denovo.cfm.
17. American College of Radiology. Data Science Institute. Accessed February 28, 2024. https://aicentral.acrdsi.org/.
18. Wu E, Wu K, Daneshjou R, Ouyang D, Ho DE, Zou J. Medical AI evaluation. Updated April 23, 2021. Accessed August 5, 2024. https://ericwu09.github.io/medical-ai-evaluation/.

PART V

Case Studies

PART OUTLINE

CHAPTER 22

Response to COVID With Artificial Intelligence–Assisted Radiologic Diagnosis

Reid Fursmidt ■ Michael M. Gilbert Bodell ■ Robert Short

KEY POINTS

- The COVID-19 pandemic showed that AI can be both rapidly implementable and accurate.
- Numerous teams from around the globe independently built advanced AI-based tools to assist radiologists' detection and diagnosis of COVID-19 pneumonia.
- Most AI models for COVID-19 pneumonia are based on deep learning approaches, which can be challenging to elucidate and comprehend.

GLOSSARY OF TERMS AND DEFINITIONS

Convolutional neural network (CNN): A type of artificial neural network commonly used for image and video analysis. CNNs are designed to automatically and adaptively learn spatial hierarchies of features from input data. They have revolutionized the field of computer vision and are widely used in various applications such as image classification, object detection, and segmentation.

Deep learning: A subfield of machine learning that uses artificial neural networks with multiple layers to model and solve complex problems. Deep learning algorithms can learn from large amounts of data and automatically extract features from the input data without human intervention.

Area under the curve (AUC): In the context of machine learning, AUC is a common evaluation metric used to measure the performance of a binary classification model. It represents the probability that a randomly chosen positive example will be ranked higher than a randomly chosen negative example.

Supervised learning: A type of machine learning where the algorithm is trained on a labeled dataset, where the correct output is provided for each input. The goal of supervised learning is to learn a mapping function from the input to the output.

Unsupervised learning: A type of machine learning where the algorithm is trained on an unlabeled dataset and the goal is to discover patterns and relationships in the data. Unsupervised learning can be used for tasks such as clustering, dimensionality reduction, and anomaly detection.

Feature vector: A vector of numerical values that represents the features or attributes of an object or data point. Feature vectors are commonly used in machine learning to represent the input data.

Cross validation: A method used to evaluate the performance of a machine learning model by partitioning the data into training and validation sets. Through this technique, the model is iteratively constructed and evaluated using various resampling and sample splitting methods of the given dataset. From this approach, one can assess the algorithm's generalizability and capability to perform accurately on new, unseen data. Cross-validation helps maximize the use of data, which can be especially helpful in smaller datasets.

Introduction

For some time now, there have been several attempts to utilize artificial intelligence (AI) to interpret various diagnostic imaging. In 2018, a prominent paper from Google-owned Verily brought this topic to the forefront, showcasing the power of AI to redefine the diagnostic landscape. At the time, Verily's AI algorithm demonstrated its capability to diagnose pneumonia with an impressive area under the curve (AUC) of 0.931 utilizing test data. However, its generalizability and external validity showed a significantly lower external performance with an AUC of 0.815.[1] Since then, the field of AI in diagnostic radiology has expanded greatly, and its use has become even more robust. A great case study of AI's utility in medical diagnosis was its extensive deployment by various research teams worldwide during the COVID-19 pandemic to diagnose COVID-19 pneumonia, highlighting its potential as a powerful tool for clinicians.[2–6]

Few were as successful as a combined group coming out of Yongzhou, China, University of Pennsylvania, and Massachusetts General Hospital, who examined AI versus radiologists in distinguishing COVID-19 pneumonia versus other causes of pneumonia.[7] Looking back during the pandemic, resource scarcity in conjunction with the heterogeneity of disease made diagnosing COVID-19 difficult and many patients were presumed to be infected solely on clinical suspicion. However, COVID-19, like all pulmonic diseases, displays a range of radiologic patterns that include peripheral, bilateral ground-glass opacities, consolidation, and septal thickening.[8–10] These features of COVID-19 pneumonia mimic many other pathological processes and, unfortunately, show low specificity in distinguishing COVID-19 from other types of pneumonia.[11] The lack of specific findings and overlap with so many other diseases provided an excellent use case for the implementation of AI to examine its prowess at diagnosing COVID-19 pneumonia.

The study design at a base level was rather simple—retrospectively examine AI performance versus that of a radiologist in diagnosing COVID-19 pneumonia using chest CT in a known patient population with reverse transcription–polymerase chain reaction (RT-PCR) results indicating COVID-19 infection. The study combined data from 10 hospitals mostly located in China, but also from the United States. The cohort included nearly 1200 patients and, like traditional AI implementation, relied heavily on proper segmentation and disease identification. Fig. 22.1 illustrates the basic AI development pipeline for image analysis. The process commenced with the collection of segmented input images, which were then fed into the AI model. The AI model used a complex system of decision trees and networks to analyze the images and generate a probability score, indicating the likelihood of COVID-19 infection.

To properly develop any AI tool that analyzes images, the first requirement is proper segmentation. Segmentation can be likened to sorting a pile of mixed-up puzzle pieces into groups that belong together. Just as separating the pieces by color, shape, and pattern makes it easier to assemble the puzzle correctly, segmenting an image into meaningful parts makes it easier for an AI algorithm to understand and analyze it. Without proper segmentation, the AI algorithm may be trying to identify patterns or features in the wrong areas of the image, leading to incorrect or unreliable results. In this case study, segmentation was performed based on attenuation, like a

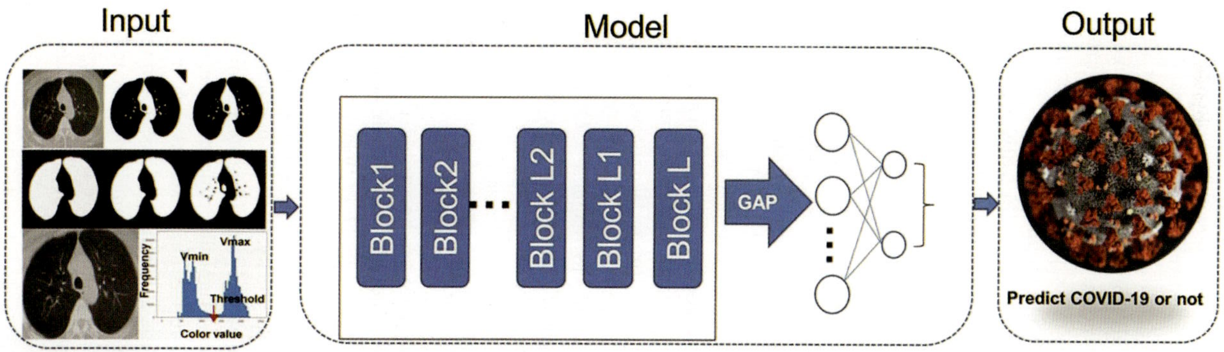

Fig. 22.1 Overview of an artificial intelligence (AI)-based approach to diagnosing COVID-19 pneumonia. The process begins with input images that are segmented based upon certain criteria (e.g., noise above background, manual delineation). The segmented images then go into a trained AI algorithm (referred to as model in image) that has learned the areas of interest within each image and the features important for classification as positive or negative. Lastly, the model outputs a prediction score for the case having COVID-19 or not. (From Wang S, Kang B, Ma J, et al. A deep learning algorithm using CT images to screen for Corona Virus Disease (COVID-19). *Eur Radiol*. 2021;31:6096–6104. License: https://creativecommons.org/licenses/by/4.0/. No changes were made to this image.)

signal-to-noise ratio, to easily eliminate the background. From there, the team used manual contour segmentation when appropriate as subtracting the background is not entirely reliable given the heterogeneity of image and pixel quality in thousands of images.

Following lung segmentation, a model was developed using radiologists' annotations to identify disease. Unlike traditional 80:20 cross validation, this research team employed a 7:2:1 split for their training, validation, and test set respectively. In other words, 70% of the data were used to train the model, 20% were used to validate the model, and the last 10% were used to determine how successful the model was versus that of actual radiologists. In addition, the research team utilized data augmentation techniques such as flipping, varying brightness and contrast levels, and scaling, to increase the model's robustness and prevent it from overfitting to nonessential features that may not be specific to COVID-19 pneumonia.

The AI model they employed was built upon EfficientNet B4 architecture. EfficientNet B4 is a deep learning–based algorithm that utilizes a convolutional neural network (CNN), which mimics the way humans process visual information. CNNs are designed to recognize patterns in images by analyzing their features at different levels of complexity. For example, at the first level, the network may recognize basic shapes and colors, whereas at a deeper level, it may identify more complex features such as texture and contours.

EfficientNet B4 takes this approach further by using a technique called neural architecture search to automatically design the network architecture that is most efficient in terms of accuracy and computational resources. This technique results in a more optimized network that can perform image recognition tasks much faster and with higher accuracy than other conventional CNNs. However, CT images are not two-dimensional, but rather composed of multiple layers. To account for this difference, the researchers implemented an additional neural network that can pool slices of a patient's CT images together. This approach more closely mimics the way humans analyze CT images and allows the AI algorithm to take into account the full set of images from each patient.

In the study, six radiologists were able to diagnose COVID-19 pneumonia versus non-COVID-19 pneumonia with an average accuracy of 85%. The AI algorithm alone outperformed the radiologists with an accuracy of 96%. Notably, when the researchers provided AI assistance to the radiologists, their accuracy significantly increased to 90% ($P < .001$). The AI assistance also improved the sensitivity and specificity from 79% to 88% ($P < .001$) and from 88% to 91% ($P = .001$), respectively.

The AI algorithm's superior performance can be attributed to its ability to identify patterns and make predictions based on a large amount of data. In this case, the AI algorithm was able to learn from the training set to identify COVID-19 pneumonia. However, it is important to note that the test set, although "independent", was sourced from the same hospitals with similar populations. Nonetheless, this study in many ways highlights the benefit AI can provide clinicians in increasing accuracy, sensitivity, and specificity. It also importantly provides the framework for which most clinicians see AI working alongside radiologists. For many, AI is often seen as a job usurper, but when it comes to medicine, diagnosing patients, and making clinically relevant decisions, AI is highly unlikely to be the sole decision maker. As such, its most likely implementation is to complement existing workflows and aid in diagnosis as seen in this study.

Yet this one successful venture during the pandemic is not isolated. In fact, quite the opposite is true. Several other studies and case examples have reported high accuracy in differentiating COVID-19 pneumonia from other types of pneumonia through the use of their own AI-based approaches. Some of the most frequently cited studies are depicted in Table 22.1. One study from a hospital in Wuhan, China used a similar deep learning-based approach to the previous case; it showcased a probability likelihood ratio for COVID-19 pneumonia, community-acquired pneumonia, and non-pneumonia of 0.96, 0.95, and 0.98, respectively.[13] A study conducted by the NIH and published in *Nature* employed its own deep learning-based approach, utilizing 3D-based

TABLE 22.1 ■ **Brief Overview of Representative Studies About Artificial Intelligence Algorithms That Diagnose COVID-19 Pneumonia**

Author	Year of Publication	AI Model Architecture	AUC of the AI Algorithm in Diagnosing COVID-19 Pneumonia
Bai et al.[7]	2020	EfficientNet B4 deep neural network	0.96
Wang et al.[12]	2021	GoogleNet Inception v3 convolutional neural network	0.895
Li et al.[13]	2020	Supervised deep learning framework (COVNet)	0.96
Harmon et al.[14]	2020	Densnet (Dense Convolutional Network) –121 architecture adapted to utilize 3D operations	0.949
Wu et al.[15]	2020	ResNet50 architecture (Deep residual learning)	0.905
Wang et al.[16]	2020	Weakly supervised 3D deep convolutional neural network (DeCoVNet)	0.959

AI, Artificial intelligence, *AUC*, area under the curve.

analytics and achieving comparable success. However, this study was perhaps more robust and more attuned to that of everyday radiologists as they examined COVID-19 pneumonia versus CT scans for any variety of indication including acute care, trauma, and oncology. Unsurprisingly, at this point their model was able to achieve a 90.8% accuracy, with 84% sensitivity and 93% specificity in identifying COVID-19 pneumonia.[14] All three of the studies discussed were published only a year after the pandemic began, demonstrating how fast these tools can be produced and deployed. Looking toward the future, these models may be able to be implemented even faster to identify the next emergent disease.

That being said, it is important to note that each case example, and furthermore every publication that features AI, has its own set of confounding variables and biases worthy of discussion. The most pressing question is how these AI algorithms learn and train that enables diagnostic predictions. Deep learning is often seen as a "black box" by which there is limited information one can draw upon as to how the model is built and works. Therefore some AI diagnostic algorithms may be built on subtleties that are superfluous or unintentional, or simply do translate to other populations. For instance, the AI algorithm could be cued to detect patients from particular CT scanners that are more likely to have patients with COVID-19 rather than the presence of COVID-19 pneumonia itself. A way to combat the lack of explainability as seen in all three studies discussed is to build heat maps to reflect where the AI is "focused" per se (Fig. 22.2).

These heat maps serve as an internal validation that the programs are focused on what is important as it relates to the pathology. Suffice to say, it is extremely important that researchers recognize the potential for biases when building these deep learning AI-based platforms and more importantly design ways that allow for verification of their models' results.

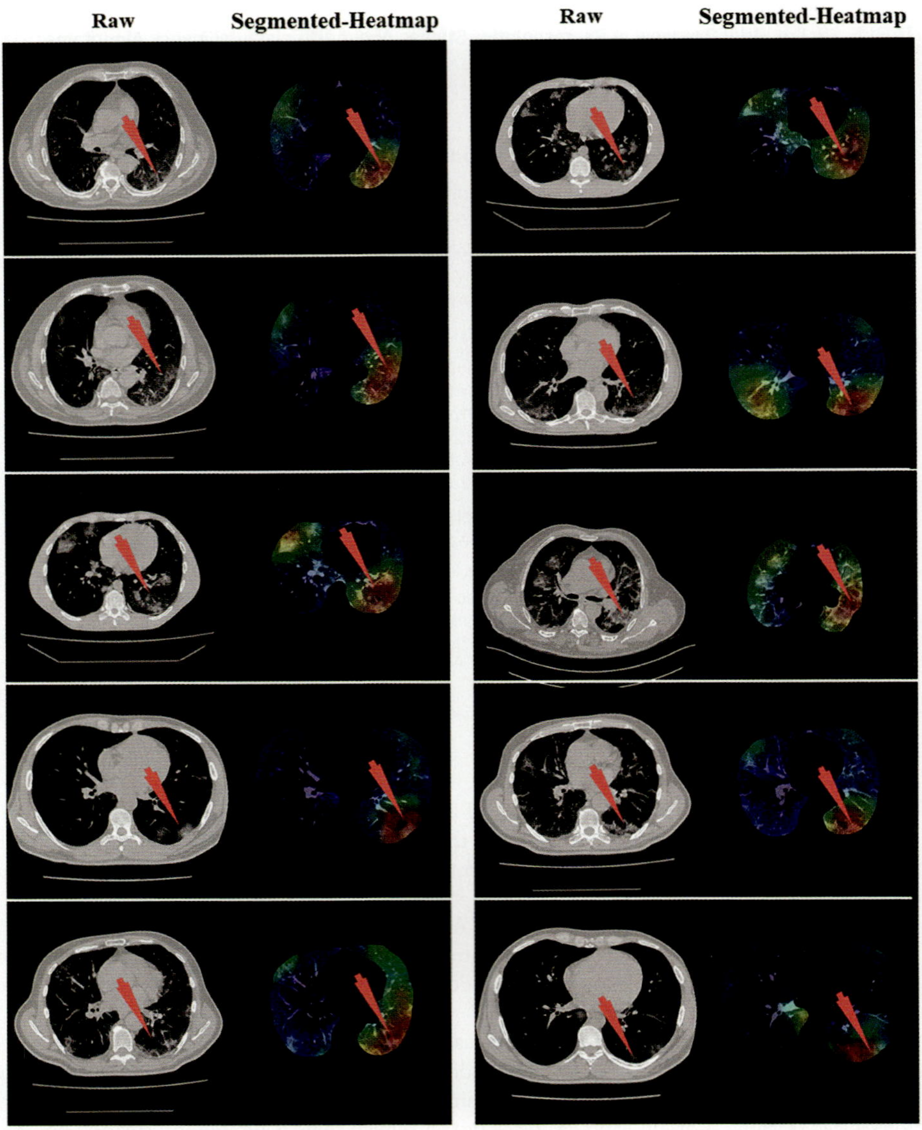

Fig. 22.2 Representative examples of attention heat maps. The left column shows the raw image taken from the CT scanner, and the right column shows the segmented lung with an overlaid heat map. The *red arrow* in both columns highlights the area of lung damage in this database of COVID-19 patients. In this heat map, the different colors represent the areas of interest marked by the AI algorithm, with the scale being from *blue* (cold) representing a lower value up to *red* (hot) representing a higher value. Overall, the *red* color on the heat map correlates well with the areas of lung damage.[17] (From Agarwal M, Agarwal S, Saba L, et al. Eight pruning deep learning models for low storage and high-speed COVID-19 computed tomography lung segmentation and heatmap-based lesion localization: a multicenter study using COVLIAS 2.0. *Comput Biol Med*. 2022;146:105571.)

In conclusion, AI stands to revolutionize diagnostic radiology and has proven to be an effective tool in diagnosing diseases. The rapid and diffuse concurrent application of AI during the COVID-19 pandemic showcased its potential as a powerful tool for clinicians. The success of AI algorithms in identifying COVID-19 pneumonia has demonstrated that it can significantly increase accuracy, sensitivity, and specificity, highlighting its benefits for clinicians in diagnosis. Although there are still questions about how AI learns and trains to predict, the future looks bright for AI. It will potentially aid in identifying emergent diseases faster than ever before, and it will continue to complement existing workflows by working alongside radiologists and providing additional support to clinicians.

References

1. Zech JR, Badgeley MA, Liu M, Costa AB, Titano JJ, Oermann EK. Variable generalization performance of a deep learning model to detect pneumonia in chest radiographs: a cross-sectional study. *PLoS Med.* 2018;15(11):e1002683.
2. Belfiore MP, Urraro F, Grassi R, et al. Artificial intelligence to codify lung CT in Covid-19 patients. *Radiol Med.* 2020;125:500–504.
3. Jin C, Chen W, Cao Y, et al. Development and evaluation of an artificial intelligence system for COVID-19 diagnosis. *Nat Commun.* 2020;11(1):5088.
4. Murphy K, Smits H, Knoops AJ, et al. COVID-19 on chest radiographs: a multireader evaluation of an artificial intelligence system. *Radiology.* 2020;296(3):E166–E172.
5. Borkowski AA, Viswanadhan NA, Thomas LB, Guzman RD, Deland LA, Mastorides SM. Using artificial intelligence for COVID-19 chest X-ray diagnosis. *Fed Pract.* 2020;37(9):398.
6. Baltazar LR, Manzanillo MG, Gaudillo J, et al. Artificial intelligence on COVID-19 pneumonia detection using chest xray images. *PLoS ONE.* 2021;16(10):e0257884.
7. Bai HX, Wang R, Xiong Z, et al. Artificial intelligence augmentation of radiologist performance in distinguishing COVID-19 from pneumonia of other origin at chest CT. *Radiology.* 2020;296(3):E156–E165.
8. Duzgun SA, Durhan G, Demirkazik FB, Akpinar MG, Ariyurek OM. COVID-19 pneumonia: the great radiological mimicker. *Insights Imaging.* 2020;11(1):1–15.
9. Choi H, Qi X, Yoon SH, et al. Extension of coronavirus disease 2019 on chest CT and implications for chest radiographic interpretation. *Radiol Cardiothorac Imaging.* 2020;2(2):e200107.
10. Araujo-Filho JDAB, Sawamura MVY, Costa AN, Cerri GG, Nomura CH. COVID-19 pneumonia: what is the role of imaging in diagnosis? *J Bras Pneumol.* 2020;46:e20200114.
11. Bai HX, Hsieh B, Xiong Z, et al. Performance of radiologists in differentiating COVID-19 from non-COVID-19 viral pneumonia at chest CT. *Radiology.* 2020;296(2):E46–E54.
12. Wang S, Kang B, Ma J, et al. A deep learning algorithm using CT images to screen for Corona Virus Disease (COVID-19). *Eur Radiol.* 2021;31:6096–6104.
13. Li L, Qin L, Xu Z, et al. Using artificial intelligence to detect COVID-19 and community-acquired pneumonia based on pulmonary CT: evaluation of the diagnostic accuracy. *Radiology.* 2020;296(2): E65–E71.
14. Harmon SA, Sanford TH, Xu S, et al. Artificial intelligence for the detection of COVID-19 pneumonia on chest CT using multinational datasets. *Nat Commun.* 2020;11(1):4080.
15. Wu X, Hui H, Niu M, et al. Deep learning-based multi-view fusion model for screening 2019 novel coronavirus pneumonia: a multicentre study. *Eur J Radiol.* 2020;128:109041.
16. Wang X, Deng X, Fu Q, et al. A weakly-supervised framework for COVID-19 classification and lesion localization from chest CT. *IEEE Trans Med Imaging.* 2020;39(8):2615–2625.
17. Agarwal M, Agarwal S, Saba L, et al. Eight pruning deep learning models for low storage and high-speed COVID-19 computed tomography lung segmentation and heatmap-based lesion localization: a multicenter study using COVLIAS 2.0. *Comput Biol Med.* 2022;146:105571.

CHAPTER 23

Arterys Artificial Intelligence: Inception, Development, Growth

Marvee Espiritu ■ John Axerio-Cilies

Part 1: Founding of Arterys—Pre Artificial Intelligence

In the winter of 2010, Fabien Beckers, PhD and entrepreneur, developed sleeping problems. He was diagnosed with sleep apnea and was informed that the best course of treatment would be a highly invasive maxillomandibular advancement surgery (MMA), which was not without risks. The success rate of soft tissue surgical interventions was a paltry 50%, and Beckers wanted assurance that this surgical intervention would cure his sleep apnea. Given his physics background, he approached John Axerio-Cilies, a PhD candidate at Stanford with a concentration in computational fluid dynamics (CFD) to attempt to model his upper airway and predict his postsurgical air structural mechanics. Patient-specific simulations in the early 2010s were starting to be in vogue, along with terms like "Big Data" and "Precision Medicine."

Taking inspiration from Beckers' own medical experience, Beckers and Axerio-Cilies identified a potential commercial opportunity to market patient-specific simulations of fluid (air and blood) and structure (soft tissue and bone) interactions in the human body to aid physicians in optimizing patient care. Such a predictive tool could remove the subjectivity of whether a surgical intervention would be appropriate; beyond improving care at the patient level, it could also provide a much-needed tool for payor prior authorization. After an 8-month exercise in understanding the market and elucidating the clinical unmet needs, it was clear that for any such product/solution, a high-fidelity medical imaging scan, primarily CT scan, would be required. In the case of sleep apnea, a CT scan is not standard of care and it would take decades of research and evidence to prove that such a scan is medically necessary.

It was at that point that Axerio-Cilies and Beckers decided to interview 100 physicians, including radiologists, to identify the role of advanced computational processing on a standard-of-care MRI or CT scan in providing additional insights to referring physicians. During this market research phase, Beckers and Axerio-Cilies met Dr. Albert Hsiao and Dr. Shreyas Vasanawala at Stanford who had developed an early prototype of a technology called "4D Flow MRI" that possessed the ability to noninvasively measure arterial and venous blood flow. With Beckers in business, Axerio-Cilies in engineering, and Hsiao/Vasanawala in medicine, the four entrepreneurs realized that they could create a company to commercialize this technology to the masses. In late 2011, Arterys was founded.

The four co-founders decided to gear the company and its technology towards cardiac imaging, specifically, measuring blood flow through all four cardiac chambers and the major arteries. Such a tool was indispensable in complex cases, such as congenital heart disease, where ultrasound was and still is currently the standard of care but had limited capability to accurately visualize and quantify complex flow dynamics. Structural heart disease affects over 80 million people annually and was a large, potentially addressable market.

Part 2: Product Development

Fundraising in 2012 proved to be very difficult because a medical imaging software venture for such a niche market like cardiac MRI was not attractive. Artificial intelligence (AI) was nonexistent (the seminal 2012 Hinton deep learning paper had yet to be published), and venture capital funding was primarily going to social media and dating apps (Facebook, WhatsApp, etc.). Nevertheless, the four co-founders were able to close a Series Seed funding round of $2 million to receive regulatory clearance for a yet-to-be-created 4D Flow software. In early 2013, the first engineers were hired from Calgary because that city had a concentration of very specialized medical imaging visualization and processing software developers, specifically a company called Calgary Scientific. As some imaging studies were larger than 20 GB in size with 30,000+ MR images, Axerio-Cilies realized that in order to efficiently process and visualize several gigabyte imaging studies, large graphical processing units (GPUs) would be required yet were not readily available in hospitals. In order to surmount this obstacle, they would leverage the newly created cloud computing environments and stream all the imaging data to the cloud. Several GPUs would be required to render and process the seven-dimensional (3D + time + three components of flow) dataset of a single patient.

Since Arterys was one of the first companies that would require hospitals to send Digital Imaging and Communications in Medicine (DICOM) images to the cloud for a clinical use case in late 2013, they were met with disdain at IT security review meetings. Comments from hospital IT personnel such as, "we will never send our data to the cloud" were commonplace, and the team needed to overcome this challenge or risk going out of business. A decision was made to divide the development team such that half the team was responsible for creating an "edge device" that would de-identify all data and act as a gateway between the hospital network and public cloud. Therefore only de-identified images and metadata would be sent to the cloud. Physicians would still be able to login via the Arterys website and see protected health information (PHI) because their browser would pull PHI from the edge device on-premises and de-identified pixels from the public cloud while reconciling both in 5 milliseconds. This capability was a breakthrough milestone for the company that allowed them to go all in on cloud and set them up for the dawn of machine learning, specifically deep learning.

Over the next 3 years Arterys focused solely on bringing out the most advanced 7D viewer ever created in a browser (Fig. 23.1).

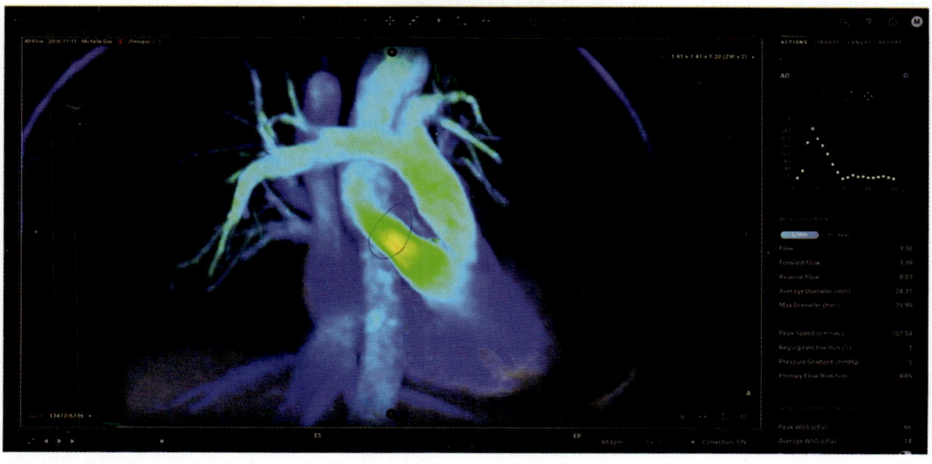

Fig. 23.1 Screenshot of Arterys software showing a cardiac 4D Flow dataset being viewed and processed in the web browser.

The first United States Food and Drug Administration (FDA) regulatory clearance for blood flow visualization and quantification was achieved in 2014, and the company partnered with GE Healthcare in 2015 to commercialize this technology (referred to at the time as Viosworks). A specialized MRI pulse sequence needed to be developed by GE Healthcare engineers, and the first clinical sites started using 4D Flow upon the release of the product in 2017.

Part 3: Pioneering AI

By mid-2014, journal articles delineating the power of "deep learning" in medical applications were being published. Nonmedical computer vision applications (detection and segmentation) of deep learning showed great promise (e.g., AlexNet architecture to identify cats in images on the internet). Beckers and Axerio-Cilies realized that they had to fully commit to the AI revolution or risk being left behind by the competition.

In 2015, they hired their first machine learning developer who, in turn, hired a team of machine learning scientists and engineers to bring to market the first FDA-cleared deep learning algorithm. At the time, no other company had attempted this feat.

Segmentation of the cardiac ventricles was a suitable first use-case for AI in the Arterys product because it was a task performed by highly specialized cardiac imagers that was time consuming (typically tens of minutes) and error prone. AI could completely automate the segmentation of the ventricles to provide key measures such as ventricular function, mass, and cardiac output. Prior to deep learning, techniques such as active contours (i.e., snakes) were employed in the early versions of the product; such methods were susceptible to leakage (segmentations incorrectly extending beyond the myocardial boundary) and cumbersome to correct. Fully convolutional networks (FCNs), a variant of convolutional neural networks (a specific type of deep learning), were used to rapidly advance the state-of-the-art in automated segmentation at the time. However, FCNs are limited by their computational cost, which increased the monetary cost and degraded the user experience of production systems. To combat this shortcoming, Arterys developed a novel architecture based on the ENet architecture that was four times faster and ran with six times less memory than the previous state-of-the-art segmentation architecture while still maintaining excellent clinical accuracy.

One of the most challenging aspects of commercial success for any AI application in radiology is product-market fit, which was and is truly difficult to achieve, even in 2023. Determining how a radiologist can interact efficiently with AI while also achieving higher diagnostic accuracy is extremely challenging. The user interface needed to be optimized in such a way to allow users to accept, reject, modify, and add contours that were pregenerated automatically by AI. Not all AI in radiology needs an interface for AI interaction (triage, for example, does not), but AI for interpretation and quantification typically requires an interface. Once Arterys determined the end user interface, they created requirements for the software that would then lead to requirements for the machine learning algorithm, which in turn would lead to the validation protocol required for regulatory clearance, which would further lead to the data required to achieve the desired marketing claims. It was truly a reverse waterfall technique, and if anything in that chain changed during product development and testing, it could prove to be catastrophic.

Once the machine learning algorithm was determined, ground truth data needed to be collected. The Arterys "secret sauce" was that it would deploy postprocessing software to its installed base with no automation, thereby allowing users to manually detect, segment, and quantify the imaging data for routine clinical use. Since all these annotations were performed in a browser, all sessions would be saved, giving Arterys all raw DICOM data with accompanying contours that could be used for machine learning model training purposes. Arterys at the time did not have to purchase data. When it came time to validate and test the machine learning models, Arterys hired four expert cardiac imagers to manually segment the same cohort of patients (encompassing thousands of images of the heart), providing a consensus read dataset. Dice scores (Sørensen-Dice coefficient) were used to compare model performance, and Arterys was able to prove with statistical significance that its deep learning model could achieve the same level of accuracy as any expert in the field; this achievement was a major milestone for the company and the healthcare industry as a whole.

The most common clinical trial (i.e., clinical assessment) protocol to prove equivalency (or preferably benefit) to a radiologist was to perform a reader study on retrospective data. A reader study is one in which a cohort of radiologists would read a set of patient studies with and without the help of AI and then compare an outcome measure (typically time and accuracy). This sort of protocol was very common for CADx (computer-aided diagnosis) and CADe (computer-aided detection) medical devices. Such protocols were very common for FDA Class II medical devices. Given that a majority of the deep learning algorithms employed by Arterys in 2016 were for segmentation tasks, no such clinical trial or reader study was required to get their FDA clearance; just standalone performance for a hold-out validation set was sufficient at this point in time.

In 2016, Arterys successfully received their first US FDA clearance of a deep learning algorithm, a true pioneering moment for the AI in radiology industry. This event generated considerable attention, which was utilized to raise additional capital (Series B – $30 million) in order to expand AI in radiology beyond cardiac MRI.

Arterys continued investing heavily in its AI capabilities and started experimenting with different techniques and processes from a business, technical, and operational perspective with the goal of automating the radiologist workflow as much as possible. Data availability and ground truth annotation/consensus soon proved to be the major challenge. Raw medical imaging files were being sourced not only from routine use of the Arterys application but also from open-source repositories and licensed from data vendors. At the time, there were no ethical restrictions related to acquiring raw imaging data, because it was very common for hospitals to have patients sign a consent allowing their de-identified images to be given to third parties (for research or commercial purposes). Roughly 90% of the time spent by the machine learning team was around data curation and model testing. Engineers would complain that they were "data engineers" and not "machine learning scientists." Certain applications, for instance, segmentation of lesions on prostate MR, produced very poor consensus amongst the experts. Arterys attempted to utilize crowd-sourcing companies to generate labels, but only extremely simple tasks proved effective. A majority of these approaches failed to provide reliable labels; there were no shortcuts to the time and capital needed to create a high-quality machine learning model. On average, about 18 months of development was required to commercialize a machine learning model, with a cost of approximately $1 million per model. The Cardio AI application from Arterys has 7 machine learning (ML) models, which cost $10 million to develop. A majority of this cost can be attributed to data purchasing, data labeling, machine learning scientist salaries, multi-reader multi-case (MRMC) clinical assessments, and regulatory filings.

Part 4: Clinical Application Expansion

In 2015, Arterys expanded the 4D flow clinical application to be part of a comprehensive cardiac MRI software solution referred to as Cardio AI. This decision was necessary due to the fact that the three major original equipment manufacturer magnetic resonance imaging vendors (namely Siemens, GE, Philips) did not have the necessary hardware and pulse sequences required to generate such high-fidelity temporal and spatial data. The market for 4D Flow had not been developed, and it would take a decade for this to become a >$10 million opportunity. Conversely, conventional cardiac MRI postprocessing was a market that had been around for over a decade and was estimated to be $30 million in size. Therefore additional modules such as ventricular function based on steady-state free precession (SSFP) images, 2D phase contrast, perfusion for blood flow estimation, delayed enhancement for scar quantification, and tissue characterization (T1, T2, T2*) were added to round out the comprehensive cardiac package.

In 2016, a systematic market analysis was performed to identify clinical applications where AI could truly achieve product market fit. Clinical pain points were identified, which then translated to clinical unmet needs and value proposition statements. From there, functional and nonfunctional software requirements were generated very much following the Biodesign playbook (book published in 2010 by Yock et al.). All of the potential areas for AI integrating seamlessly into the clinical workflow were identified. Ultimately, a list of 100+ ideas spanning modality (CT, MR, x-ray, ultrasound, mammography, tomography), body parts (head, chest, musculoskeletal, heart), and pathologies (cardiovascular disease, cancer, neurodegenerative disease) were ranked according to 15+ criteria (scored from 1–10). Examples of such criteria included market size (total addressable market), positive return on investment, clinical need, clinical deviation avoidance, regulatory clearance pathway, willingness to buy, short time to market, and red/blue ocean. The graphic in Fig. 23.2 was created to show across several modalities the inverse correlation between volume, number of models on the market and integration needs versus reimbursement amount, complexity of analysis, and tolerance for a second viewer creating workflow changes.

The top four choices for expansion beyond cardiac MRI included chest CT detection of lung nodules, liver MR detection and quantification of liver lesions, mammography/tomography detection of breast lesions, and x-ray detection of skeletal pathologies.

In 2017, Arterys began internal research and development to create these clinical applications in house; however, they did not have the capital necessary (in the order of $10 million each) to bring these applications into the market. At the time, the company revenue was not large enough to raise a $100+ million funding round. By 2018, venture capital for deep learning radiology companies was at its peak, and several companies on the market were developing similar applications. There was no need to compete; instead, a cash-conscious partnership approach was favored. Enter the dawn of the AI marketplace.

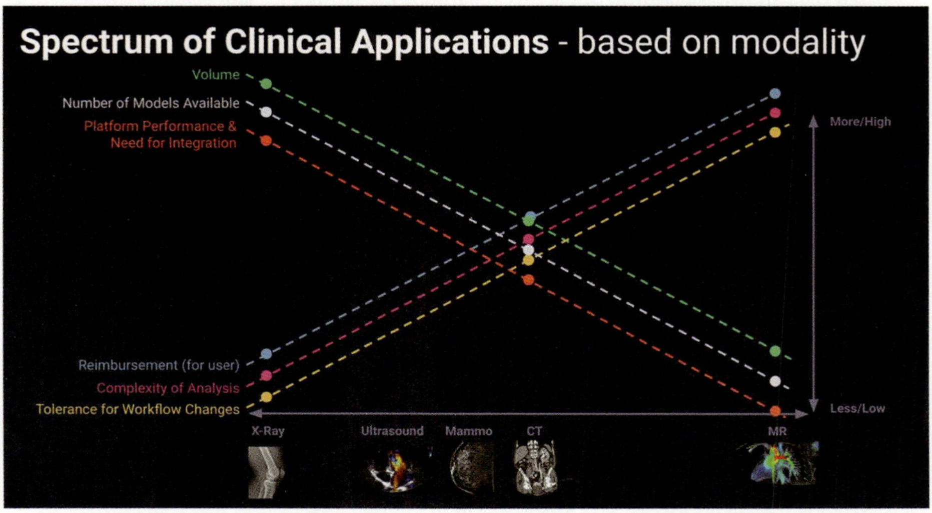

Fig. 23.2 Inverse correlation between volume, number of models on the market and integration needs versus reimbursement amount, complexity of analysis, and tolerance for a second viewer creating workflow changes.

Part 5: Platform, Scale, and Acquisition

By 2019, Arterys knew that they did not want to compete on a model-by-model or clinical app–by–clinical app niche level. Instead, they wanted to offer the market the most comprehensive set of clinical AI (whether developed in house or third party developed) hosted on the most advanced medical imaging platform ever created. Such a platform needed to firstly support any form of AI (for triage, interpretation, reporting, and population health), secondly have fast turnaround (2 minutes or less for a large CT/MRI, measured from image sent from scanner to AI result notification), thirdly render 7D 20 GB data at 60 frames per second in a browser on a 3 Mpbs internet connection, and fourthly have deep and completely customizable integrations (specifically with picture archiving and communication systems [PACS], radiology information systems [RIS], electronic medical records [EMR]), and reporting systems such as PowerScribe and 3M™ M*Modal Fluency). Tens of millions of dollars were utilized to build this platform, and shortly thereafter, the AI marketplace was launched, thereby allowing any third-party developer the ability to deploy their model within the Arterys network of provider institutions. These third parties were not only independent radiology AI vendors, but also included academic research labs and individual independent developers that wanted to contribute especially in the early detection of COVID. A software development kit (SDK) was developed to enable deployment of models in hours as opposed to months on legacy PACS platforms.

The AI marketplace approach allowed Arterys to test the hypothesis and iterate on ideas quickly without devoting tens of millions of dollars on a "bet." Arterys realized that they, together with a majority of radiology AI vendors, were not successful at picking bets. Having a product management tool like the AI marketplace gave the Arterys team the ability to make data-driven investment decisions based on real-time usage of the AI products. Another factor that played a role in moving toward a platform strategy versus going deep in any specific clinical application was that it was becoming more and more difficult to obtain FDA clearance for an AI algorithm. By 2020, the FDA was much more informed on the clinical protocols and trials that were necessary to validate AI models, including detailed scrutiny of the training as well as validation data. US-based data showing performance across subgroups including race and scanner manufacturer were also required.

From 2020 to 2022, Arterys continued to deploy advanced clinical applications focused on neuro AI, breast AI, cardio AI, lung AI, and chest and musculoskeletal AI across hundreds of institutions both in Europe and the United States. Billions of images were being centrally collected on the Arterys platform. Such a scale allowed Arterys to gain traction not only in the provider segment, but also for life sciences companies that saw value in leveraging the Arterys platform and machine learning capabilities to co-develop, deploy, annotate, validate, and achieve regulatory clearance for machine learning applications.

Separately, since its inception in 2015, the company Tempus AI, Inc. had known the value of multimodal data and a platform for powering precision medicine. The company had invested billions of dollars developing diagnostic tests and AI-powered insights based on next-generation sequencing (e.g., DNA, RNA, full transcriptome) and clinical data from the EMR. One of the missing pieces to creating a multimodal dataset with morphologic data was Arterys. Arterys provided Tempus AI with the radiologic imaging backbone (e.g., data, platform, applications, and know-how) to truly understand and optimize the full patient journey allowing patients the ability to live longer and healthier lives. In late 2022, Tempus AI acquired Arterys and a new dawn of multimodal AI was incepted. In 2023, generative pretrained transformers (GPT) were used to create large language models that, in the future, will be used to power the next generation of AI radiology insights.

Bringing to market a successful clinical product in radiology has required solving challenges that changed year after year over the past decade. They included finding access to raw imaging data, annotating the data with consensus interpretations, receiving FDA clearance after successful validation of clinical studies, deploying the application in a nonintrusive manner that streamlined workflow, generating financial return on hospital investment, and achieving reimbursement from payors for AI. Looking forward, Arterys believes that multimodal AI, combining clinical + genomic + disparate imaging data, will be the next frontier to provide value to the patient care pathway.

CHAPTER 24

Viz.ai—Pioneering Artificial Intelligence in Healthcare

David Golan ■ Yuval Duchin

Clinical Background

The year 2015 was a pivotal year for stroke care, marked by several clinical trials that demonstrated the impact of mechanical thrombectomy in the treatment of acute ischemic stroke with large vessel occlusion (LVO).

Mechanical thrombectomy involves the use of a catheter-based device to remove blood clots from the blocked blood vessels in the brain. It has been shown to be highly effective in restoring blood flow to the brain and improving patient outcomes.

The most notable of these trials is the 2015 Multicenter Randomized Clinical Trial of Endovascular Treatment for Acute Ischemic Stroke in the Netherlands (MR CLEAN), which demonstrated a significant improvement in functional outcomes for patients treated with mechanical thrombectomy compared to those treated with standard medical therapy alone.[1] Other trials have since confirmed the findings of the MR CLEAN trial, including the 2015 Endovascular Treatment for Small Core and Anterior Circulation Proximal Occlusion with Emphasis on Minimizing CT to Recanalization Times (ESCAPE) trial and the 2015 Solitaire With the Intention for Thrombectomy (SWIFT-PRIME) trial.[2,3]

These trials collectively provide strong evidence for the efficacy and safety of mechanical thrombectomy in the treatment of acute stroke. As a result, mechanical thrombectomy has become the standard of care for eligible patients. The American Heart Association and American Stroke Association have recommended the use of mechanical thrombectomy for patients with acute ischemic stroke who meet certain criteria.[4]

Time is a critical factor in the treatment of ischemic stroke, with every minute that passes without treatment resulting in the average loss of 1.9 million neurons in the brain (Fig. 24.1).[5] In fact, studies have shown that every minute of delay in treatment results in a 4.2-day loss of healthy life.[6] Therefore timely treatment is crucial to prevent or minimize brain damage and improve outcomes for stroke patients.

However, stroke treatment can be complicated and time-consuming, involving a complex workflow that often results in delays and undertreatment. The workflow typically involves several steps, including patient recognition and assessment, diagnostic imaging, and treatment administration. Delays can occur at each step, with the potential to add up and result in a significant delay in treatment.

For example, delays in recognizing stroke symptoms and activating emergency medical services (EMS) can result in delayed arrival to the hospital, which can impact treatment eligibility and outcomes.[7] Delays in diagnostic imaging and interpretation can also result in delayed treatment, as can delays in accessing or administering the appropriate treatment.

Despite efforts to improve stroke systems of care, delays in treatment continue to be a major challenge. Studies have shown that many stroke patients receive suboptimal care, with only a small percentage of eligible patients receiving thrombolytic or mechanical thrombectomy treatment within the recommended time frame.[8,9]

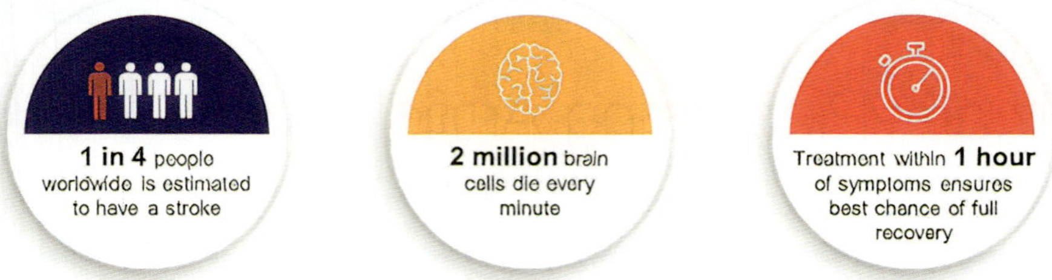

Fig. 24.1 Key metrics associated with acute ischemic stroke.

To address these challenges, efforts are underway to improve stroke systems of care, including the development of stroke centers, the use of telestroke technology, and the implementation of standardized stroke protocols.[10,11] However, there is still much work to be done to improve the timeliness and effectiveness of stroke treatment and ensure that all eligible patients receive the care they need to optimize outcomes.

Viz.ai Founding

Dr. Chris Mansi, a neurosurgeon from Britain and a student at Stanford University's Graduate School of Business, teamed up with Dr. David Golan, an expert in machine learning and a post-doctoral fellow at Stanford, to found Viz.ai. The impetus for the company arose from Dr. Mansi's work with acute trauma patients, where he observed that despite his expertise in the surgical theater, his performance was overshadowed by complex care coordination pathways causing significant delays and inefficiencies in patient care. Dr. Golan, too, experienced similar frustrations firsthand when he was hospitalized at Stanford with a suspected stroke in 2015.

Dr. Mansi and Dr. Golan recognized that critical findings were often slow to be identified and communicated across the convoluted networks of healthcare providers involved in patient care. They also saw a path forward to a solution: advances in computer vision, cloud computing, and mobile applications provided a potential solution to this challenge—a system that could leverage artificial intelligence to identify acute findings in real time and communicate them directly to care teams via the cloud, streamlining communication and synchronizing care (Fig. 24.2).

Product Development

When developing artificial intelligence (AI) solutions for healthcare, three main factors must be taken into account: utility, feasibility, and clinical impact.

Utility: To evaluate the utility of an AI solution, it is required to identify the main beneficiaries of the AI solution and understand what action or intervention can be taken based on the AI outcome to improve medical care. One must verify that such action actually exists and evaluate the ability and incentives to intervene.

Viz.ai identified that within the acute setting of ischemic stroke there exists an intervention that, if taken within a short time window, will result in very high utility for all beneficiaries. Namely, by allowing fast detection and seamless communication and coordination between all the caregivers, a life-saving treatment such as thrombectomy can be delivered within a short time window. Viz.ai identified high utility for many beneficiaries. For hospital administration, faster and coordinated stroke treatment reduces hospitalization days and saves costs. For clinicians, faster and coordinated stroke treatment advances better patient outcomes. And most importantly, for

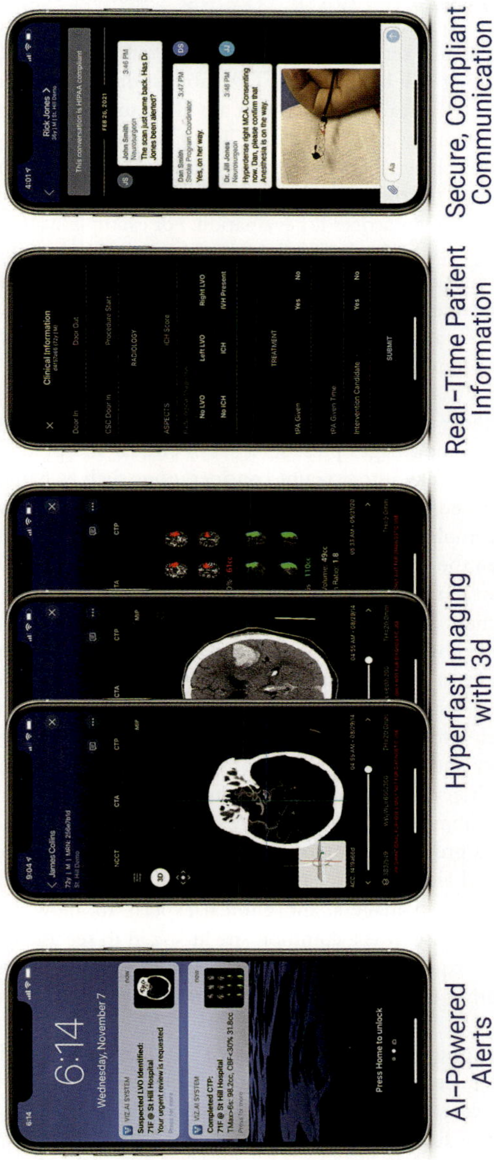

Fig. 24.2 Key components of the Viz LVO solution.

patients, faster intervention translates to better outcomes in terms of saved lives and lower chance of disability.

Feasibility: The feasibility of an AI solution usually refers to data availability, implementation costs, deployment challenges, clinical uptake, and maintenance over time.

Data availability: AI solutions usually depend on large amounts of high-quality data. The data need to be retrieved, preprocessed, and cleaned. It is crucial to carefully label the data and design the training, validation, and test sets. Furthermore, consideration should be given to regulatory issues such as the dataset that will be used for FDA submission and whether the data cover the different demographic and technical subgroups that are likely to benefit from the AI solution.

Due to the high dimensionality and high variability of clinical data, even the process of truthing and labeling the data to achieve high-quality and consistent ground truth is not trivial. Creating an agreed-upon ontology for the ground truthing process is crucial for designing the correct algorithm and setting the correct matrices for evaluation. For example, at Viz.ai, creating a ground truth dataset for LVO required multiple discussions with clinical experts to refine the ontology and define the different types of LVO including defining exactly which type of LVO Viz.ai will detect. Specifically, LVO is defined by the anterior location of the occlusion (such as internal carotid artery [ICA], ICA-T, and M1 occlusions; Fig. 24.3). Due to the variable nature of brain artery morphologies, it is often not straightforward to define the exact type of the LVO. Having a clear definition of the LVO types allowed Viz.ai to clearly set the matrices for evaluation and effectively communicate these matrices with the FDA.

Collecting medical data and images presents a set of ethical and practical challenges. When collecting the data, one must take into account considerations such as patient privacy, legal consent for using the data for medical device development, signing agreements with hospitals on data usage, HIPAA/GDPR compliance, and verifying that the data collected adequately represent different subgroups within the population. To address these challenges, early on Viz.ai employed a full-time legal consultant to verify the compliance to regulations, data privacy, security, and legal issues around data collection. Viz.ai has endeavored to collect data for development from large healthcare institutions where usually the population is relatively more diverse and the chance of under-representation of any subgroup is lower. To comply with patients' privacy, Viz.ai developed from day one an in-house system to anonymize the collected data and invested a great deal in securing the data to a high level.

Due to the complexity and interdependency of the data operation, Viz.ai chose to develop all the data operation in-house so it can closely monitor and design the datasets used for algorithm development and submission. Early on, Viz.ai employed a full-scale operation of data collection by developing a proprietary annotation platform for CT scans and employing clinical experts for labeling and cleaning the data. In addition, Viz.ai insisted on integrated teams of algorithm developers, data managers, and clinical experts to allow a tight feedback cycle between their different expertise. It is a common site at Viz.ai to see an algorithm developer sit side by side with a clinical expert and a data manager discussing clinical cases and on occasions annotating the data together to achieve a better understanding of the data and refine the data preparation pipeline.

Implementation costs and clinical uptake: When implementing an AI solution, one needs to evaluate what the system setup that the AI solution will run on will be, how this system will be deployed, and at what cost. Additionally, one must consider how the AI output will get back into the clinical workflow at the intervention time window and to all the stakeholders. Early on, Viz.ai decided to solve these challenges using cloud computing and mobile phone technology in its AI solution. Cloud computing solutions allow scaling and lower cost of deployment, although there is a high initial cost in building the required infrastructure and convincing stakeholders to adopt this solution. This approach, which was innovative in 2016–2018, is now the standard in most AI solutions. The clinical uptake was designed to lean on mobile devices, which allows Viz.

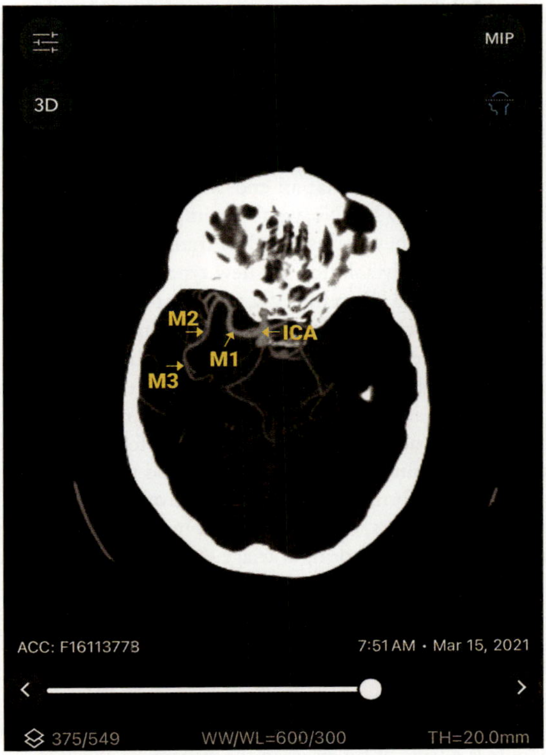

Fig. 24.3 Demonstration of the internal carotid artery and middle cerebral artery component vessels (M1, M2, M3) that can be impacted by a large vessel occlusion. Internal Carotid Artery (ICA),

ai to capitalize on the rapid improvement in smartphone technologies and communication. For example, content delivery networks (CDNs), built and optimized for rapid delivery of media to end users, could be leveraged for faster streaming of CT angiography (CTA) scans to mobile devices. Thus large CTA scans, which may be up to 0.5 Gb, could be downloaded and viewed in seconds, instead of minutes, resulting in better clinical performance and user experience. Using cloud technology combined with mobile technology allowed Viz.ai to create an AI solution that is scalable, easy to deploy, effective in serving its users within the tight time window required, and easy to monitor and maintain over time.

Clinical impact: When developing an AI solution, it is beneficial to evaluate the overall effect of the solution on clinical care, patient outcome, and care standards. Such evaluation can help identify if this solution is actually useful. In the case of stroke, the answer was very clear due to the devastating outcome of a stroke that is not treated within a short period of time. As mentioned before, on average, every minute of delay in treatment results in a 4.2-day loss of healthy life. Therefore an efficient solution that will decrease the time to treatment will result in better clinical care, better compliance to care standards, and better patient outcomes. Time is literally brain.

Algorithm Development

Once the business requirements were defined using the above framework, Viz.ai researchers started to develop the algorithmic solution to detect LVO on CTA. Deep learning algorithms usually require a large amount of data to be able to learn to detect something like an LVO. Unfortunately, such data can be expensive, scarce, and highly variable. The term "big data" does not necessarily translate to large amounts of data that can be readily used in the healthcare context given the high dimensionality and variance of the data; there will almost always be small subgroups within the data that are considered as special cases relative to the textbook definitions. In that sense, Viz.ai data can be defined as highly dimensional and highly variable data rather than purely big data. At the time, Viz.ai researchers determined that an end-to-end deep learning algorithm, where the input is CTA and the output is LVO Yes/No, would be impractical. Another pitfall of end-to-end deep learning algorithms is that they are usually less transparent, less interpretable, and harder to debug; in addition, often the only solution for new types of data is to retrain the entire deep learning model with additional data. Therefore Viz.ai chose to use a hybrid solution of a decision pipeline that involves classical machine learning models in combination with deep learning algorithms at certain stages of the pipeline. Classical machine learning models usually require less data and are more robust to data variability. Deep learning approaches are found to be more suitable at pipeline stages where more data are available and for tasks like image segmentation or denoising. Combining these different approaches (image preprocessing, followed by a deep learning model, followed by several classical machine learning approaches and post processing), allowed Viz.ai to achieve a very high algorithm performance, even with relatively small amounts of data.

To ensure high utility for the users, it is crucial to set metrics that represent the utility for the user as closely as possible. When monitoring a triage AI application, there are multiple metrics that can and should be monitored:

- Sensitivity—the probability of alerting on a positive (LVO) case. Low sensitivity will result in many false negatives.
- Specificity—the probability of not alerting on a negative (non-LVO) case. Low specificity will result in many false positives.
- Positive Predictive Value (PPV)—the probability that an alerted case is indeed positive. Low PPV may hurt the trust of the users in the system.
- Negative Predictive Value (NPV)—the probability that a case that was not alerted on is indeed negative.
- Accuracy—the number of correct predictions divided by total predictions.
- Processing time—the time it takes the system to process a case. A long processing time may reduce the clinical utility of the system.
- Coverage—the percentage of cases that should be processed by the AI application that are indeed processed by the AI application. Scans may not be processed due to a wide range of reasons including implementation problems and image quality.
- Up-time—although not directly related to the performance of the AI system, up-time measures the amount of time the system is available.

Within these metrics, Viz.ai decided to focus on sensitivity, specificity, and PPV, as they were found to drive clinical impact, user satisfaction, and user engagement. Specifically, PPV was found to be highly correlated with user satisfaction because in the stroke setting, when an alarm goes off whenever an LVO is detected, there is a real risk for the user to develop alarm fatigue in case of multiple false alarms (false positives). This situation might lead to reduced trust in the AI product and result in reduced clinical utility. Early on, Viz.ai therefore put a lot of effort into improving the PPV of its product to improve the clinician utility while ensuring a high sensitivity to keep the utility high for patients.

Regulatory Approval

The intention of Viz.ai was to bring their new product to the US market, which requires regulatory approval from the Food and Drug Administration (FDA). Most software-as-a-medical-device

(SaMD) products are approved via a pathway known as the 510(k) pathway (referred to as being "cleared"). Simply put, the company should identify an existing device that has received regulatory approval from the FDA (known as the "predicate device") and argue that the new, suggested product is similar enough in its clinical function and technological method of operation.

In 2017, when Viz.ai first engaged with the FDA, there were no directly applicable predicate devices. The closest types of devices were:

1. Computer-Aided Detection (CADe) devices are intended to assist users—typically radiologists—by identifying indication to a presence of clinically significant abnormalities, such as lesions on mammography scans or pulmonary nodules on chest CT scans. The FDA is typically concerned about how the outputs of such devices might influence the overall accuracy of the radiologist (the "reader") reading such studies. Toward that end, the FDA typically requires, for clearing CADe devices, not only standalone evidence that an algorithm works, but also proof that the reader+device combination yields better results than just the reader, with the concern being that the device might create false confidence and result in deteriorated performance. This superiority is typically demonstrated by showing an increase in the area under the curve (AUC) in a "reader study"—a study where a large number of readers review a large number of scans, with and without the output of the device in question, which allows for comparison of the reader accuracy with and without the device in question.

   When considering this option, Viz.ai faced two challenges. First of all, reader studies are long and costly; as such, many young companies wish to find alternative ways to bring their products to market. Second and more importantly, Viz.ai leadership identified that the key issue with identifying LVOs on CTA scans is not necessarily accuracy, but rather the time to getting the right scan in front of the right physician as fast as possible. The product designed by Viz.ai was designed not only to accurately detect LVOs but also to improve the speed by which these scans were escalated throughout the healthcare system.
2. Image manipulation software: they are typically semiautomatic tools used for functions such as segmenting specific anatomic structures or abnormalities. For example, a software device can allow a technologist to click on a cerebral hyperdensity (e.g., hematoma) and will then automatically segment it and provide measurements. Typically, the FDA does not require a reader study for these types of devices and proof for the accuracy of the performance of the software is sufficient for clearance. The reason is, from the FDA's perspective, these devices are operated *after* a diagnosis was made and are therefore not likely to influence the reader's diagnosis.

Viz.ai's product was different and did not fit into either category. On the one hand, it was not CADe, as it was not intended to enhance the accuracy of a radiologist. Moreover, it was aimed to flag findings to specialist doctors (stroke specialists such as a vascular neurologist or a neurointerventionalist) who may be associated with a different hospital. It was therefore not suitable for the CADe category. On the other hand, the device was aimed to flag, or alert, on a finding before a diagnosis was made, hence it did not fit into the image manipulation category.

Seeing the potential benefit of the suggested device but recognizing that no applicable predicate device existed, the FDA made an appealing suggestion to Viz.ai: seek regulatory approval via the *de novo* pathway (referred to as being "granted a *de novo* request"). This pathway is for new, novel devices whose type has not previously been classified. Together, the FDA and Viz.ai worked to define a new category of medical devices: computer-aided triage (CADt) devices. These devices analyze scans and provide an alert for specific findings. In that sense, they are clinical diagnostic decision support (CDDS) tools that help identify suspected abnormalities but rely on a physician to make a clinical diagnosis. There were several important caveats regarding this new category of device:

1. These devices are not diagnostic. The device is therefore not allowed to mark the finding on the image. It merely flags a specific scan as "suspected."

BOX 24.1 ■ Indications for Use of ContaCT.

ContaCT is a notification-only, parallel workflow tool for use by hospital networks and trained clinicians to identify and communicate images of specific patients to a specialist, independent of standard of care workflow. ContaCT uses an artificial intelligence algorithm to analyze images for findings suggestive of a prespecified clinical condition and to notify an appropriate medical specialist of these findings in parallel to standard of care image interpretation. Identification of suspected findings is not for diagnostic use beyond notification. Specifically, the device analyzes CT angiogram images of the brain acquired in the acute setting, and sends notifications to a neurovascular specialist that a suspected large vessel occlusion has been identified and recommends review of those images. Images can be previewed through a mobile application. Images that are previewed through the mobile application are compressed and are for informational purposes only and not intended for diagnostic use beyond notification. Notified clinicians are responsible for viewing noncompressed images on a diagnostic viewer and engaging in appropriate patient evaluation and relevant discussion with a treating physician before making care-related decisions or requests. ContaCT is limited to analysis of imaging data and should not be used in lieu of full patient evaluation or relied upon to make or confirm diagnosis.

The underlined text emphasizes key components.

2. There should be sufficient evidence that the device provides a significant acceleration as compared to the standard of care.
3. The sensitivity and specificity of the algorithm should be demonstrated to be significantly higher than 80%.

Moreover, CADt devices are clearly indicated to operate in parallel with the standard of care. This specification is made clear by the indications for use of Viz LVO, which was called ContaCT when it was granted a de novo request (Box 24.1).

First Steps in the Real World

Once FDA approval was obtained, the Viz.ai team quickly signed multiple deals with various hospitals and hospital systems. As more and more hospitals sought to purchase and implement the Viz.ai device, it became clear that different hospital systems were suffering from different problems, had different business goals, and were structured differently. Some examples of these different needs included:

- A large healthcare system, launching a quality improvement program for its stroke-related metrics, aimed to reduce their door-to-needle and door-to-groin time metrics.
- A small site with a single stroke neurologist wanted to best support that neurologist and enhance her availability.
- A large healthcare center wanted to get more patients transferred from spoke hospitals that were not thrombectomy capable.

As Viz.ai gained prominence and reputation, customers started reaching out, asking for advice on anything from how to optimize their program to how to configure their CT scanners. It became clear that to fully deliver the value of the Viz.ai products, a much deeper bond needed to be created between Viz.ai and the hospitals it was serving.

Clinical Studies

From day 1, Viz.ai sought to establish the clinical utility of its platform beyond doubt. This endeavor served multiple purposes—first and foremost to build the company's confidence that the developed products were indeed delivering an impact on patient care, which was Viz.ai's *raison d'etre*. Moreover, these studies could be leveraged to further prove the value proposition and justify a price point for the products. Lastly, one unique feature of healthcare sales, compared to sales in other industries, is the strong reliance of customers on published, peer-reviewed research papers.

Viz.ai has collaborated on and supported a wide range of studies, and there have also been many independent clinical studies showing the real-world clinical impact of Viz.ai.[12–24] One of these studies clearly demonstrated the impact of Viz.ai on stroke workflow duration (Fig. 24.4).[18]

Reimbursement Via the NTAP Program

The innovative nature of the Viz.ai solution, together with the overwhelming clinical evidence collected in a short period of time, drove Viz.ai to apply for the New Technology Add-on Payment (NTAP) program—an initiative of the Centers for Medicare & Medicaid Services (CMS) in the United States. The program was created to provide additional reimbursement for new medical technologies that have been approved by the FDA and are used in the hospital setting.

To qualify for NTAP, the new technology must meet two main criteria:

- Newness: the technology must be new and not be substantially similar to any other technology that is already available on the market. As such, the technology must represent a significant advancement in medical treatment.
- Substantial clinical impact: the technology must demonstrate that it offers substantial clinical improvement over existing technologies. As such, the technology must have been shown to provide better patient outcomes or to be more effective than existing treatments.

Viz.ai leveraged being granted a *de novo* request to demonstrate its technology satisfied the newness criterion and publications from real-world clinical studies to demonstrate the substantial clinical impact criterion.

At the end of a long process, CMS chose to provide reimbursement for the Viz LVO product, a decision that created significant excitement in the stroke and radiology AI communities (Fig. 24.5). The new reimbursement code created a strong financial incentive for hospitals to adopt AI technology, resulting in an increase in the rate of adoption of Viz.ai's software across the United States. A detailed analysis of the NTAP process and the specific decision regarding Viz.ai was provided in the "Out of Pocket" blog.[25]

Where Viz.ai Is Today: Healthcare's "System of Action"

The focus of Viz.ai's LVO solution on addressing the main pain points in the stroke workflow combined with excellent execution in terms of AI performance, implementation, and demonstration of clinical impact resulted in its customer base quickly growing to over 1200 hospitals within just 4 years. Viz.ai also obtained CE Mark in Europe in 2021, which helped fuel expansion globally. In parallel, Viz.ai is expanding beyond stroke and now offers a wide range of solutions for other workflows within hospital systems (Fig. 24.6).

The same methodologies and platforms that were used to develop and implement AI solutions for LVO were used to develop and implement multiple additional AI solutions for healthcare. To date, these solutions can be categorized into six categories:

- **Neurovascular Suite:** this suite includes AI solutions to detect and facilitate treatment workflow for LVO, intracranial hemorrhage, subdural hemorrhage, and aneurysm. It has also incorporated CT perfusion analysis. As mentioned before, the adoption of this solution and its clinical impact have been extremely significant.
- **Vascular Suite:** this suite includes AI solutions to detect and facilitate treatment workflow for pulmonary embolism, the heart's right and left ventricle diameter measurements, aortic dissection, and aortic aneurysm. Due to the proven performance of these solutions, together with Viz.ai's footprint in the healthcare system, Viz.ai has been selected as the AI partner-of-choice for the groundbreaking Pulmonary Embolism—Thrombus Removal with Catheter-Directed Thrombolysis (PE-TRACT) trial.

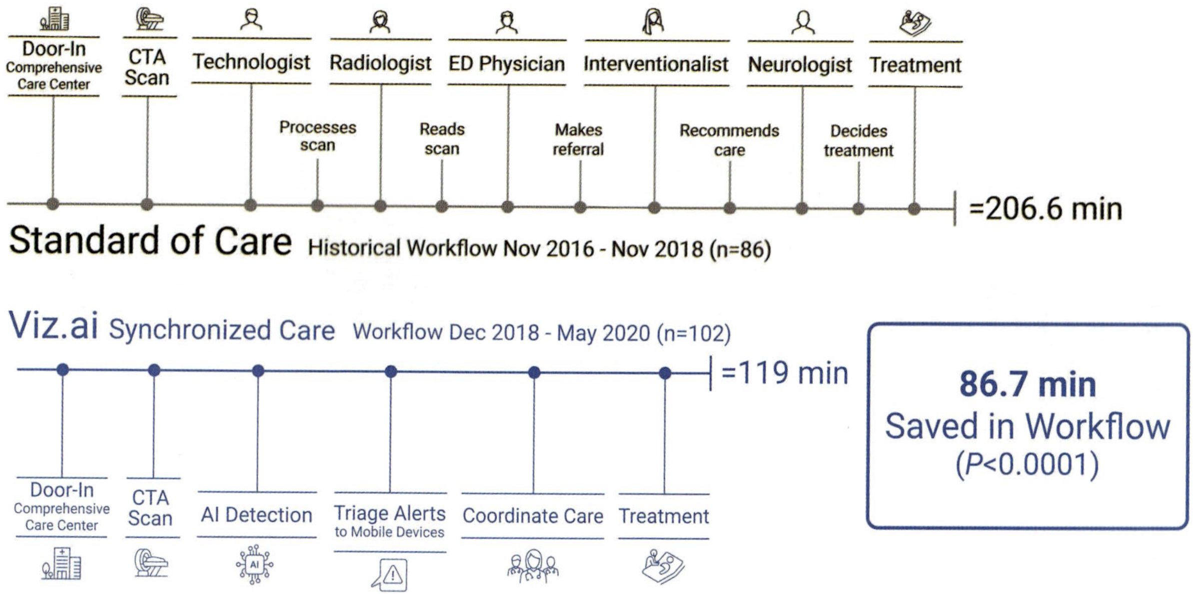

Fig. 24.4 Demonstration of impact of Viz.ai on stroke workflow duration. (From Hassan AE, Ringheanu VM, Preston L, Tekle WG. Artificial intelligence–parallel stroke workflow tool improves reperfusion rates and door-in to puncture interval. *Stroke Vasc Interv Neurol*. 2022;2(5):e000224.)

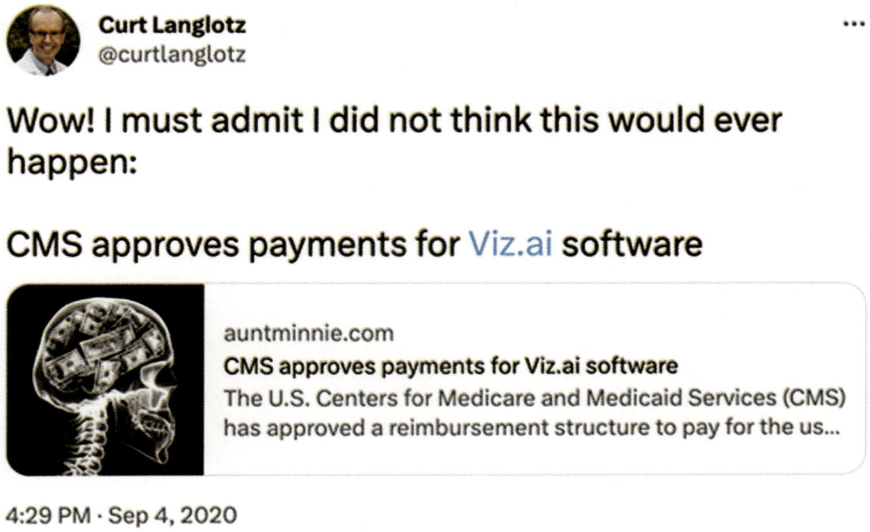
Curt Langlotz
@curtlanglotz
Wow! I must admit I did not think this would ever happen:
CMS approves payments for Viz.ai software
auntminnie.com
CMS approves payments for Viz.ai software
The U.S. Centers for Medicare and Medicaid Services (CMS) has approved a reimbursement structure to pay for the us...
4:29 PM · Sep 4, 2020

Fig. 24.5 A reaction to the CMS approval of NTAP for the Viz LVO device.

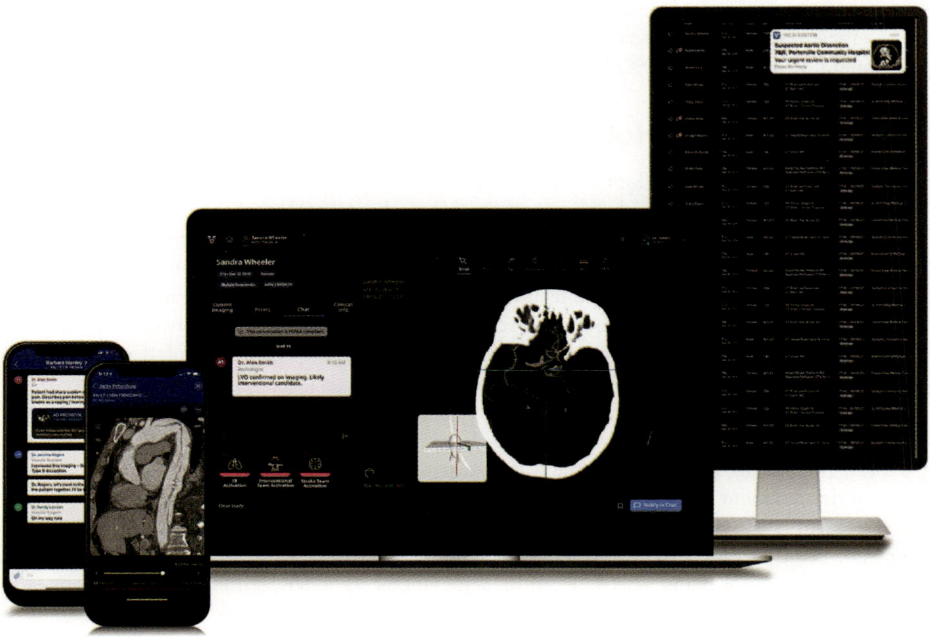

Fig. 24.6 Demonstration of different Viz.ai products.

- **Cardiology Suite:** Viz.ai identified that the same methodologies and platform used for its neurovascular applications could be applied to cardiology. As a result, Viz.ai developed a new AI algorithm to automatically analyze electrocardiograms (ECGs), a routine test, to detect signs of hypertrophic cardiomyopathy (HCM). This device has since been granted a *de novo* request under a regulation for cardiovascular machine learning–based notification software. More applications are under development.
- **Radiology platform:** The clinical uptake of Viz.ai AI solutions was initially designed to lean on mobile devices. Although it was an excellent choice for serving healthcare intervention teams like the stroke response team or pulmonary embolism response team, radiologists desired desktop capabilities and integration with their existing workflow. To meet radiologists' needs and to increase the clinical uptake of Viz.ai AI solutions by radiologists, Viz.ai has now developed a platform for visualization and communication dedicated to radiologists. The platform allows seamless integration between the workflows of radiologists and interventionalists, and streamlines the communication between them.
- **Viz Trauma**: Viz.ai capabilities are tailored for trauma care providers to expedite patient care and improve outcomes. Trauma teams can review patient scans with a hyperfast 3D-capable image viewer with dynamic scrolling, maximum intensity projection (MIP) images, custom window width and window level, and alternate views. Alerts are delivered as soon as possible, allowing teams to see and prioritize work appropriately, and receive immediate updates as patient status changes with bi-directional electronic health record integration.
- **Viz RECRUIT:** Early on, Viz.ai noticed that clients were using Viz.ai AI solutions to identify, coordinate, and recruit patients for various clinical trials. As a result, Viz.ai developed a specialized platform that capitalized on its AI and communication capabilities to automatically identify eligible clinical trial candidates, connect the research team, and help accelerate clinical trial enrollment. Viz.ai's vast and growing customer base also allows for efficient clinical trial recruitment, which has been shown to speed up clinical trial enrollment by more than 200%.[26]

What the Future Holds

The rapid development and adoption of Viz.ai solutions attest to the value of augmenting healthcare systems and care teams with AI-powered care coordination. We believe that the adoption of these types of solutions will accelerate in the coming years, covering multiple care pathways for many critical diseases. As has already occurred in stroke, we hope these solutions will become the standard of care across the board and facilitate earlier treatments that result in improved patients' outcomes. Furthermore, we believe that these solutions will provide significantly better healthcare equality, as disease detection and care coordination are provided by the Viz.ai platform regardless of the patient or caregiver locations.

Viz.ai envisions a future where its platform becomes an ecosystem that consists of multiple AI solutions where part of them are developed organically in-house and the rest by its ecosystem partners. Integrating partners into the Viz.ai platform allows even further accelerated pace of solution development and deployment.

The world is currently at the beginning of an AI revolution. Each year, we will see better and more powerful AI algorithms in multiple areas such as image segmentation, object detection, natural language processing, text generation, large language models, reinforcement learning, and more. Harnessing the growing power of these AI technologies, together with a disciplined product development within the framework of healthcare, will advance Viz.ai's mission to increase access to life-saving treatments for all patients worldwide.

References

1. Berkhemer OA, Fransen PS, Beumer D, et al. A randomized trial of intraarterial treatment for acute ischemic stroke. *N Engl J Med.* 2015;372(1):11–20. http://doi.org/10.1056/NEJMoa1411587.
2. Goyal M, Demchuk AM, Menon BK, et al. Randomized assessment of rapid endovascular treatment of ischemic stroke. *N Engl J Med.* 2015;372(11):1019–1030. http://doi.org/10.1056/NEJMoa1414905.
3. Saver JL, Goyal M, Bonafe A, et al. Stent-retriever thrombectomy after intravenous t-PA vs. t-PA alone in stroke. *N Engl J Med.* 2015;372(24):2285–2295. http://doi.org/10.1056/NEJMoa1415061.
4. Powers WJ, Rabinstein AA, Ackerson T, et al. Guidelines for the early management of patients with acute ischemic stroke: 2019 update to the 2018 guidelines for the early management of acute ischemic stroke: a guideline for healthcare professionals from the American Heart Association/American Stroke Association. *Stroke.* 2019;50(12):e344–e418. http://doi.org/10.1161/STR.0000000000000211.
5. Saver JL. Time is brain–quantified. *Stroke.* 2006;37(1):263–266. http://doi.org/10.1161/01.STR.0000196957.55928.ab.
6. Lees KR, Bluhmki E, von Kummer R, et al. Time to treatment with intravenous alteplase and outcome in stroke: an updated pooled analysis of ECASS, ATLANTIS, NINDS, and EPITHET trials. *Lancet.* 2010;375(9727):1695–1703. http://doi.org/10.1016/S0140-6736(10)60491-6.
7. Fonarow GC, Zhao X, Smith EE, et al. Door-to-needle times for tissue plasminogen activator administration and clinical outcomes in acute ischemic stroke before and after a quality improvement initiative. *JAMA.* 2014;311(16):1632–1640. http://doi.org/10.1001/jama.2014.3203.
8. Adeoye O, Albright KC, Carr BG, et al. Geographic access to acute stroke care in the United States. *Stroke.* 2014;45(10):3019–3024. http://doi.org/10.1161/STROKEAHA.114.006293.
9. Smith EE, Schwamm LH. Endovascular clot retrieval therapy: implications for the organization of stroke systems of care in North America. *Stroke.* 2015;46(6):1462–1467. http://doi.org/10.1161/STROKEAHA.115.008385.
10. Meretoja A, Strbian D, Mustanoja S, Tatlisumak T, Lindsberg PJ, Kaste M. Reducing in-hospital delay to 20 minutes in stroke thrombolysis. *Neurology.* 2012;79(4):306–313. http://doi.org/10.1212/WNL.0b013e31825d6011.
11. Schwamm LH, Pancioli A, Acker JE, et al. Recommendations for the establishment of stroke systems of care: recommendations from the American Stroke Association's Task Force on the Development of Stroke Systems. *Stroke.* 2005;36(3):690–703. http://doi.org/10.1161/01.STR.0000158165.42884.4F.
12. Ali I, Salazar-Marioni S, Abdelkhaleq R, et al. Abstract TMP14: machine learning-enabled detection of unruptured cerebral aneurysms improves detection rates and clinical care. *Stroke.* 2023;54(Suppl_1). ATMP14–ATMP14. http://doi.org/10.1161/str.54.suppl_1.TMP14.
13. Colasurdo M, Shalev D, Robledo A, et al. Validation of an automated machine learning algorithm for the detection and analysis of cerebral aneurysms. *J Neurosurg.* 2023;139(4):1002–1009. http://doi.org/10.3171/2023.1.JNS222304.
14. Elijovich L, Dornbos III D, Nickele C, et al. Automated emergent large vessel occlusion detection by artificial intelligence improves stroke workflow in a hub and spoke stroke system of care. *J Neurointerv Surg.* 2022;14(7):704–708. http://doi.org/10.1136/neurintsurg-2021-017714.
15. Figurelle ME, Meyer DM, Perrinez ES, et al. Viz.ai implementation of stroke augmented intelligence and communications platform to improve indicators and outcomes for a comprehensive stroke center and network. *AJNR Am J Neuroradiol.* 2023;44(1):47–53. http://doi.org/10.3174/ajnr.A7716.
16. Golan D, Shalitin O, Sudry N, Mates J. AI-powered stroke triage system performance in the wild. *J Exp Stroke Transl Med.* 2020;12(3):1–4.
17. Hassan AE, Ringheanu VM, Rabah RR, Preston L, Tekle WG, Qureshi AI. Early experience utilizing artificial intelligence shows significant reduction in transfer times and length of stay in a hub and spoke model. *Interv Neuroradiol.* 2020;26(5):615–622. http://doi.org/10.1177/1591019920953055.
18. Hassan AE, Ringheanu VM, Preston L, Tekle WG. Artificial intelligence–parallel stroke workflow tool improves reperfusion rates and door-in to puncture interval. *Stroke Vasc Interv Neurol.* 2022;2(5):e000224. http://doi.org/10.1161/SVIN.121.000224.
19. Hassan AE, Ringheanu VM, Tekle WG. The implementation of artificial intelligence significantly reduces door-in-door-out times in a primary care center prior to transfer. *Interv Neuroradiol.* 2023;29(6):631–636. http://doi.org/10.1177/15910199221122848.

20. Karamchandani RR, Helms AM, Satyanarayana S, et al. Automated detection of intracranial large vessel occlusions using Viz.ai software: Experience in a large, integrated stroke network. *Brain Behav.* 2023;13(1):e2808. http://doi.org/10.1002/brb3.2808.
21. Matsoukas S, Morey J, Lock G, et al. AI software detection of large vessel occlusion stroke on CT angiography: a real-world prospective diagnostic test accuracy study. *J Neurointerv Surg.* 2023;15(1):52–56. http://doi.org/10.1136/neurintsurg-2021-018391.
22. Murray NM, Unberath M, Hager GD, Hui FK. Artificial intelligence to diagnose ischemic stroke and identify large vessel occlusions: a systematic review. *J Neurointerv Surg.* 2020;12(2):156–164. http://doi.org/10.1136/neurintsurg-2019-015135.
23. Stanton RJ, Wang LL, Smith MS, et al. Differences in automated perfusion software: do they matter clinically? *Stroke Vasc Interv Neurol.* 2022;2(6):e000424. http://doi.org/10.1161/SVIN.122.000424.
24. Yahav-Dovrat A, Saban M, Merhav G, et al. Evaluation of artificial intelligence-powered identification of large-vessel occlusions in a comprehensive stroke center. *AJNR Am J Neuroradiol.* 2021;42(2):247–254. http://doi.org/10.3174/ajnr.A6923.
25. Krishnan N. Viz.ai and why workflow >tech. Out-Of-Pocket. Updated September 30, 2020. Accessed July 19, 2024. https://www.outofpocket.health/p/viz-ai-and-why-workflow-tech.
26. Jankowitz B, Davies J, Schirmer C, et al. E-022 Viz recruit ICH volume increased the screening rate and enrollment in ENRICH. *J Neurointerv Surg.* 2021;13(Suppl 1):A75–A76. http://doi.org/10.1136/neurintsurg-2021-SNIS.118.

INDEX

Note: Page numbers followed by "*f*" indicate figures, "*t*" indicate tables, and "*b*" indicate boxes.